Introduction to Nutrition and Metabolism

Second edition

Introduction to Nutrition and Metabolism

Second edition

DAVID A. BENDER

Department of Biochemistry and Molecular Biology
University College London

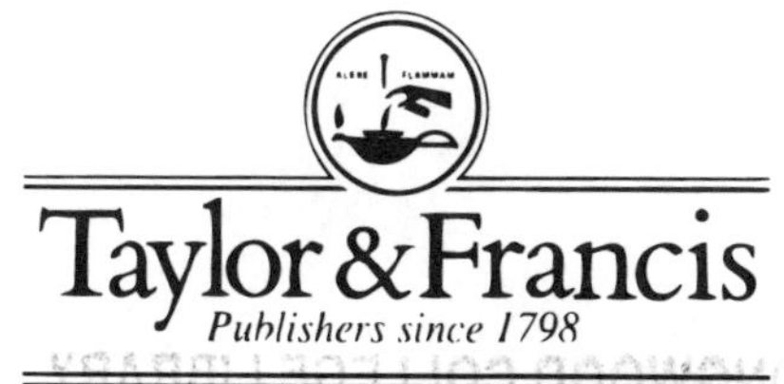

UK Taylor & Francis Ltd, 1 Gunpowder Square, London, EC4A 3DE
USA Taylor & Francis Inc., 1900 Frost Road, Suite 101, Bristol, PA 19007

British Library Cataloguing in Publication Data

A catalogue record for this book is available from the British Library.

ISBN 0-7484-0782-0 (cased)
ISBN 0-7484-0781-2 (paperback)

Library of Congress Cataloging Publication data are available

Cover design by Jim Wilkie

Typeset in Times 10/12pt by Santype International Limited, Salisbury, UK

Printed in Great Britain by T. J. International Ltd, Padstow, UK

Contents

Preface to the second edition

The food we eat has a major effect on our physical health and psychological well-being. An understanding of the way in which nutrients are metabolized, and hence of the principles of biochemistry, is essential for an understanding of the scientific basis of what we would call a prudent or healthy diet.

My aim in the following pages is both to explain the conclusions of the many expert committees which have deliberated on the problems of nutritional requirements, diet and health over the years, and also the scientific basis on which these experts have reached their conclusions. Much of what is now presented as 'facts' will be proven to be incorrect in years to come. This book is intended to provide a foundation of scientific knowledge and understanding from which to interpret and evaluate future advances in nutrition and health sciences.

Nutrition is one of the basic sciences that underlie a proper understanding of health and human sciences and the ways in which man and his environment interact. In its turn, the science of nutrition is based on both biochemistry and physiology on one hand, and the social and behavioural sciences on the other. This book contains such biochemistry as is essential to an understanding of the science of nutrition.

In a book of this kind, which is an introduction to nutrition and metabolism, it is neither possible nor appropriate to cite the original scientific literature which provides the (sometimes conflicting) evidence for the statements made. The bibliography lists sources of more detailed information. In turn, these will lead the reader into research review essays, and from there into the original research literature.

My colleagues have provided helpful comments: I am especially grateful to Barbara Banks, Professor of Physiology at UCL; Peter Campbell, emeritus

Professor of Biochemistry at UCL; Derek Everard, emeritus Reader in Biochemistry at Chelsea College, University of London; for their constructive criticisms of the first edition of this book, and to Bill Coulson, Senior Lecturer in Biochemistry at UCL, for many helpful discussions of the problems students face in understanding the material we teach.

I am also grateful to those of my students whose perceptive questions have helped me to formulate and clarify my thoughts. This book is dedicated to those who will use it as a part of their studies, in the hope that they will be able, in their turn, to advance the frontiers of knowledge, and help their clients, patients and students to understand the basis of the advice they offer.

David A. Bender
London, June 1996

1

Why Eat?

An adult eats about a tonne of food a year. This book attempts to answer the question 'Why?' – by exploring the need for food and the uses to which food is put in the body. Some discussion of chemistry and biochemistry is obviously essential in order to investigate the fate of food in the body, and why there is a continual need for food throughout life. Therefore, in the following chapters various aspects of biochemistry and metabolism will be discussed. This should provide not only the basis of our present understanding, knowledge and concepts in nutrition, but also, more importantly, a basis from which to interpret future research findings and evaluate new ideas and hypotheses as they are formulated.

We eat because we are hungry. Why have we evolved complex physiological and psychological mechanisms to control not only hunger, but also our appetite for different types of food? Why do meals form such an important part of our life?

1.1 The need for energy

There is an obvious need for energy to perform physical work. Work has to be done to lift a load against the force of gravity, and there must be a source of energy to perform that work. As discussed in Chapter 7, the energy used in various activities can readily be measured, as can the metabolic energy yield of the foods that are the fuel for that work (see Table 1.1). This means that it is possible to calculate a balance between the intake of energy, as metabolic fuels, and the body's energy expenditure. Obviously, energy intake has to be appropriate for the level of energy expenditure; as discussed in Chapters 7 and 8, neither excess intake nor a deficiency is desirable.

Quite apart from this visible work output, the body has a considerable requirement for energy, even at rest. Only about one-third of the average person's energy expenditure is for obvious work (see §7.1.3). Two-thirds is required for maintenance of the body's functions, homeostasis of the internal environment, and metabolic integrity. This energy requirement, the basal metabolic rate (BMR, see §7.1.3.1), can be measured by the output of heat when the subject is completely at rest.

Part of this basal energy requirement is obvious: the heart beats to circulate the blood; respiration continues; there is considerable electrical activity in nerves and muscles, whether they are 'working' or not; and the kidneys expend a considerable amount of energy during the filtration of waste products from the bloodstream. All of these processes require a metabolic energy source. Less obviously, there is also a requirement for energy for the wide variety of biochemical reactions occurring all the time in the body: laying down reserves of fat and carbohydrate; turnover of tissue proteins; transport of substrates into, and products out of, cells; and the production and secretion of hormones and neurotransmitters.

1.1.1 Units of energy

Energy expenditure is measured by the output of heat from the body (see §7.1). The unit of heat used in the early studies was the calorie – the amount of heat required to raise the temperature of 1 g of water by 1°C. The calorie is still used to some extent in nutrition; in biological systems the kilocalorie, kcal (sometimes written as 'Calorie', with a capital C) is used. One kilocalorie is 1000 calories (10^3 cal), and hence the amount of heat required to raise 1 kg of water through 1°C.

Correctly, the joule (J) is used as the unit of energy. The joule is an SI unit, named after James Prescott Joule, who first showed the equivalence of heat, mechanical work and other forms of energy. In biological systems the kilojoule (kJ, $=10^3$ J = 1000 J) and megajoule (MJ, $=10^6$ J = 1 000 000 J) are used.

To convert between calories and joules:

1 kcal = 4.186 kJ (normally rounded off to 4.2 kJ)

1 kJ = 0.239 kcal (normally rounded off to 0.24 kcal)

As discussed in §7.1.3, average energy expenditure of adults is between 7.5 and 10 MJ day^{-1} for women and 8 to 12 MJ day^{-1} for men.

1.2 Metabolic fuels

The dietary sources of metabolic energy (the metabolic fuels) are carbohydrates, fats, protein and alcohol. The metabolism of these fuels results in the production of carbon dioxide and water (and also urea in the case of protein; see §10.3.1.4). They can be converted to the same end-products chemically, by burning in air. Although the process of metabolism in the body is more complex, it is a fundamental law of chemistry that, if the starting material and end-products are the same, the energy yield is the same, regardless of the route taken. Therefore, the energy yield of foodstuffs can be determined by measuring the heat produced when they are burnt in air, making allowance for the extent to which they are digested and absorbed from foods. The energy yields of the metabolic fuels in the body, allowing for metabolic efficiency, are shown in Table 1.1.

1.2.1 The need for carbohydrate and fat

Although there is a requirement for energy sources in the diet, it does not matter unduly how that requirement is met. There is no requirement for a dietary source of carbohydrate – as discussed in §7.7, the body can make as much carbohydrate as it requires from proteins. Similarly, there is no requirement for a dietary source of fat, apart from the essential fatty acids (see §6.3.1.1), and there is certainly no requirement for a dietary source of alcohol.

Although there is no requirement for fat in the diet, fats do have nutritional importance:

- It is difficult to eat enough of a very low-fat diet to meet energy requirements. As shown in Table 1.1, the energy yield of 1 g of fat is more than twice that of 1 g of carbohydrate or protein. It would be necessary to eat a considerably larger amount of a very low-fat diet to meet energy needs from carbohydrate and protein alone; indeed, it is unlikely that it would be possible to eat a sufficient bulk of food to meet energy requirements from a diet that was devoid of fat. The problem in Western countries is an undesirably high intake of fat, contributing to the development of obesity (see Chapter 8) and the diseases of affluence (see Chapter 2).
- Four of the vitamins, A, D, E and K (see Chapter 12), are fat soluble, and are found in fatty and oily foods. More importantly, because they are absorbed dissolved in fat, their absorption requires an adequate intake of

Table 1.1 The energy yield of metabolic fuels

	kcal g^{-1}	kJ g^{-1}
Carbohydrate	4	17
Protein	4	16
Fat	9	37
Alcohol	7	29

1 kcal = 4.186 kJ or 1 kJ = 0.239 kcal.

fat. On a very low-fat diet the absorption of these vitamins will be inadequate to meet requirements.

- There is a requirement for small amounts of the essential fatty acids. These are constituents of fats which are required for specific functions; they cannot be formed in the body, so they must be provided in the diet (see §6.3.1.1).
- In many foods much of the flavour (and hence the pleasure of eating) is carried in the fat.
- Fats lubricate food and make it easier to chew and swallow.

1.2.2 The need for protein

Unlike fats and carbohydrates, there is a requirement for protein in the diet. In a growing child this need is obvious. As the child grows, and the size of its body increases, so there is an increase in the total amount of protein in the body.

Adults also require protein in the diet. There is a continual small loss of protein from the body, for example in hair, shed skin cells, enzymes and other proteins secreted into the gut and not completely digested, and so on. More importantly, there is turnover of tissue proteins, which are continually being broken down and replaced. Although there is no change in the total amount of protein in the body, an adult with an inadequate intake of protein will be unable to replace this loss, and will lose tissue protein. Protein turnover and requirements are discussed in Chapter 10.

1.2.3 The need for minerals and vitamins

In addition to metabolic fuels and protein, the body has a requirement for a variety of mineral salts, in very much smaller amounts. Obviously, if a metal or ion has a function in the body, it must be provided by the diet, since the different elements cannot be interconverted. Again, the need is obvious for a growing child; as the body grows in size, so the total amounts of minerals in the body will increase. In adults there is a turnover of minerals in the body, and losses must be replaced from the diet.

There is a requirement for a different group of nutrients, also in very small amounts – the vitamins. These are relatively complex organic compounds that have essential functions in metabolic processes. They cannot be synthesized in the body, and so must be provided by the diet. There is turnover of the vitamins, so there must be replacement of the losses. Vitamins and minerals are discussed in Chapter 12.

1.3 Hunger and appetite

Human beings have evolved an elaborate system of physiological and psychological mechanisms to ensure that the body's needs for metabolic fuels and nutrients are met.

As shown in Figure 1.1, there are hunger and satiety centres in the brain, which stimulate us to begin eating (the hunger centres in the lateral hypothalamus), or to stop eating when hunger has been satisfied (the satiety centres in the ventromedial hypothalamus). A great deal is known about the role of these brain centres in controlling food intake, and there are drugs that modify responses to hunger and satiety. Such drugs can be used to reduce appetite in the treatment of obesity (see §8.3.3.9) or stimulate it in people with anorexia (see §9.2.1.1).

The hypothalamic hunger and satiety centres control food intake very precisely. Without conscious effort, most people can regulate their food intake to match energy expenditure very closely; they neither waste away from lack of metabolic fuel for physical activity nor lay down excessively large reserves of fat. Even people who have excessive reserves of body fat, and can be considered to be so overweight or obese as to be putting their health at risk (see §8.2.2), balance their energy intake and expenditure relatively well, considering that the average intake is a tonne of food a year; the most obese people weigh about 250 kg (compared with average weights between 60 and 100 kg), and it takes many years to achieve such a weight.

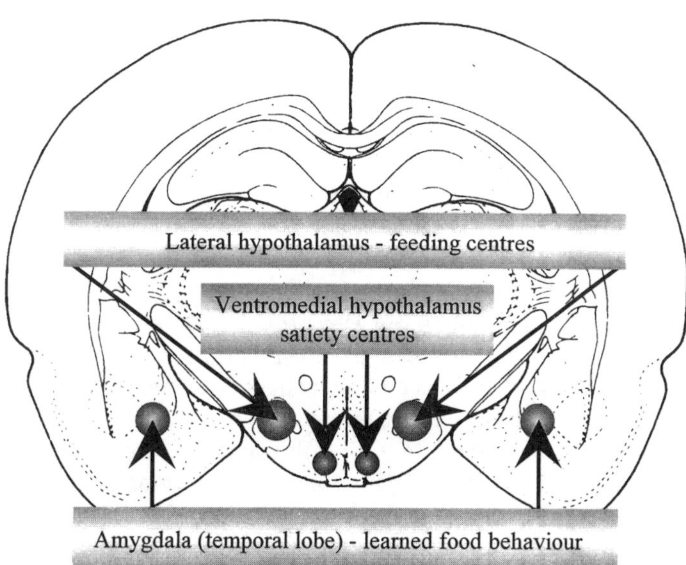

Figure 1.1 Appetite control centres in the brain.

In addition to hunger and satiety, which are basic physiological responses, food intake is controlled by appetite, which is related not only to physiological need but also to the pleasure of eating: flavour and texture, and a host of social and psychological factors.

1.3.1 Taste and flavour

Taste buds on the tongue can distinguish five basic sensations: salt, savouriness, sweet, bitter and sour.

Salt (correctly the mineral sodium) is essential to life, and wild animals will travel great distances to a salt lick. Like other animals, human beings have evolved a pleasurable response to salty flavours, which ensures that physiological needs are met. However, there is no shortage of salt in developed countries and, as discussed in §2.4.4, average intakes of salt are considerably greater than requirements and may pose a hazard to health.

The sensation of savouriness is distinct from that of saltiness and is sometimes called *umami* (the Japanese for savoury). It is largely due to the presence of free amino acids in foods. Stimulation of the umami receptors of the tongue is the basis of flavour enhancers such as monosodium glutamate, which is an important constituent of traditional oriental condiments, and is widely used in manufactured foods.

The other instinctively pleasurable taste is sweetness. The evolutionary reason for this is less clear than the response to salt, but it can be argued that ripe fruits are sweet (the process of ripening is largely one of converting starches to sugars) and, in general, fruits are better sources of nutrients when they are ripe.

Sourness and bitterness are instinctively unpleasant sensations. Learnt behaviour will overcome the instinctive aversion, but this is a process of learning or acquiring tastes, not an innate or instinctive response. It is likely that the aversion to bitterness evolved as a protection against poisonous compounds found in some plants, many of which are bitter. The aversion to sourness is presumably the converse of the pleasurable reaction to sweetness – sour unripe fruit is a poorer source of nutrients.

In addition to the sensations of taste provided by the taste buds on the tongue, a great many flavours can be distinguished by the sense of smell. Again, some flavours and aromas (fruity flavours, fresh coffee and, at least to a non-vegetarian, the smell of roasting meat) are pleasurable, tempting people to eat and stimulating their appetite. Other flavours and aromas are repulsive, warning us not to eat the food. Again, this can be seen as a warning of possible danger; the smell of decaying meat or fish tells us that it is not safe to eat.

Like the acquisition of a taste for bitter or sour foods, a taste for foods with what would seem at first to be an unpleasant aroma or flavour can also be acquired. Here things become more complex – a pleasant smell to one person may be repulsive to another. Some people enjoy the smell of cooked cabbage and sprouts; others can hardly bear to be in the same room. The durian fruit is a highly prized delicacy in South East Asia, yet to the uninitiated it smells of sewage or faeces – hardly an appetizing aroma.

1.3.2 *Why do people eat what they do?*

People have different responses to the same taste or flavour. This may be explained in terms of childhood memories, pleasurable or otherwise. An aversion to the smell of a food may protect someone who has a specific allergy or intolerance (although sometimes people have a craving for the foods to which they are intolerant). Most often we simply cannot explain why some people dislike foods that others eat with great relish.

Various factors may influence why people choose to eat particular foods:

1.3.2.1 *The availability and cost of food*

In developed countries the simple availability of food is not likely to be a constraint on choice. There is a wide variety of foods available, and when fruits and vegetables are out of season at home they are imported; frozen, canned or dried foods are widespread. By contrast, in developing countries the availability of food is a major constraint on what people choose. Little food is imported, and what is available will depend on the local soil and climate. Even in normal times the choice of foods may be very limited, while in times of drought there may be little or no food available at all, and what little is available will be very much more expensive than most people can afford.

Even in developed countries, the cost of food may be important, and for the most disadvantaged members of the community, poverty may impose severe constraints on the choice of foods. In developing countries, cost is the major problem. Indeed, even in times of famine, food may be available, but it is so expensive that few people can buy it.

1.3.2.2 *Religion, habit and tradition*

Religious and ethical considerations are important in determining the choice of foods. Observant Jews and Muslims will eat meat only from animals that have cloven hooves and chew the cud. The terms *kosher* in Jewish law and *hallal* in Islamic law both mean clean; the meat of other animals, which are scavenging animals, birds of prey and detritus-feeding fish, is regarded as unclean (*traife* or *haram*). We now know that many of these forbidden animals carry parasites that can infect human beings, so these ancient prohibitions are based on food hygiene.

Hindus will not eat beef. The reason for this is that the cow is far too valuable, as a source of milk, dung (as manure and fuel) and as a beast of burden, for it to be killed just as a source of meat.

Many people refrain from eating meat as a result of humanitarian concern for the animals involved. Vegetarians can be divided into a variety of groups, according to the strictness of their diet:

- ovolactovegetarians will eat eggs and milk, but not meat
- lactovegetarians will eat milk, but not eggs
- vegans will eat only plant foods, and no foods of animal origin

Perhaps the strictest of all vegetarians are the Jains (originally from Gujarat in India), whose religion not only prohibits the consumption of meat, but extends the concept of the sanctity of life to insects and grubs as well – an observant Jain will not eat any vegetable that has grown underground, lest an insect was killed in digging it up.

Foods that are commonly eaten in one area may be little eaten elsewhere, even though they are available, simply because people have not been accustomed to eating them. To a very great extent, eating habits as adults continue the habits learnt as children.

Haggis and oatcakes are rarely eaten outside Scotland, except as speciality items; black pudding is a staple of northern British breakfasts, but is rarely seen in the south-east of England. Until the 1960s, yogurt was almost unknown in Britain, apart from a few health food 'cranks' and immigrants from eastern Europe; many British children believe that fish is available only as rectangular fish fingers, whereas children in inland Spain may eat fish and other seafood three or four times a week. The French mock the British habit of eating lamb with mint sauce – and the average British reaction to such French delicacies as frogs' legs and snails in garlic sauce is one of horror. The British eat their cabbage well boiled; the Germans and Dutch ferment it to produce sauerkraut.

This regional and cultural diversity of foods provides one of the pleasures of travel. As people travel more frequently, and become (perhaps grudgingly) more adventurous in their choice of foods, so they create a demand for different foods at home, and there is an increasing variety of foods available in shops and restaurants.

A further factor that has increased the range of foods available has been immigration of people from a variety of different backgrounds, all of whom have, as they have become established, introduced their traditional foods to their new homes. It is difficult to realize that in the 1960s there was only a handful of Tandoori restaurants in the whole of Britain, that Balti cooking was unknown until the 1990s, or that pizza was something seen only in southern Italy and a few specialist restaurants.

Some people are naturally adventurous, and will try a new food just because they have never eaten it before. Others are more conservative, and will try a new food only when they see someone else eating it safely and with enjoyment. Others are yet more conservative in their food choices; the most conservative eaters 'know' that they do not like a new food because they have never eaten it before.

1.3.2.3 *Luxury status of scarce and expensive foods*

Foods that are scarce or expensive have a certain appeal of fashion or style; they are (rightly) regarded as luxuries for special occasions rather than everyday meals. Conversely, foods that are widespread and cheap have less appeal. In the nineteenth century, salmon and oysters (which are now relatively expensive luxury foods) were so cheap that the Articles of apprentices in London specified that they should not be given salmon more than three times a week, and oysters were eaten by the poor. Conversely, chicken and trout, which were expensive luxury foods in the 1950s, are now widely available, as a result of changes in farming practice, and they form the basis of inexpensive meals. As farming practices change, so salmon is again becoming an inexpensive meal, and venison is no longer the exclusive preserve of the wealthy landed gentry or poachers.

1.3.2.4 *The social functions of food*

Human beings are essentially social animals, and meals are important social functions. People eating in a group are likely to eat better, or at least to have a wider variety of foods and a more lavish and luxurious meal, than people eating alone. Entertaining guests may be an excuse to eat foods that we know to be nutritionally undesirable, and perhaps to eat to excess. The greater the variety of dishes offered, the more people are likely to eat. As we reach satiety with one food, so another, different, flavour is offered to stimulate appetite. Studies have shown that, faced with only one food, people tend to reach satiety sooner than when a variety of different foods is on offer. This is the difference between hunger and appetite: even when we are satiated, we can still 'find room' to try something different.

Conversely, and more importantly, many lonely single people (and especially the bereaved elderly) have little incentive to prepare meals and no stimulus to appetite. Although poverty may be a factor, apathy (and often, in the case of widowed men, ignorance) severely limits the range of foods eaten, possibly leading to undernutrition. When these problems are added to the problems of infirmity, ill-fitting dentures (which make eating painful) and arthritis (which makes handling many foods difficult), and the difficulty of carrying food home from the shops, it is not surprising that we include the elderly among those vulnerable groups of the population who are at risk of undernutrition.

In hospitals and other institutions there is a further problem. People who are unwell may have low physical activity, but they have higher than normal requirements for energy and nutrients, as a part of the process of replacing tissue in convalescence (see §10.1.2.2) or as a result of fever or the metabolic effects of cancer (see §9.2.1.4). At the same time, illness impairs appetite, and a side effect of many drugs is to distort the sense of taste, depress appetite or cause nausea. It is difficult to provide a range of exciting and attractive foods under institutional conditions, yet this is what is needed to tempt the patient's appetite.

2

Diet and Health: the Diseases of Affluence

The World Health Organization defines health as 'a state of complete mental, physical and social well-being, and not merely the absence of disease or infirmity'. One of the factors essential for the attainment of health is a diet that is both adequate and appropriate. An adequate diet is one that provides adequate amounts of metabolic fuels and nutrients to meet physiological needs and prevent the development of deficiency diseases. To achieve an adequate diet is a minimum objective, albeit one to which many in developing countries aspire. An appropriate diet is one which not only meets physiological needs, but does so in a balanced way, without causing any health problems which may be associated with an excessive intake of one or more nutrients or types of food. As discussed in §12.1 and §12.2.3.2, intake of some nutrients at higher levels than those required to prevent the development of deficiency may confer health benefits.

Human beings have evolved in a hostile environment in which food has always been scarce. It is only in the past half-century or less that food has become available in large amounts – and even then it is only in western Europe, North America and Australasia that there is a surplus of food. Food is still desperately short in much of Africa, Asia and Latin America, and indeed much of eastern Europe has inadequate food. Even without all too frequent droughts, floods and other disasters, there is scarcely enough food produced worldwide to feed all the people of the world. Although world food production has more than kept pace with population growth over the past three decades, so that most countries now have more food available per head of population than in the 1960s, the world population is projected to increase from the present 5.5 billion to 8.5 billion by 2025, and it is unlikely that food production can be increased to the same extent.

This means that any discussion of the problems of diet and health must distinguish between the problems of undernutrition and those associated with affluence and the availability of plentiful supplies of food at prices that people can readily afford.

2.1 Problems of deficiency

On a global scale, overall lack of food is the problem. Up to 300 million people are at risk from protein-energy malnutrition in developing countries; this is discussed in Chapter 9. Deficiency of individual nutrients is also a major problem. Here the total amount of food may be adequate to satisfy hunger, but the quality of the diet is inadequate:

- Vitamin A deficiency (see §12.2.1.3) is the single most important cause of childhood blindness in the world, with some 14 million pre-school children worldwide showing clinical signs of deficiency, and 190 million people at risk of deficiency.
- Deficiency of vitamins B_1 (see §2.2.5.1) and B_2 (§12.2.6.1) continues to be a major problem in large areas of Asia and Africa.
- Deficiency of iodine affects many millions of people living in upland areas over limestone soil; in some areas of central Africa, Brazil and the Himalayas more than 90 per cent of the population may have goitre because of iodine deficiency (see §12.3.3.3). Where children are iodine deficient both *in utero* and postnatally, the result is severe intellectual impairment (goitrous cretinism).
- Iron deficiency anaemia affects many millions of women in both developing and developed countries (see §12.3.2.3).

Deficiency of other vitamins and minerals also occurs, and can still be an important cause of ill health and disease, as discussed in Chapter 12. Sometimes this is the result of an acute exacerbation of a marginal food shortage, as in the outbreaks of the niacin deficiency disease, pellagra, reported in East and southern Africa during the 1980s (see §12.2.7.1); sometimes it is a problem of immigrant populations living in a new environment, as with the incidence of rickets and osteomalacia among Asians living in northern Europe (see §12.2.2.4).

The problems of undernutrition are discussed in Chapter 9, protein deficiency in Chapter 10 and vitamin and mineral deficiencies in Chapter 12.

2.2 Diseases of affluence

This chapter is concerned with the role of diet and nutrition in the so-called *diseases of affluence*; the health problems of developed countries, associated with a superabundant availability of food. Diet is, of course, only one of the differences between life in the developed countries of western Europe, North America and Australasia, and that in developing countries; there are a great many other differences in environment and living conditions. Despite the problems to be discussed in this chapter, which are major causes of premature death, people in developed countries have a greater life expectancy than those in developing countries.

It can be assumed that human beings and their diet have evolved together. Certainly, we have changed our crops and farm animals by selective breeding over the past 10 000 years, and it is reasonable to assume that we have evolved by natural selection to be suited to our diet. The problem is that evolution is a slow process, and there have been major changes in food availability in developed countries over the past century. As recently as the 1930s (very recent in evolutionary terms) it was estimated that up to one-third of households in Britain could not afford an adequate diet. Malnutrition was a serious problem, and the provision of 200 ml of milk daily to schoolchildren had a significant beneficial effect on their health and growth.

Foods that were historically scarce luxuries are now commonplace and available in surplus. Sugar was an expensive luxury until the middle of the nineteenth century; traditionally, fat was also scarce, and every effort was made to save and use all the fat (dripping) from a roast joint of meat.

Together with this increased availability of food, there has been an increase in average lifespan in the developed countries over the past century. This can be attributed to several factors: increased medical knowledge and better medical treatment; reliable supplies of clean drinking water and improved sewage disposal; and eradication of the diseases of hunger. Superimposed on this improvement has been the rise of new diseases. The major causes of death in developed countries today are heart disease, high blood pressure, strokes and cancer. These are not just diseases of old age, although it is true to say that, the longer people live, the more likely they are to develop cancer. Heart disease is a major cause of premature death, striking a significant number of people aged under 40. This is not solely a Western phenomenon. As countries develop, so people in the prosperous cities begin to show a Western pattern of premature death from these same diseases.

Table 2.1 shows the types of study that have yielded the evidence that diet is a significant factor in the development of the diseases of affluence. Diet is not the sole cause, since these diseases are due to interactions of multiple factors, including heredity, a variety of environmental factors, smoking and exercise (or the lack of it). Nonetheless, diet is a factor that is readily amenable to change. Individuals can take decisions about diet, smoking and exercise, whereas they can do little about the stresses of city life, environmental pollution or the other problems of industrial society, and nothing, of course, to change their heredity.

The major change in the diet over the past century has been an increase in the total amount of food available, and particularly in the amount of fat and sugar eaten. Most people now eat less dietary fibre than 100 years ago; in general, people eat more highly refined cereal products, and are less reliant on cereals and vegetables. Meat is now eaten most days of the week, rather than being a 'Sunday treat'.

Table 2.1 Types of evidence linking diet and diseases of affluence

Changes in diet with changes in disease incidence over time	Obviously diet is only one of many factors that have changed over the last 2 to 4 generations
International correlations between disease incidence and diet	Based on national food availability data, not individual records of consumption; assume equal reliability of information about food and disease incidence from different countries
Migration studies	Many factors other than diet change as people migrate
Case-control studies	Diet histories of patients and matched controls; gives information of present diet, but not lifetime diet history
Case–control studies with biochemical assessment of nuritional status	More useful than simple diet history for specific nutrients, but reflects only recent intake; disease may affect food (and hence nutrient) intake, as well as nutrition affecting the disease process
Prospective studies	Very large numbers of people have to be followed for many years
Prospective studies with biochemical assessment of nutritional status	Very large numbers of people have to be followed for many years, very large numbers of samples have to be analysed; if samples are to be stored and analysed in a case–control manner then problems of stability in storage may arise
Modified prospective studies	Where the probability of, or time until, recurrence is known with reasonable precision (e.g. in cancer of breast, larynx or bladder) then nutritional status and diet of patients can be assessed at first presentation, and these patients followed. This method still suffers from problems of ignorance of diet at the time of initiation of the disease process, and from confounding effects of disease on food and nutrient intake
Animal studies	Can give insight into mechanisms, and hence the likelihood that nutritional intervention may be beneficial, but generally rely on peculiar dietary conditions to induce disease, or specific chemically-induced tumours
Intervention studies	All the problems of prospective studies, plus requirement for long-term compliance of subjects

There are thus two separate, but related, questions to be considered:

- Is diet a factor in the aetiology of diseases of affluence, which are major causes of premature death in developed countries?
- Might changes in average Western diets reduce the risk of developing cancer and cardiovascular disease?

The epidemiological evidence linking dietary factors with the diseases of affluence shows that, in countries or regions with, for example, a high intake of saturated fat, there is a higher incidence of cardiovascular disease and some forms of cancer than in regions with a lower intake of fat. It does not show that people who have been living on a high fat diet will necessarily benefit from a relatively abrupt change to a low fat diet. Indeed, in many intervention studies, in which large numbers of people have been persuaded to change their diets, the results over a period of 10 to 20 years have been disappointing. Overall, premature death from cardiovascular disease is reduced, but the total death rate remains unchanged, with an increase in suicide, accidents and violent death. Nevertheless, the epidemiological data are irrefutable. People who have lived on what we can call a prudent diet (as discussed in §2.4) are significantly less at risk of death from the diseases of affluence than those whose intakes of fat (and especially saturated fat), salt and sugar are higher, and of dietary fibre, fruit and vegetables lower. The aim therefore must be to inculcate what are considered to be prudent and appropriate dietary habits at an early age.

2.3 Food safety: additives and contaminants

The first general food laws anywhere in the world were passed in Britain in 1860. They were intended to stamp out widespread adulteration of common foods: diluting flour with chalk dust; mixing sugar with 'sugar of lead' (lead acetate, a poisonous compound), added because it was cheap and sweet tasting, while sugar was expensive; diluting milk and alcoholic beverages with water.

Since then there has been considerable progress, and all countries have comprehensive regulations on food safety and hygiene, covering all aspects of food production, manufacture, sale, preparation and serving. There are lists of those compounds that may legally be added to food during manufacture or processing, based on exhaustive testing for safety. Compounds not included in the list of permitted additives may not be added to foods.

2.3.1 Food additives

Food additives may be colours and flavours, preservatives to prevent spoilage, or processing aids to maintain the texture, appearance and stability of the food. They may be naturally occurring compounds, such as colours extracted from various plants, or they may be synthetic chemicals, or chemically synthesized compounds that are identical to those occurring in nature (and hence called *nature identical*). What they all have in common is that they have been tested, and have been found to be safe, as far as anyone can tell, causing no adverse effects in experimental animals or human beings. On the very few occasions when potentially hazardous effects of a food additive have been suspected, it has been withdrawn from use with great haste, sometimes even before the hazard has been established as a real one.

2.3.2 *Food contamination*

Contamination of foods poses a more serious problem because it occurs accidentally. Where we know or believe that specific compounds that might enter the food chain are hazardous, strict limits are set on the concentration that may be permitted in foods. This is generally based on estimates of the amounts likely to be consumed from foods, and the **acceptable daily intake** is set at 1 per cent of the lowest level at which any adverse effect can be detected. Food manufacturers, the Ministry of Agriculture, Fisheries and Food (and equivalent government departments in other countries) and the public health services maintain a close watch on possible contamination of foods, and there are mechanisms to ensure that contaminated foods are withdrawn and destroyed rapidly. Foods being imported are subject to inspection and checks at ports to ensure safety and freedom from contamination by chemicals or toxin-producing microorganisms.

Similarly, the Central Public Health Laboratory in Britain (and equivalent laboratories in other countries) monitors all reported cases of infectious **food poisoning**, and provides, together with Medical Officers of Health and Trading Standards Officers, a system for tracing, withdrawing and ordering the destruction of foods found to be contaminated with harmful bacteria or fungi. Where particular foods are especially likely to contain potentially dangerous numbers of harmful bacteria, as for example the presence of *Salmonella* spp. in eggs and poultry, or *Listeria* spp. in soft cheeses, the Department of Health issues special advice. Thus, eggs should be cooked, not eaten raw or partially cooked. Frozen poultry should be thoroughly defrosted before cooking, so as to ensure adequate heating of the interior, and hence destruction of the bacteria. The developing foetus is especially susceptible to infection with *Listeria*, and pregnant women are specifically advised to avoid soft cheeses which may carry an unacceptable burden of these bacteria.

2.4 Guidelines for healthy eating and nutritional goals

There is general agreement among nutritionists and medical scientists about changes in the average Western diet that would be expected to reduce the prevalence of the diseases of affluence, and most countries have published nutritional guidelines and dietary advice. Changing diets in the way suggested below is not a guarantee of immortality, and indeed some of the evidence is conflicting. As new data are gathered, old data reinterpreted, and the results of long-term studies become available, it is inevitable that opinions as to what constitutes a prudent or desirable diet will change. It will be essential to have an understanding of the underlying physiology and biochemistry of nutrition, the way in which nutrients are metabolized and interact with each other and with a host of metabolic and regulatory systems in the body, in order to be able to evaluate this new information.

2.4.1 Energy intake

Obesity involves both an increased risk of premature death from a variety of causes and increased morbidity from conditions such as varicose veins and arthritis (see §8.2). On the other hand, people who are significantly underweight are also at increased risk of illness as a result of undernutrition (see Chapter 9). Therefore, it is possible to define a range of **desirable or ideal weight** relative to height, based on life expectancy (see §8.1).

For people whose body weight is within the desirable range, energy intake should be adequate to maintain a reasonably constant body weight, with an adequate amount of exercise. Energy expenditure in physical activity and appropriate levels of energy intake are discussed in §7.1.3.

The metabolic fuels are fats, carbohydrates, protein and alcohol. Table 2.2 shows the average percentage of energy intake from each of them in the diets of adults in Britain in the 1990s, compared with the guidelines for a prudent diet. The percentage of energy intake derived from the different metabolic fuels can be calculated from the energy yield per gram, and the amount consumed, estimated from weighed diet records and food composition tables (see Appendix II).

2.4.2 Fat intake

Dietary fat includes not only the obvious fat in the diet (the visible fat on meat, cooking oil, butter or margarine spread on bread), but also the hidden fat in foods. This latter may be either the fat naturally present in foods (e.g. the fat between the muscle fibres in meat; the oils in nuts, cereals and vegetables) or fat used in cooking and manufacture of foods.

Table 2.2 The percentage of energy from different metabolic fuels in the average British diet, compared with dietary guidelines

	Average	Range	Guidelines	Desirable change (%)
Carbohydrate	43	30–55	53	+23
Fat	40	27–50	30	−25
Protein	15	9–20	15	–
Alcohol	3	0–28	see Table 2.10	

Table 2.3 The percentage of energy from different types of fat in the average British diet, compared with dietary guidelines

	Average	Range	Guidelines	Desirable change (%)
Total fat	40	27–50	30	−25
Saturated	17	10–23	10	−41
Mono-unsaturated	12	8–17	12	0
Polyunsaturated	6	3–12	6	0
Trans-unsaturated	2	—	2	0
Carbohydrate	43	30–55	53	+23
Protein	15	9–20	15	0
Alcohol	3	0–28	see Table 2.10	

Table 2.3 shows intakes of fat as a percentage of energy intake in the average diet. As well as the total amount of fat (the first row of the table), it also shows intakes of saturated and unsaturated fats separately. The chemical difference between saturated and unsaturated fats is discussed in §6.3.1.1; it is relevant here since, as discussed in §2.4.2.1, both the total amount of fat in the diet and the proportion of that fat which is saturated or unsaturated are important in considering the role of diet in the diseases of affluence. As a general rule, animal foods (meat, eggs and milk products) are rich sources of saturated fats, whereas oily fish and vegetables are rich sources of unsaturated fats (see Table 2.5).

There are two problems associated with a high intake of fat:

- The energy yield of fat (37 kJ per g) is more than twice that of protein (16 kJ per g) or carbohydrate (17 kJ per g). This means that foods high in fat are also concentrated energy sources. It is easier to have an excessive energy intake on a high fat diet, and hence a high fat diet can be a factor in the development of obesity (see Chapter 8).
- Studies in many countries have shown that the average intake of fat is statistically correlated with premature death from a variety of conditions, including especially atherosclerosis and ischaemic heart disease, and cancer of the colon, breast and uterus.

The concentration of cholesterol (see §6.3.1.3) in plasma, and specifically cholesterol in plasma low density lipoproteins (LDL) is related to the development of atherosclerosis and ischaemic heart disease. The main dietary factor which affects the concentration of cholesterol in plasma is the intake of fat. Both the total amount of fat and also the relative amounts of saturated and unsaturated fats affect the concentration of cholesterol in LDL. High intakes of total fat, and especially saturated fat, are associated with undesirably high concentrations of LDL cholesterol. Relatively low intakes of fat, with a high proportion as unsaturated fat, are associated with a desirable lower concentration of LDL cholesterol.

From the results of epidemiological studies, it seems that diets providing about 30 per cent of energy from fat are associated with the lowest risk of ischaemic heart disease. Above 35 per cent of energy intake from fat, there is an increase in serum cholesterol to above what is regarded as the normal or desirable range (over 5.2 mmol per L). There is no evidence that a fat intake below about 30 per cent of energy intake confers any additional benefit, although a very low fat diet is specifically recommended as part of treatment for some types of hepatitis, malabsorption and hyperlipidaemia.

As shown in Table 2.3, the average intake of fat in Britain is almost 40 per cent of energy. This means that there is a need for a considerable decrease in fat intake to meet the goal of 30 per cent of energy from fat. Table 2.4 shows the foods that are especially high in fat. From this table, it is relatively easy to

Table 2.4 Foods that are especially high in fat

	Fat (g per 100 g)[a]
Nuts	50–64
Meat	
Bacon rashers	30–36
Duck	25
Pork	20–24
Lamb	19–30
Sausages	17–25
Bacon joint	19
Beef	11–23
Chicken	14
Milk products	
Double cream	48
Cheddar cheese	34
Stilton cheese	26
Edam cheese	24
Single cream	21
Full cream milk	3.8
Fish[b]	
Herring	20
Salmon	20
Halibut	4
Cod	1
Eggs	11

[a] Assuming that foods have not been fried in oil or fat.

[b] The fat content of canned fish will depend on whether it is canned in oil, water or a sauce.

Table 2.5 Types of fat spreads

	Content	Fat (%)
Butter	Traditional churned butter, sometimes called sweetcream butter; may be salted or unsalted	80–82
Lactic butter	Made from cream with the addition of lactic bacteria to give a sharp taste; usually unsalted or lightly salted	80–82
Hard margarine	Hardened animal and vegetable oils, mainly used for baking	80
Soft margarine	Mainly vegetable oils, spreads easily	80
Pufa margarine	Mainly sunflower, corn or soya bean oils, for a high content of polyunsaturated fatty acids	80
Dairy spreads	Blended cream and vegetable oil, spreads easily	72–75
Reduced fat spreads	Mainly vegetable oils, may be some animal or dairy fat	60–70
Low fat spreads	May contain dairy fat and vegetable oils, not suitable for cooking use	37–40
Very low fat spreads	May contain dairy fat and vegetable oils, not suitable for cooking use	20–25
Extremely low fat spreads	Made with fat substitutes (e.g. Simplesse, a modified protein) to replace almost all of the fat, not suitable for cooking use	5

Butter and margarine are legally defined, and hence low fat substitutes cannot legally be called margarine. Low fat spreads contain less fat, and hence more water, than margarine. They may also be whipped, so as to be lighter. They are intended for spreading, and are not suitable for cooking use.

work out which foods should be eaten in smaller quantities in order to reduce the total intake of fat.

As an aid to reducing fat intake, low-fat versions of foods traditionally high in fat are available. Some of these are meat products which make use of leaner (and more expensive) cuts of meat for the preparation of sausages, hamburgers and pies. Low-fat minced meat (containing about 10 per cent fat by weight, instead of the more usual 20 per cent) is widely available in supermarkets, although it is, of course, more expensive, and low-fat cheeses and pâtés are also available, as are salad dressings made with little or no oil. There are also low-fat spreads to replace butter or margarine (Table 2.5). Skimmed and semi-skimmed milk are now widely available, providing very much less fat than full cream milk, although full cream milk is an important source of vitamins A and D, especially for children.

A more recent advance has been the development of compounds that will replace fat more or less completely, while retaining the texture and flavour of traditional fatty foods. Two such compounds are Simplesse, which is a modified protein used in low-fat spreads (see Table 2.5), and not suitable for cooking, and Olestra, which is a fatty acid ester of sucrose (and hence chemically related to fats (see §6.3.1), but not absorbed) which is stable to cooking and can be used to prepare fat-free potato crisps, and so on.

2.4.2.1 *The type of fat in the diet*

Both the total amount of fat in the diet and also the type of fat are important in the development of the diseases of affluence. The fatty acids that make up the dietary fats can be classified chemically as being saturated or unsaturated. The different types of fat have different actions in the body, so there is a need for an understanding of the chemistry of foods. The chemistry of fats and fatty acids is discussed in §6.3.1. In saturated fatty acids there are only single bonds between the carbon atoms that make up the molecule, while in unsaturated fatty acids there may be one (mono-unsaturated) or more (polyunsaturated) double bonds between carbon atoms. In general, fats that contain mainly saturated fatty acids are hard at room temperature, whereas those that contain mainly unsaturated fatty acids are oils at room temperature. Table 2.6 shows the main sources of different types of fats in the average diet, and Table 2.7 shows the relative amounts of saturated, mono-unsaturated and polyunsaturated fatty acids in different types of cooking oil and fat.

Most studies of fat intake, heart disease and plasma cholesterol have shown that it is mainly saturated fats which pose a hazard to health, whereas unsaturated fatty acids have a beneficial effect, lowering LDL cholesterol, reducing the coagulability of blood platelets and reducing the risk of heart disease.

Therefore, the recommendation is to reduce intake of saturated fats considerably more than just in proportion with the reduction in total fat intake.

Table 2.6 Sources of different types of fat in the average British diet[a]

	Total	Saturated	Mono-unsaturated	Polyunsaturated
Meat and meat products	24	23	31	17
Butter and margarine	16	17	11	20
Milk and cheese	15	23	12	2
Cakes, biscuits, etc[b]	13	14	—	—
Vegetables[c]	11	6	12	24
Eggs	4	3	5	4
Fish	3	2	3	4

[a] The figures show the percentage of the total intake of different types of fat obtained from various foods in the average diet. They thus combine both the fat content of different foods and the amounts of various foods that people eat.

[b] The relative amounts of different types of fat in baked and other cooked foods will depend on the fat or oil used in cooking.

[c] The figures for vegetables include vegetable oils used in cooking.

Table 2.7 The percentage of saturated and unsaturated fatty acids in different types of cooking oil and fat

	Saturated	Mono-unsaturated	Polyunsaturated
Butter	64	33	3
Hard margarine[a]	38	49	13
Soft margarine[a]	33	44	23
Pufa margarine[a]	20	17	63
Lard	45	45	10
Coconut oil	91	7	2
Cottonseed oil	27	22	51
Corn oil	17	31	52
Olive oil	15	74	11
Palm oil	47	44	9
Peanut (arachis or groundnut) oil	20	50	30
Soya bean oil	15	25	60
Sunflower oil	14	34	52

[a] These are 'typical' values; the precise composition of the mixture of vegetable oils used in making margarines will vary from one type to another. Similarly, 'mixed vegetable oil' may well have a variable composition, containing different amounts of the various oils listed here.

Total fat intake should be 30 per cent of energy intake, with no more than 10 per cent from saturated fats (compared with the present average of 17 per cent of energy from saturated fat; see Table 2.3). The present average intakes of 6 per cent of energy from polyunsaturated fats and 12 per cent from monounsaturated fats match what is considered to be desirable, on the basis of epidemiological studies. About 2 per cent of energy intake is accounted for by the *trans*-isomers of unsaturated fatty acids (see §3.7.1.1), and it is considered that this should not increase.

2.4.3 *Carbohydrate intake*

If the total energy intake is to remain constant, but the proportion supplied by fat is to be reduced from the present average of about 39 per cent to about 30 per cent, and the proportion supplied by protein is to remain at about 15 per cent, then, obviously, the proportion supplied by carbohydrates will increase. The guideline is that 55 per cent of energy should come from carbohydrates.

Carbohydrates can be divided into two main groups: starches and sugars (this is a chemical term for a variety of carbohydrates, one of which is sucrose, cane or beet sugar; see §6.2.1). The guideline is that the proportion of energy that is derived from starches should be increased, and that from sugars reduced. Table 2.8 shows the average intakes of carbohydrate as a percentage

Table 2.8 The percentage of energy from different types of carbohydrate in the average British diet, compared with dietary guidelines

	Average	Range	Guidelines	Desirable change (%)
Total carbohydrate	43	30–55	53	+23
Starch	24	—	38	+58
Total sugars	19	—	15	−21
Sucrose	14	—	10	−29
Lactose	3	—	3	0
Glucose	2	—	2	0
Fat	40	27–50	30	−25
Protein	15	9–20	15	0
Alcohol	3	0–28	see Table 2.10	

of energy intake, and Table 2.9 shows those foods that are the main sources of carbohydrate in the diet.

2.4.3.1 *Sugars in the diet*

Dietary sugars can be considered in two groups:

- Intrinsic sugars in foods, contained within plant cell walls
- Extrinsic sugars, which are free in solution in the food and not contained within plant cell walls

Extrinsic sugars consist of the sugars released into solution when fruit juice is prepared, sugar and honey added to foods, and the lactose in milk. Milk is an excellent source of a variety of nutrients, most notably calcium (see §12.3.1)

Table 2.9 Sources of carbohydrate in the average British diet[a]

Source	Total carbohydrate	Sugars
Cereal products (including bread)	46	23
Bread	22	—
Fruit and vegetables	27	14[b]
Sugar, confectionery and jams	13	29
Soft drinks	7	17
Milk and milk products	6	13[c]

[a] The figures show the percentage of the total intake of carbohydrate (column 2) and sugars (column 3) obtained from various foods in the average diet. They thus combine both the carbohydrate content of different foods and the amounts of various foods that people eat.

[b] Mainly intrinsic sugars within plant cell walls.

[c] This includes both lactose in milk and sugar added to fruit yogurt, etc.

and vitamin B_2 (see §12.2.6). Apart from people who are intolerant of lactose (the sugar of milk, see §6.2.2.2), there is no evidence that lactose is associated with any health hazards. It is the non-milk extrinsic sugars that give cause for concern, and for which a reduction in intake is considered desirable.

Although there are various different sugars in the diet, the ones that cause most concern are sucrose (cane or beet sugar, a disaccharide of glucose and fructose; see §6.2.1.2) and honey (which is a mixture of glucose and fructose). There is some evidence that a high intake of sugar is a factor in the development of maturity onset diabetes and atherosclerosis, although the evidence is less convincing than for the adverse effects of a high intake of saturated fats. There is strong evidence for a harmful effect of sugar in the development of obesity and dental caries.

Sugar added to foods is a source of additional energy, but provides no nutrients. It makes many foods more palatable, and hence increases consumption. It may thus have a significant role in the development of obesity (see Chapter 8). This added sugar is mainly sucrose, although glucose syrups and mixtures of glucose and fructose are also widely used in food manufacturing.

Extrinsic sugars have a major role in the development of dental caries. Sucrose and other sugars encourage the growth of those bacteria that form dental plaque, and provide a metabolic substrate for the production by other bacteria of the acid which attacks dental enamel. Other factors are also important in the development of dental caries, including general oral hygiene and, perhaps most importantly, the intake of fluoride (see §12.3.5.1). The use of fluoride-containing toothpaste, and the addition of fluoride to drinking water, have led to a very dramatic decrease in dental decay since the 1960s, despite high intakes of sucrose.

The guideline is that 10–11 per cent of energy intake should be from non-milk extrinsic sugars. This can readily be achieved by reducing consumption of soft drinks, sweets, sugar added to foods, jams and honey, and so on.

2.4.3.2 *Undigested carbohydrates (dietary fibre)*

The residue of plant cell walls is not digested by human enzymes, but provides bulk in the diet (and hence in the intestines). It is measured by weighing the fraction of foods that remains after treatment with a variety of digestive enzymes. This is what is known as dietary fibre. It is a misleading term, since not all the components of dietary fibre are fibrous; some are soluble and form viscous gels.

Different compounds are grouped together under the heading of 'dietary fibre'. Chemically, the important compounds are polysaccharides (complex carbohydrates) other than starch (see §6.2.1.5), and a relatively recent development has been the specific measurement of these non-starch polysaccharides in foods.

The two methods of analysis give different results. Measurement of non-starch polysaccharides in the diet gives average intakes in Britain of 11–13 g per day, compared with an intake of dietary fibre of about 20 g per day, as measured by the less specific method. Non-starch polysaccharides are found only in foods of vegetable origin, and vegetarians have a higher intake than omnivores.

Dietary fibre has little nutritional value in its own right, since it consists of compounds that are not digested or absorbed to any significant extent. Nevertheless, it is a valuable component of the diet, and some of the products of fermentation of dietary fibre by colonic bacteria can be absorbed and utilized as metabolic fuel.

Diets low in fibre are associated with the excretion of a small bulk of faeces, and frequently with constipation and straining while defecating. This has been linked with the development of haemorrhoids, varicose veins and diverticular disease of the colon. These diseases are more common in Western countries, where people generally have a relatively low intake of non-starch polysaccharide, than in parts of the world where the intake is higher.

Some components of dietary fibre bind potentially undesirable compounds in the intestinal lumen, and so reduce their absorption; this may be especially important with respect to colon cancer. Compounds believed to be involved in causing or promoting cancer of the colon occur in the contents of the intestinal tract, both because they are present in foods and as a result of bacterial metabolism in the colon. They are bound by non-starch polysaccharides, and so cannot interact with the cells of the gut wall, but are eliminated in the faeces. In addition, the products of intestinal bacterial fermentation, of both non-starch polysaccharides and starch that is resistant to digestion in the small intestine, include compounds such as butyric acid, which has an inhibitory effect on the proliferation of tumour cells and is hence potentially valuable in terms of anticancer activity.

Epidemiological studies show that diets high in fibre are associated with a low risk of colon cancer. However, such diets also contain relatively large amounts of fruit and vegetables, and are therefore also rich in vitamins C and E and in carotene, which also have some protective action against the development of cancer (see §2.5.3). Furthermore, since they contain more fruit and vegetables, and less meat, such diets are also generally relatively low in saturated fats, and there is some evidence that a high intake of saturated fats is a separate risk factor for colon cancer.

A diet rich in fibre may help to lower blood cholesterol, and hence reduce the risk of atherosclerosis and coronary heart disease. This is because the bile salts, which are required for the absorption of fats (see §6.3.2), are formed in the liver from cholesterol and are secreted in the bile. Normally the greater part of bile salts secreted is reabsorbed; when the diet is rich in fibre, bile salts are bound, and so cannot be reabsorbed. This means that more bile salts have to be synthesized, using more cholesterol.

A total intake of about 18 g of non-starch polysaccharides per day is recommended (equivalent to about 30 g per day of dietary fibre). In general this should come from fibre-rich foods – whole grain cereals and wholemeal cereal products, fruits and vegetables – rather than supplements. This is because, as well as the fibre, these fibre-rich foods are valuable sources of a variety of nutrients. There is no evidence that intakes of fibre over about 30 g per day confer any benefit, other than in the treatment of bowel disease. Above this level of intake it is likely that people would reach satiety (or at least feel full, or even bloated) without eating enough food to satisfy energy needs (see §8.3.3.6). This may be a problem for children fed on a diet that is very high in fibre; they may be physically full but still physiologically hungry.

2.4.4 Salt

There is a physiological requirement for the mineral sodium, and salt (sodium chloride, NaCl) is the major dietary source of sodium. One of the basic senses of taste is for saltiness – a pleasant sensation (see §1.3.1). However, average intakes of salt in Western countries are considerably higher than the physiological requirement for sodium. Most people are able to cope with this excessive intake adequately by excreting the excess. However, people with a genetic predisposition to develop high blood pressure are sensitive to the amount of sodium in their diet. One of the ways of treating dangerously high blood pressure (hypertension) is by a severe restriction of salt intake. It is estimated that about 10 per cent of the population are salt sensitive, and epidemiologically there is a relationship between sodium intake and the increase in blood pressure that occurs with increasing age.

The problem in terms of public health and dietary advice to the population at large (as opposed to specific advice to people known to be at risk of, or suffering from, hypertension) is one of extrapolating from clinical studies in people who have severe hypertension, and who benefit from a severe restriction in salt intake, to the rest of the healthy population. It is not clear whether a modest reduction in salt intake will benefit those salt-sensitive individuals who might go on to develop severe hypertension. Nevertheless, it is prudent to recommend reducing the average intake of salt by about one-quarter, to a level that meets requirements for sodium without providing so great an excess over requirements as is seen in average diets at present. This can be achieved quite easily by reducing the amount of salt added in cooking, tasting food before adding salt at the table, and reducing the intake of salty snack foods. Low-sodium salt substitutes (*light salt*), containing mixtures of sodium and potassium chlorides, are available. They can be used in place of ordinary salt to help reduce the intake of sodium.

2.4.5 Alcohol

A high intake of alcoholic drinks can be a factor in causing obesity, both as a result of the energy yield of the alcohol itself and also because of the relatively high carbohydrate content of many alcoholic beverages. People who satisfy much of their energy requirement from alcohol frequently show vitamin deficiencies, because they are meeting their energy needs from drink, and therefore not eating enough foods to provide adequate amounts of vitamins and minerals. Deficiency of vitamin B_1 is a problem among heavy drinkers (see §12.2.7.1).

In moderate amounts, alcohol has an appetite-stimulating effect, and may also help the social aspect of meals. Furthermore, there is good epidemiological evidence that modest consumption of alcohol is protective against atherosclerosis and coronary heart disease. However, alcohol has harmful effects in excess, not only in the short term, when drunkenness may have undesirable consequences, but also in the longer term.

Habitual excess consumption of alcohol is associated with long-term health problems, including loss of mental capacity, liver damage and cancer of the oesophagus. Continued abuse can lead to physical and psychological addiction. The infants of mothers who drink more than a very small amount of alcohol during pregnancy are at risk of congenital abnormalities, and heavy alcohol consumption during pregnancy can result in the foetal alcohol syndrome: low birth weight and lasting impairment of intelligence, as well as congenital deformities. The guidelines on alcohol intake, the prudent upper limits of habitual consumption, are summarized in Table 2.10, and the alcohol content of beverages in Table 2.11. Daily consumption of more than 3 to 7 units (2 to 5 units for women) is considered hazardous, and over 7 units per day (5 units per day for women) dangerous, by the Royal College of Physicians.

2.4.6 *Food labelling and nutritional information*

In order to permit consumers to make informed choices of foods, to achieve these goals discussed above, there are clear regulations on the information that

Table 2.10 Prudent limits of alcohol consumption (in units of alcohol)[a]

	Men		Women	
	Weekly	Daily	Weekly	Daily
Low risk	<21	<3	<14	<2
Prudent upper limit[b]		3–4		2–3
Hazardous	28–50	4–7	21–35	3–5
Harmful	>50	>7	>35	>5

[a] 1 unit = 8 g of alcohol; see Table 2.11.
[b] A daily limit is preferred, because of the hazards associated with binge drinking.

Table 2.11 The alcohol content of beverages

	% alcohol by volume	Amount for 1 unit
Beer and cider	4–6	$\frac{1}{2}$ pint (300 ml)
Table wine	9.5–12.5	1 glass (100 ml)
Vermouth, aperitifs	15–18	
Port and sherry	18–20	
Liqueurs	20–40	
Spirits	35–45	1 single (25 ml)
Proof spirit, UK	57.07	
Proof spirit, USA	50	

must, or may, be provided on food labels, and the format in which the information must be presented.

By law, food labels must contain a list of the ingredients of the food, in the order of the quantities present. Food additives may be listed by either their chemical names or numbers in the list of permitted additives (the 'E-' numbers). The weight or volume of the contents must also be shown on the label; where this is a size which has been registered with the appropriate authority of the European Union, the weight or volume is preceded by a small letter 'e'. The name and address of the manufacturer must also be printed on the label.

Nutritional labelling involves giving further information: the energy yield, and the content of fat, protein and carbohydrate; the proportion or amount of saturated and unsaturated fats in the foods; and the proportion of the total carbohydrate present as starches and sugars. This detailed nutritional labelling is not yet obligatory in the European Union (although it is compulsory in the USA), but if the information is provided, it must be in a standard format. If *any* nutritional claims are made, then full nutritional information must be given, in the prescribed form.

Claims for the vitamin and mineral content of foods must similarly be made in a standard format, and may only be made if the food in question provides a significant percentage of requirements. The content of vitamins and minerals must be shown as both the amount present and as the percentage of the reference intake (see §12.1.1.2). Within the European Union, labels must show the nutrient content per unit weight of the food; in the USA the information must be presented per standard serving.

2.5 Free radicals and antioxidant nutrients

As discussed in §3.2.2.2, free radicals are highly reactive, unstable molecular species. They exist for only extremely short periods of time, of the order of nanoseconds (10^{-9} s) or less, before reacting with another molecule. However, in the process a new radical is generated, so that radicals initiate self-perpetuating chain reactions.

2.5.1 Sources of oxygen radicals

In biological systems the most damaging radicals are those derived from oxygen – the so-called reactive oxygen species. They arise in the body in four main ways:

- As a result of normal oxidative metabolism, and especially reactions involving the reoxidation of reduced flavin coenzymes (see §5.3.1).
- As a part of the action of macrophages in killing invading microorganisms. This means that infection can lead to a considerable increase in the total radical burden in the body. As discussed in §9.3.1, this may be an important factor in the protein-energy deficiency disease, kwashiorkor.
- As a result of non-enzymic reactions of a variety of metal ions in free solution (and especially iron and copper) with oxygen. Normally such reactive metal ions are not present in free solution to any significant extent, but are bound to transport proteins (in plasma) or storage proteins and enzymes (in cells).
- As a result of exposure to ionizing radiation – X-rays, the radiation from radioactive isotopes (see §3.1.1) and ultraviolet radiation from sunlight.

2.5.2 Tissue damage by oxygen radicals

Radicals may interact with any compounds present in the cell, and the result may be initiation of cancer, inheritable mutations, atherosclerosis and coronary heart disease or autoimmune disease. The most important, and potentially damaging, such interactions are:

- With DNA in the nucleus, causing chemical changes in the nucleic acid bases (see §10.2.1) or breaks in the DNA strand. This damage may result in heritable mutations if the damage is to ovaries or testes, or the induction of cancer in other tissues.
- With individual amino acids in proteins. This results in a chemical modification of the protein, which may therefore be recognized as foreign by the immune system, leading to the production of antibodies that will also react with the normal unmodified body protein. This may be an important factor in the development of autoimmune disease.
- With unsaturated fatty acids in cell membranes. If the damage is severe enough, it will result in lysis of the membrane and cell death. Less severe damage does not kill the cell, but oxidation of unsaturated fatty acids leads to the formation of very reactive dialdehydes. These react especially with DNA, causing chemical modification, and hence may result in either heritable mutations or initiation of cancer.

- With unsaturated fatty acids in plasma lipoproteins. Oxidative damage to plasma lipoproteins leads to activation of macrophages, and eventually to the initiation of the development of atherosclerotic plaque.

2.5.3 *Antioxidant nutrients and non-nutrients: protection against radical damage*

Apart from avoidance of exposure to ionizing radiation, there is little that can be done to prevent the formation of radicals, since they are the result of normal metabolic processes and responses to infection. However, there are mechanisms to minimize the damage done by radical action. Since the important radicals are oxygen radicals, and the damage done is oxidative damage, the protective compounds are known collectively as antioxidants.

Three vitamins have important antioxidant actions. In each case they are capable of reacting with a radical and, because of their chemical structure, forming a stable radical that persists for long enough to undergo a chemical reaction to quench the chain reaction. Vitamin E (see §12.2.3) acts to inactivate the products of radical damage to unsaturated fatty acids in membranes and plasma lipoproteins. There is a fairly convincing body of evidence to suggest that intakes of vitamin E considerably higher than those required to prevent deficiency, and probably higher than can be achieved from normal diets, may have significant protective action against the development of atherosclerosis and cardiovascular disease, and some forms of cancer. Vitamin C (see §12.2.13) reacts with the vitamin E radical, regenerating active vitamin E, and forming a stable radical that is reduced back to active vitamin C enzymically. β-Carotene (see §12.2.1.2) can also form stable radicals, and may have beneficial effects in preventing the development of some forms of cancer.

Several minerals, including especially selenium (see §12.3.2.5), copper (§12.3.2.2) and zinc (§12.3.2.6), are required for the formation of enzymes that remove reactive oxygen species, and so provide protection. Although deficiency of these minerals may increase radical damage (see §9.3.1), there is no evidence that intakes above amounts required to meet requirements will provide any further protection.

Other compounds that are not nutrients, but are formed in the body as normal metabolites, also provide protection against radical damage. Such compounds include uric acid (the end-product of the metabolism of the purines) and the coenzyme ubiquinone (see §5.3.1.2). This latter is sometimes marketed as vitamin Q, but it can be synthesized in the body, and there is no evidence that it is a dietary essential, nor that an increase above the amount that is normally present in tissues confers any benefit.

In addition to these protective nutrients and normal metabolites, a considerable variety of compounds that are naturally present in plant foods also have antioxidant action. Some non-nutrients present in plant foods also have other potentially protective effects, altering the metabolism of potentially carcinogenic compounds by either reducing the rate at which they are activated in the body or increasing the rate at which they are metabolized to forms that are excreted.

Collectively these beneficial (and sometimes also hazardous) non-nutrients in plant foods are known as phytochemicals. They are not classified as nutrients because they do not have a clear function in the body, and deficiency does not lead to any specific lesions. Nevertheless, they are important in the diet and they provide a sound basis for increasing intake of fruits and vegetables, quite apart from the beneficial effects of increased intake of dietary fibre, vitamins and minerals, and reduced intake of fat (and especially saturated fat) that would be the result.

2.6 Is there any need for nutritional supplements?

Average intakes of vitamins and minerals in developed countries are more than adequate to meet requirements, and deficiency diseases are rarely, if ever, caused simply by an inadequate intake. The main nutritional problems in developed countries are associated with an excessive intake of food, and especially saturated fats and sugars, not with inadequate intakes of nutrients. There is no evidence that supplements of vitamins and minerals will increase a child's intelligence or ability to learn, although if the child were marginally deficient then supplements would, of course, be beneficial. Nevertheless, there is an ever-growing market for vitamin and mineral supplements, as well as a whole host of compounds of dubious nutritional value.

The potential benefits of vitamin E at levels above what might be achieved from a normal diet were discussed in §2.5.3. In addition, there are three nutrients that do give cause for concern, even in developed countries, and where supplements are recommended for specific population groups:

- Some 10–15 per cent of women suffer a greater loss of iron in menstruation than can be replaced from the diet. They are therefore at risk of iron deficiency and will benefit from iron supplements (see §12.3.2.3).
- Spina bifida and neural tube defects affect some 0.75 per 1000 live births, and there is excellent evidence that supplements of folic acid of 400 μg per day reduce the incidence very considerably (see §12.2.10.2). This is above the level that could be achieved from a normal diet, so again supplements are recommended. Although it might seem that the supplements are required only in pregnancy, to protect the developing foetus, the problem is that the neural tube closes (and hence the damage, if any, is done) 27 days after conception – before the mother knows that she is pregnant. Therefore, the advice is that all women who might be about to become pregnant should take folic acid supplements.
- There are very few dietary sources of vitamin D (see §12.2.2), and it is unlikely that people who are housebound and elderly, who have little exposure to sunlight, will be able to achieve an adequate intake without the use of supplements or enriched foods.

Vitamin and mineral supplements which provide about the reference intake of the various nutrients (itself an amount greater than average requirements; see §12.1.1) may be regarded as a sensible insurance policy by people whose diet is inadequate. Although they may not be beneficial, at least they will do no harm. However, preparations are available that provide very large amounts of individual vitamins, minerals or amino acids. Here the effects of supplements are pharmacological or drug-like, rather than nutritional. However, because they are nutrients, they are subject to food laws and hence are freely available, rather than the laws governing the sale of medicines, which require clear evidence of efficacy and safety. The possible pharmacological actions of some vitamins and minerals, and the dangers of excessive intakes, are discussed in Chapter 12.

The basic guidelines for a prudent diet can be summarized as follows:

- Eat as wide a variety of foods as you can.
- Read the labels on food packaging (§2.4.6). These will generally give you a great deal of information, but read the small print containing the nutrition information on the side of the package as well as the bold flash on the front which claims that the contents are *low in fat* or *low in sugar*.
- Eat at least one meal of fish a week (§6.3.1.1).
- Eat five servings of fruit or yellow or green vegetables each day (§2.5.3).
- Try eating vegetarian dishes instead of meat now and again.
- Eat wholemeal bread and whole grain cereal products in preference to refined cereals (§2.4.3.2).
- Trim visible fat off meat and grill meat rather than frying it (§2.4.2).
- Buy low-fat mince, sausages, burgers, etc. (§2.4.2).
- Use vegetable oils and margarine rich in polyunsaturated fats in preference to saturated cooking fats and butter (§2.4.2.1).
- Use low fat spreads rather than butter or margarine (§2.4.2).
- Use semi-skimmed or skimmed milk instead of full cream milk (§2.4.2), but not for young children.
- Use yogurt rather than cream (§2.4.2) – but be warned that fruit-flavoured yogurts contain high levels of sugar.
- Reduce your intake of sugar (§2.4.3.1) – use non-nutritive sweeteners in beverages and low calorie lemonades made with non-nutritive sweeteners (see §8.3.3.8).
- Do not add salt to food unless you have tasted it and know you need to add it, and do not add salt when cooking vegetables (§2.4.4).
- Drink alcohol in moderation, if at all – and try to have an alcohol-free day now and again (§2.4.5).

3

The Chemical Basis of Life

In order to understand the basis of the dietary guidelines discussed in Chapter 2, to interpret and evaluate new evidence of health risks and benefits from changes in diet, and appreciate the way in which nutrition is important for the maintenance of the normal integrity and functions of the body, it is necessary to understand the chemistry and metabolism of the body. This chapter reviews the basic principles of chemistry that are important for an understanding of nutrition and metabolism, and the structures of biologically and metabolically important compounds.

3.1 Elements and atoms

The basic unit of chemical structure is the atom. There are 112 different chemical elements known, of which 96 occur naturally, the remainder being the products of nuclear reactions. Only a few of these 112 elements are important in biological systems. Each element has a characteristic atomic composition, but the underlying structure of all atoms is similar.

An atom consists of a nucleus, which has a positive electric charge, surrounded by a cloud of electrons, which have a negative electric charge. The number of positively charged particles (protons) in the nucleus is equal to the number of electrons surrounding the nucleus, so that an atom has no net electrical charge.

The simplest element is hydrogen, which consists of a single proton, accompanied by a single electron. The different elements are characterized by the number of protons in the nucleus, which in turn determines the number of electrons surrounding the nucleus. This is the atomic number of that element. Each element has a unique atomic number.

As well as protons, the nuclei of most elements contain uncharged particles, the most important of which are the neutrons. The mass of a neutron is almost the same as that of a proton (which is 1.67×10^{-24} g; the mass of an electron is only 1/1840 of that of a proton (i.e. 9×10^{-28} g), and can be considered to be negligible). A relative atomic mass or weight is assigned to each element, based on the number of protons and neutrons in the nucleus, with one unit of mass for each proton or neutron. Table 3.1 lists some of the elements that are important in biological systems, together with their atomic numbers and relative atomic masses.

For convenience when writing chemical formulae, one or two letter abbreviations of the names of the elements are used. Some are obvious and simple – for example, H for hydrogen, C for carbon and Ca for calcium; others are less obvious. This is because two or more different elements could have the same abbreviation. In such cases the abbreviations are based on the old Latin names of the elements. Thus, copper is Cu, from *cuprum*, to avoid confusion with cobalt, which is Co; iron is Fe (*ferrum*), sodium is Na (*natrium*), potassium is K (*kalium*) and lead is Pb (*plumbum*).

Table 3.1 The biologically important elements

Element	Symbol	Atomic number	Atomic mass
Carbon	C	6	12.01
Hydrogen	H	1	1.008
Oxygen	O	8	16.00
Nitrogen	N	7	14.00
Phosphorus	P	15	30.98
Aluminium	Al	13	26.97
Calcium	Ca	20	40.08
Chlorine	Cl	17	35.46
Chromium	Cr	24	52.01
Cobalt	Co	27	58.94
Copper	Cu	29	63.57
Fluorine	F	9	19.00
Iodine	I	53	126.91
Iron	Fe	26	55.85
Lead	Pb	82	207.21
Lithium	Li	3	6.94
Magnesium	Mg	12	24.32
Manganese	Mn	25	54.93
Mercury	Hg	80	200.61
Molybdenum	Mo	42	95.95
Nickel	Ni	28	58.69
Potassium	K	19	39.09
Selenium	Se	34	78.96
Sodium	Na	11	22.97
Sulphur	S	16	32.06
Tin	Sn	50	118.70
Zinc	Zn	30	65.38

Although the composition of the nucleus is unique for any element, it is the distribution of electrons around the nucleus that determines the chemical reactivity of the atom, and hence the characteristic chemistry of that element.

Electrons are not randomly distributed around the nucleus, but occupy a series of concentric shells or orbitals. Those orbitals nearest to the nucleus are normally filled first. Elements with a higher atomic number will have more electrons surrounding the nucleus, and hence their atoms will be larger than those of elements with lower atomic numbers. The diameter of the outermost orbital of electrons around the carbon atom (atomic number = 6) is 0.154 nm, about 10^4 times larger than the nucleus.

It is the outermost electrons that participate in chemical reactions. This means that elements with a similar distribution of electrons in the outermost orbitals will have similar chemistry.

3.1.1 Isotopes

The chemistry of an element is determined by its atomic number, and therefore the electron distribution around the nucleus. Some elements exist in multiple forms, called isotopes, with differing nuclear composition. As discussed below, isotopes are widely used in biochemical, nutritional and medical research.

The nuclei of the different isotopes of any element contain the same number of protons, and therefore they have the same number of electrons, and chemically they react in the same way. However, the nuclei of the different isotopes contain different numbers of neutrons. This means that the isotopes differ from each other in their atomic mass, which can be measured.

Some isotopes are unstable, and their nuclei decay, emitting radiation. These are the radioactive isotopes, and they can be detected and measured by the radiation they emit. Other isotopes are stable; their nuclei do not decay, and they do not emit any radiation. They are detected and measured by their differing atomic mass.

In order to specify a particular isotope, the atomic mass is shown as a superscript before the abbreviation for the element. Thus, the most commonly occurring form of carbon has an atomic mass of 12, whereas the radioactive isotope has an atomic mass of 14, shown as ^{14}C to specify that this is the isotope of carbon being considered.

Some stable and radioactive isotopes (Table 3.2) are widely used in biochemical and nutritional research. A chemical compound containing one or more atoms of either a radioactive or stable isotope is labelled by that isotope. Although the presence of the isotope can be detected by measuring the radiation emitted as it decays, or its abnormal atomic mass, the labelled compound behaves chemically in exactly the same way as the unlabelled compound. Such labelled compounds can be used to follow metabolic pathways; many of the pathways that will be discussed in later chapters of this book have been established in this way. As discussed in §7.1.2, the use of water

Table 3.2 Isotopes commonly used in biochemical and nutritional research

Element	Isotope	Stability
Hydrogen[a]	^{2}H	Stable
	^{3}H	Radioactive
Carbon	^{13}C	Stable
	^{14}C	Radioactive
Oxygen	^{18}O	Stable
Nitrogen	^{15}N	Stable
Sulphur	^{35}S	Radioactive
Phosphorus	^{32}P	Radioactive
Iron	^{57}Fe	Radioactive
	^{59}Fe	Radioactive
Iodine	^{125}I	Radioactive
	^{131}I	Radioactive
Sodium	^{23}Na	Radioactive
Calcium	^{45}Ca	Radioactive
Cobalt	^{65}Co	Radioactive

[a] The isotopes of hydrogen are sometimes called: deuterium (^{2}H) and tritium (^{3}H).

labelled with the stable isotopes ^{2}H and ^{18}O has permitted measurement of average energy expenditure over a period of several weeks and has permitted revision of estimates of energy requirements. In the same way, use of proteins containing the stable isotope of nitrogen, ^{15}N, allows changes in protein turnover in the body to be followed, permitting more precise estimates of protein requirements (see §10.1).

The radiation emitted when radioactive isotopes decay may penetrate solid matter for quite a distance before it interacts with an atom. Excessive exposure to such penetrating radiation is dangerous, because the radiation can interact with body constituents, producing highly reactive free radicals (see §2.5 and §3.2.2.2), causing genetic damage, or even killing cells. Controlled exposure to small amounts of such radiation is used in X-rays and computer axial tomography (CAT) scanning to visualize internal organs, and in radiotherapy, where the aim is to exploit the damaging action of the radiation to kill the cancer cells it is focused on.

Other radioactive isotopes produce radiation with very much lower energy, which is absorbed by only a few centimetres of air, a thin layer of paper or plastic gloves. Such isotopes include ^{14}C and ^{3}H, which are commonly used in studies of metabolism. Although radioactive isotopes of carbon and hydrogen have been given to human beings in the past for experimental purposes, this is rarely done now, because, even though the radiation has very low energy, it can still cause tissue damage when taken internally. Radioactive isotopes are sometimes given to patients, for example when there is no other means of investigating a rare disease, or as a means of imaging specific glands and organs.

3.2 Compounds and molecules: the formation of chemical bonds

The electrons surrounding the nucleus of an atom occupy orbitals in a series of defined shells. The innermost shell can contain two electrons. The next can contain eight, and the third eighteen. When these three sets of orbitals are filled, so a further set begins, consisting of shells capable of containing eight and eighteen electrons. This is repeated as necessary to make up the characteristic pattern of electrons of the various elements.

The only elements whose atoms have completely filled electron shells are the inert gases (helium, argon, neon, etc.). These gases exist as isolated atoms and have little or no chemical reactivity, because of their stable outer electron configuration.

For all the other elements, isolated atoms are unstable, because they have unfilled orbitals. Isolated atoms of most elements exist only under extreme conditions, for example at very high temperatures, as in a flame.

The empty orbitals can be filled, to create a stable configuration, in two ways:

- Transfer of electrons from one atom to another to create charged particles (ions, see §3.2.1)
- Sharing of electrons between atoms, forming a covalent bond (see §3.2.2).

3.2.1 *Ions and ionic bonds*

The basis of ionic bonding is the transfer of electrons from one atom to another. The atoms of some elements can achieve a stable electron configuration by giving up one or more electrons to a suitable acceptor atom. Other elements achieve a stable electron configuration by accepting one or more electrons. The result of donation or acceptance of electrons is the formation of a charged particle – an ion.

Donation of electrons results in the formation of a positively charged ion, because there are now fewer (negatively charged) electrons surrounding the nucleus than there are (positively charged) protons in the nucleus. Elements that achieve a stable electron configuration by the donation of electrons, forming positive ions, are electropositive and metallic.

Acceptance of electrons results in the formation of a negatively charged ion, since there are now more electrons surrounding the nucleus than protons within the nucleus. Elements that achieve a stable electron configuration by the acceptance of electrons, forming negative ions, are electronegative and non-metallic.

Hydrogen occupies an interesting position. It has one electron, and can achieve stability by either donating that electron, resulting in the formation of a proton (H^+ ion) or, less commonly, accepting an electron from a donor, resulting in the formation of the H^- (hydride) ion.

The magnitude of the positive charge on a metal ion depends on the number of electrons it has donated:

- A metal with one 'spare' electron can achieve a stable configuration by donating one electron to an acceptor, so forming an ion with a single positive charge. Biologically important metals that form ions with a single positive charge include sodium (Na^+) and potassium (K^+).
- A metal with two 'spare' electrons can achieve a stable configuration by donating two electrons to an acceptor, so forming an ion with a double positive charge. Biologically important metals that form ions with a double positive charge include calcium (Ca^{2+}), magnesium (Mg^{2+}) and zinc (Zn^{2+}).
- Some metals can achieve more than one stable configuration of electrons, by leaving some of the inner electron orbitals unfilled, and thus can form more than one positively charged ion. For example, copper can form ions with single or double positive charges (Cu^+ or Cu^{2+}) and iron can form ions with two or three positive charges (Fe^{2+} or Fe^{3+}).
- A non-metallic element that lacks one electron to achieve stability can accept one electron from a donor, forming an ion with a single negative charge. Biologically important elements in this group include chlorine, which forms the chloride ion (Cl^-), fluorine (forming the fluoride ion, F^-) and iodine (forming the iodide ion, I^-).
- An element which lacks two electrons to achieve stability can accept two electrons from a donor, forming an ion with a double negative charge. Biologically important elements in this group include oxygen, which forms the oxide ion (O^{2-}) and sulphur, which forms the sulphide ion (S^{2-}).

Ions do not exist in isolation. The total number of positive and negative charges is always equal, with no net electric charge. Thus, ordinary salt is sodium chloride; its formula is shown as NaCl, although actually it consists of Na^+ and Cl^- ions. Calcium chloride is $CaCl_2 : Ca^{2+} + 2 \times Cl^-$.

3.2.2 *Covalent bonding: the formation of molecules*

In addition to achieving a stable electron configuration by an overall transfer of electrons between atoms, to form ions, atoms can achieve stability by sharing electrons. An electron shared between two atoms can be considered to spend part of its time in the empty orbitals of each atom, thus creating a stable configuration of partially occupied orbitals around the two nuclei. This sharing of electrons forms a bond between the atoms, and the result is a molecule rather than separate atoms or ions. Each atom requires to share a char-

Two atoms of hydrogen share two electrons, forming a single bond

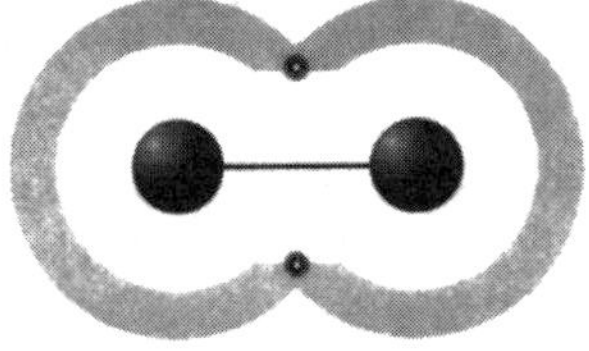

Two atoms of oxygen share four electrons, forming a double bond

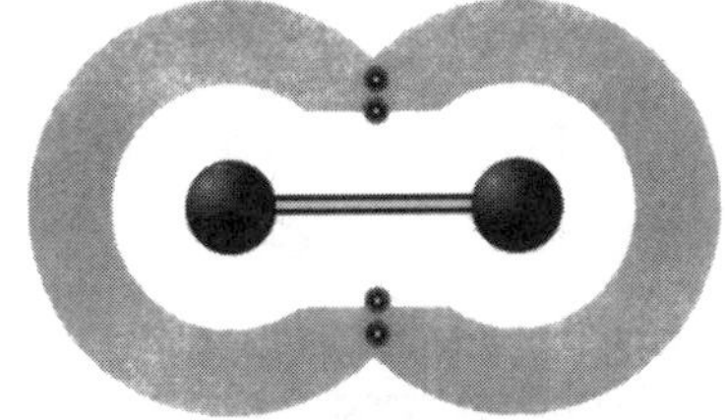

Two atoms of nitrogen share six electrons, forming a triple bond

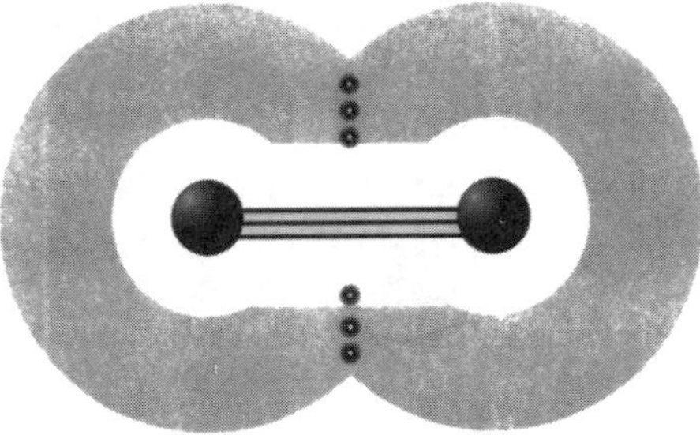

Figure 3.1 The formation of molecules of hydrogen, oxygen and nitrogen by covalent bonding.

acteristic number of electrons with other atoms to achieve a stable configuration. This means that each element forms a characteristic number of bonds to other atoms in a molecule. The number of bonds that must be formed by an element to achieve a stable electron configuration is the valency of that element. This type of chemical bond between atoms is covalent bonding, because the individual atoms making up the molecule share electrons in such a way that each achieves a share in the number of electrons required to meet its valency requirement and so complete a stable outer shell of electrons.

- Hydrogen has one electron per atom, and therefore requires to share one more to achieve a stable electron configuration. Hydrogen thus forms one bond to another atom and has a valency of 1.

- Oxygen requires to share two electrons to achieve a stable configuration; it forms two bonds to other atoms and has a valency of 2.
- Nitrogen requires to share three electrons to achieve a stable configuration; it forms three bonds to other atoms and has a valency of 3.
- Carbon requires to share four electrons to achieve a stable electron configuration; it forms four bonds to other atoms and has a valency of 4.

The simplest molecules consist of two atoms of the same kind, as occurs in the gases hydrogen, oxygen and nitrogen, forming molecules written as H_2, O_2 or N_2 (see Figure 3.1).

- Two atoms of hydrogen share two electrons, forming one bond, H—H.
- Two atoms of oxygen share four electrons, forming two bonds, O=O.
- Two atoms of nitrogen share six electrons, forming three bonds, N≡N.

Covalent bonding also occurs between atoms of different elements (see Figure 3.2). The number of bonds formed is determined by the valency of each element.

- In methane, four hydrogen atoms each share an electron with one carbon atom. The result is CH_4. Each hydrogen now has its share in four electrons, and forms one bond; the carbon has a share in eight electrons and forms four bonds, one to each hydrogen.
- In water, two atoms of hydrogen each share an electron with one atom of oxygen. The result is H–O–H (H_2O). Each hydrogen now has a share in two electrons, and forms one bond; the oxygen atom has a share in four electrons, and thus forms two bonds, one to each hydrogen.
- In carbon dioxide, two atoms of oxygen each share two electrons with an atom of carbon. The result is O=C=O (CO_2). Each oxygen now has a share in four electrons, and forms two double bonds, and the carbon has a share in eight.

3.2.2.1 *Unsaturated compounds: single, double and triple bonds*

For simple compounds of carbon and hydrogen (hydrocarbons), valency can be satisfied by a mixture of single, double and triple bonds between carbon atoms.

The simplest hydrocarbon is the gas methane (CH_4; as shown in Figure 3.2). Here, four atoms of hydrogen each share electrons with carbon, so fulfilling the valency of hydrogen (1) and that of carbon (4). The same occurs with the gas ethane (C_2H_6). Here, there is one bond formed between the two carbon atoms, and the remaining three valencies of each carbon are fulfilled by sharing electrons with hydrogen atoms: $H_3C–CH_3$.

Methane: one carbon atom shares electrons with each of four hydrogen atoms, forming 4 single bonds.

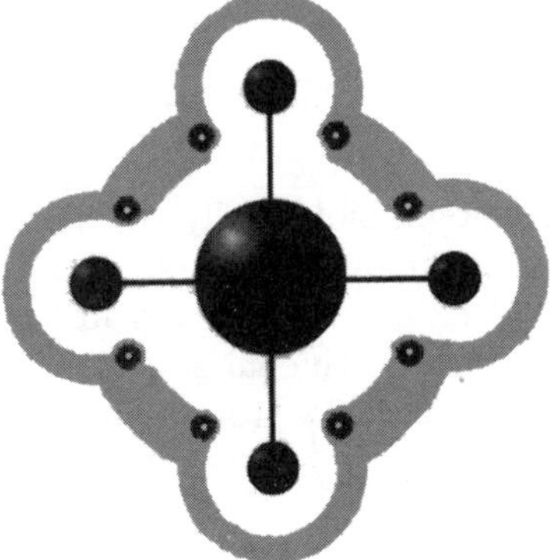

Water: one oxygen atom shares electrons with each of two hydrogen atoms, forming 2 single bonds

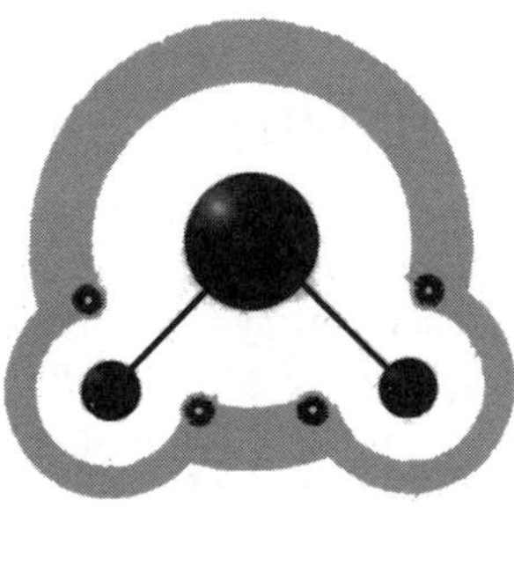

Carbon dioxide: one carbon atom shares four electrons with each of two oxygen atoms, forming 2 double bonds

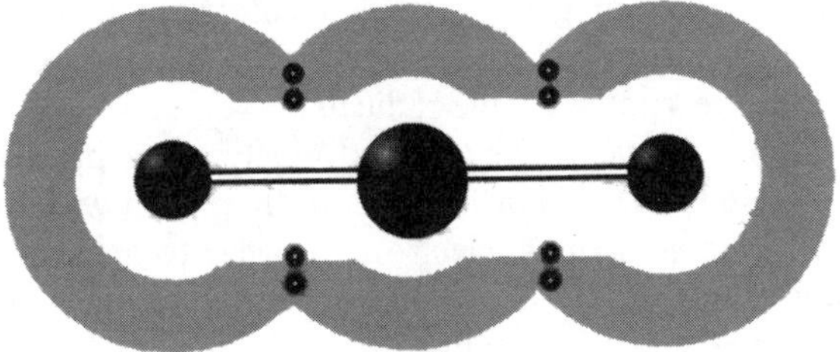

Figure 3.2 The formation of molecules of methane, water and carbon dioxide by covalent bonding.

In the gas ethene (sometimes also called ethylene, C_2H_4) a double bond is formed between the two carbon atoms, so that two of the four valencies of each carbon have been satisfied. Therefore, each carbon only needs to share electrons with two hydrogens to fulfil its valency of four: $H_2C{=}CH_2$.

In the gas ethyne (sometimes also called acetylene, C_2H_2) a triple bond is formed between the two carbon atoms, so that three of the four valencies of each carbon have been satisfied. Therefore, each carbon needs to share electrons with only one hydrogen to fulfil its valency: $HC{\equiv}CH$.

Such compounds, with carbon–carbon double or triple bonds, are known as unsaturated. Although they form stable molecules, in which all the valencies of carbon are occupied, they can react with more hydrogen, until they form a saturated compound (one in which there is only a single bond between the carbon atoms) and all the remaining valencies of the carbon are occupied by sharing electrons with hydrogen:

- Ethyne can be partially saturated with hydrogen, to form ethene:

$$HC{\equiv}CH + H_2 \rightarrow H_2C{=}CH_2\,;$$

- Ethene can react with more hydrogen, yielding the fully saturated compound ethane:

$$H_2C{=}CH_2 + H_2 \rightarrow H_3C{-}CH_3\,.$$

Triple bonds between carbon atoms are rare in biologically important molecules, but carbon–carbon double bonds are extremely important in a variety of biochemical systems. As discussed in §2.4.2.1, saturated and unsaturated fatty acids have different effects in the body, and nutritional guidelines involve not only the total amount of fat in the diet but also the proportion of saturated and unsaturated fat.

3.2.2.2 Free radicals

A compound that loses or gains a single electron, and thus has an unpaired electron in its outermost shell, is extremely unstable and very highly reactive. Such compounds are known as free radicals.

Free radicals usually exist for only extremely short periods of time, of the order of nanoseconds (10^{-9} s) or less, before they react with another molecule, either gaining or losing a single electron, in order to achieve a stable configuration. However, this reaction in turn generates another molecule with an unpaired electron. Each time a radical reacts with a molecule, while losing its unpaired electron and achieving stability, it generates another radical in turn, which is again short-lived and highly reactive. This is a chain reaction.

To show that a compound is a free radical, its chemical formula is shown with a superscript dot ($^{\bullet}$) to represent the unpaired electron; for example, the hydroxyl radical is $^{\bullet}OH$.

If two radicals react together, each contributes its unpaired electron to the formation of a new, stable bond. This means that the chain reaction, in which reaction of radicals with other molecules generates new radicals, is stopped. This is quenching of the chain reaction, or quenching of the radicals. Since radicals are generally so short-lived, it is rare for two radicals to come together to quench each other in this way.

Some radicals are relatively stable. This applies especially to those formed from molecules with aromatic rings or conjugated double-bond systems (see §3.6.1.1). A single unpaired electron can be distributed or delocalized through such a system of double bonds, and the resultant radical is less reactive and longer lived than most radicals. Compounds capable of forming relatively stable radicals are important in quenching radical chain reactions. Their radicals often have a lifetime long enough to permit two such stable radicals to come together, react with each other, and so terminate the chain. Vitamin E (see §12.2.3) and carotene (§12.2.1.2) are especially important in quenching radical reactions in biological systems. The tissue damage done by free radicals, and the main mechanisms of protection against radical damage are discussed in §2.5.

3.2.2.3 *Molecular mass and moles*

In order to consider equal amounts of compounds, it is necessary to know how many molecules of each compound are present, rather than the mass or weight of material. The relative molecular mass (M_r, sometimes called the molecular weight) of any compound is calculated from its chemical formula and the relative atomic masses of its constituent atoms (see Table 3.1). For example:

- methane = CH_4 = 1 × C(=12) + 4 × H(=4 × 1 = 4), therefore $M_r = 16$
- water = H_2O = 2 × H(=2 × 1) + 1 × O (=16), therefore $M_r = 18$
- carbon dioxide = CO_2 = 1 × C (=12) + 2 × O (=2 × 16 = 32), therefore $M_r = 44$

Since the molecules of methane, water and carbon dioxide have different masses, it is obvious that 1 g of each will contain a different number of molecules; in other words, different amounts of each compound, although there will be the same mass of each compound present. There are more molecules of water ($M_r = 18$) in a gram of water than there are molecules of carbon dioxide in a gram of carbon dioxide ($M_r = 44$). When describing chemical or biochemical reactions, it is the number of molecules that are present to react with each other that is important, not the mass of material present.

The number of molecules of different compounds is described using the term mole (abbreviated to mol, and derived from molecule). The mole is defined as the relative molecular mass of a compound, expressed in grams, and is the SI unit for the amount of substance present. Thus, for the reaction: $A + B \rightarrow C$, 1 mol of compound A reacts with 1 mol of compound B to form 1 mol of the product C.

One mole of a compound has a mass equal to the relative molecular mass in grams; thus, 1 mol of methane weighs 16 g, 1 mol of water 18 g and 1 mol of carbon dioxide 44 g. The number of moles of a compound in a given mass can be calculated from the same information; for example, 1 g of methane ($M_r = 16$) contains 1/16 mol = 0.0625 mol = 62.5 mmol.

3.3 The states of matter: solids, liquids and gases

Molecules are not stationary, but are continually moving. Indeed, the whole of chemistry depends on the fact that molecules do move around, and hence different molecules can come together to undergo chemical reactions. The extent of their movement depends mainly on the size of the molecules (and hence on their relative molecular mass), and the temperature. At higher temperatures, molecules move faster and farther from each other. In a solid, the molecules move only relatively slowly, and do not move far from each other. Because of this, a solid has a defined shape. It expands as the temperature increases, because the molecules can move slightly farther from each other. As the temperature of a solid increases, so the molecules move faster and farther from each other. Eventually they reach such a speed that the defined shape of the solid is lost: the solid has melted to a liquid. The temperature at which each compound melts is a characteristic of that particular compound and it depends on two main factors:

- *The size of the molecules* (i.e. the relative molecular mass): Larger, heavier, molecules will remain closely associated, as solids, at higher temperatures than smaller molecules.
- *The shape of the molecules*: Some molecules have a regular shape, and can interact very closely with each other. Such molecules require a greater input of energy (in the form of heat) to break away from each other and melt than do molecules that cannot fit so closely to each other. The different shapes of saturated and unsaturated fatty acids (see §6.3.1.1) mean that unsaturated fats melt at a lower temperature than do saturated fats. Indeed, unsaturated fats are liquids (oils) at ordinary temperatures, whereas saturated fats are solids.

As the temperature of a liquid increases, so the molecules move faster and further from each other, leading to an increase in volume as a liquid is heated. For example, a thermometer depends on the fact that the mercury or alcohol inside expands, and so takes up more room, as its temperature increases.

As a liquid is heated further, so it reaches the point where the molecules break away from each other altogether, and the liquid boils to form a gas. Like the temperature at which a compound melts, the temperature at which it boils is a characteristic of that compound, and depends on three main factors:

- *The size of the molecule, and hence its relative molecular mass*: As with melting, larger, heavier molecules require a greater input of energy in order to break away from the liquid.
- *Interactions between the molecules*: These may depend on the shape of the molecules, as described above for melting, or may be more complex interactions, as discussed in §3.3.1.
- *The pressure*: Boiling requires the molecules to break away from the liquid and join other molecules in the gas phase. At higher pressure, the molecules have to move faster to join the gas phase, and therefore have to be heated to a higher temperature. At a pressure of 15 lb (6.8 kg) above atmospheric pressure, water reaches a temperature of 121°C without boiling. Not only does this cook food faster (in a domestic pressure cooker), but it is also a temperature high enough to kill more or less all microorganisms within

about 15 min. This is the basis of the autoclave, which is used to sterilize surgical instruments, dressings, and so on.

3.3.1 Interactions between molecules: why water is a liquid

Both methane ($M_r = 16$) and carbon dioxide ($M_r = 44$) are gases at ordinary temperature and pressure, yet water ($M_r = 18$) is a liquid. This is because water molecules can interact with each other in a way which carbon dioxide and methane molecules cannot.

Although the formation of a covalent bond is the sharing of one or more electrons between the atoms that make up the molecule, it is not always completely even sharing. Some atoms exert a greater attraction for the shared electrons than do their partners (see Figure 3.3). This means that one atom often has a greater share of the electrons forming a covalent bond than does the other. The atom that attracts the shared electrons more strongly is said to be more electronegative than the other atom.

Oxygen is more electronegative than hydrogen. This means that in water the oxygen atom tends to attract the shared electrons more strongly than the hydrogen atoms. The result is that the oxygen atom has a slight excess of negative charge and the hydrogen atoms have a slight excess of positive charge. This is shown in Figure 3.3 as δ^- associated with the oxygen and δ^+ associated with the hydrogens, where the δ^- or δ^+ indicates a partial charge, not the full charge associated with the transfer of an electron from one atom to the other. Therefore, water has (small) positive and negative charges in the same molecule. Opposite charges attract each other, so that water can form weak bonds from the δ^- of its oxygen to the δ^+ charge of a hydrogen on

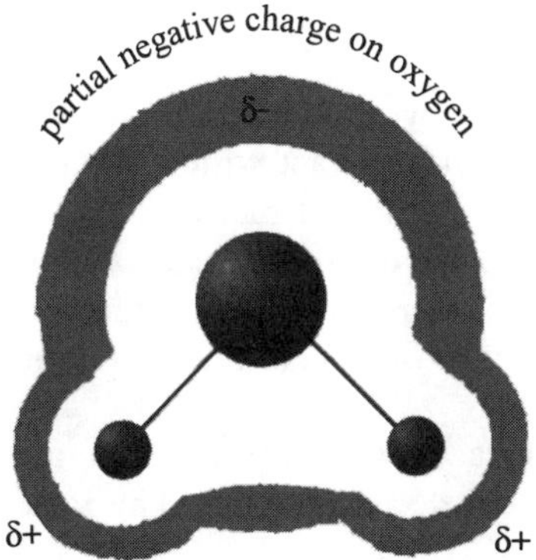

Figure 3.3 Uneven distribution of electrons in the water molecule.

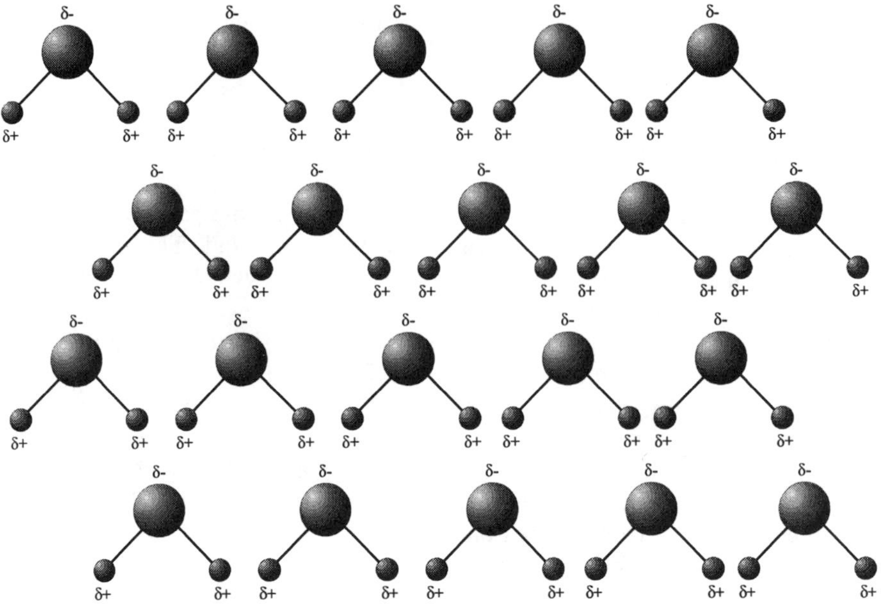

Figure 3.4 The formation of hydrogen bonds in water.

another molecule. These intermolecular bonds are hydrogen bonds (see also §3.5.1).

Because of this hydrogen bonding, water molecules require a greater input of heat in order to break away from each other and boil than would be expected from the M_r of water. Therefore, between 0 and 100°C water is a liquid, whereas carbon dioxide and methane are both gases.

3.3.1.1 *Solution in water: ions and electrolytes*

When salts that are formed by ionic bonding are dissolved in water, the ions separate from each other and interact with the water molecules, as shown in Figure 3.5. Since opposite charges attract each other, positively charged ions interact with the δ^- charges on the oxygen atoms of the water molecule, whereas negatively charged ions interact with the δ^+ charges on the hydrogen atoms of the water molecule. Such compounds dissociate or ionize when they are dissolved in water.

Compounds that ionize on solution in water are known as electrolytes, because they will carry an electric current. The ions move to the oppositely charged electric pole:

- Positively charged ions move to the negative pole. This pole is called the cathode, and ions that move to the cathode are called cations.

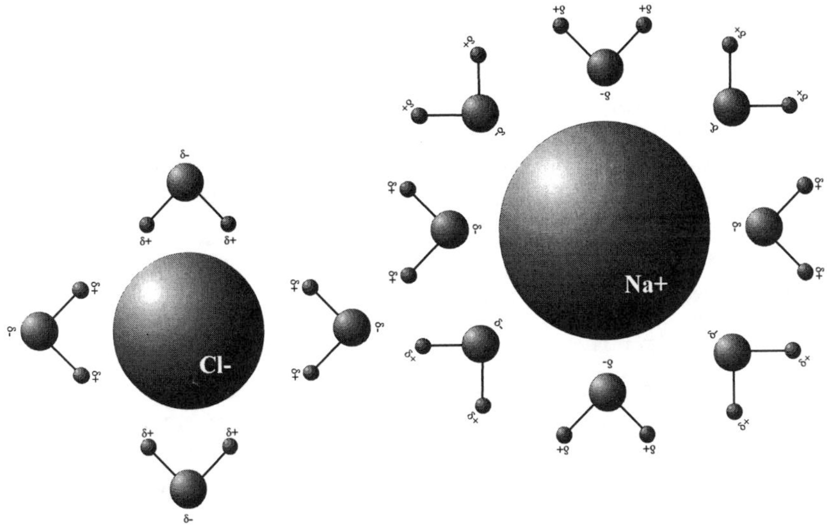

Figure 3.5 Solution of sodium chloride in water.

- Negatively charged ions move to the positive pole, which is called the anode. Such ions are called anions.

3.3.1.2 *Solution of non-ionic compounds in water*

Any compound containing atoms that are relatively electropositive or electronegative, so that there is uneven sharing of electrons in covalent bonds and the development of δ^- and δ^+ partial charges on the surface of the molecule, can interact with the partial charges on the water molecules, and so dissolve.

If a compound is dissolved in water, it apparently disappears. What has happened is that there were many molecules of the compound together making up the crystal of the solid. When it is dissolved in water, these molecules separate from each other, and become dispersed, because the molecules can interact with water molecules rather than each other. The result is a solution; water the solvent, and the compound which has dissolved to form the solution is the solute.

Although the individual molecules of the solute have been separated from each other and dispersed throughout the solution, they are still present as molecules. Dissolving a compound does not break covalent bonds that make up the molecules; it simply disperses the individual molecules uniformly throughout the solution.

3.4 Complex ions, acids and bases

Not all ions are formed by single atoms of elements donating or accepting electrons. Atoms can achieve a stable electron configuration by covalent bonding, ion formation or a mixture of the two. Many of the biologically important ions are of this type: a covalent molecule that also donates or accepts electrons to achieve a stable configuration. Examples of such ions are shown in Table 3.3.

The ammonium ion, NH_4^+, arises when ammonia gas (NH_3) dissolves in water, as a result of interaction between ammonia and water:

$$NH_3 + H_2O \rightleftharpoons NH_4^+ + OH^-$$

Here the ammonia has attracted a hydrogen ion (H^+) from the water, to form the positively charged ammonium ion (NH_4^+), and a negative hydroxyl ion (OH^-) from the rest of the water molecule. The reaction is written with arrows in both directions, because it is a readily reversible process. The solution will contain both ammonia (NH_3) and ammonium ions (NH_4^+).

A similar process, but this time with a different effect on the water molecule, occurs when carbon dioxide dissolves in water:

$$CO_2 + H_2O \rightleftharpoons H^+ + HCO_3^-.$$

In this case the carbon dioxide has interacted with a hydroxyl ion (OH^-) derived from water, to form the bicarbonate ion, leaving a hydrogen ion (H^+) to balance the charge in the solution. Again the process is reversible and the solution will contain both bicarbonate ions and un-ionized carbon dioxide.

3.4.1 *Acids, bases and salts*

When carbon dioxide dissolves in water, it interacts with water to form a bicarbonate ion (HCO_3^-) and a hydrogen ion (H^+). Compounds of this type,

Table 3.3 Some biologically important complex ions

Ion	Formula	Molecular mass
Ammonium	NH_4^+	18
Carbonate	CO_3^{2-}	60
Bicarbonate	HCO_3^-	61
Phosphate	PO_4^{3-}	95
Sulphate	SO_4^{2-}	96
Nitrate	NO_3^-	62
Acetate	CH_3COO^-	59

which dissociate when dissolved in water to give rise to hydrogen ions and an anion, are acids. Indeed, carbon dioxide is sometimes still known by its old name of carbonic acid gas.

Other examples of acids include hydrochloric acid (HCl) and acetic acid (CH_3COOH). Both of these dissociate in the same way when they dissolve in water – hydrochloric acid gives the chloride ion (Cl^-) and a hydrogen ion, while acetic acid yields the acetate ion (CH_3COO^-) and a hydrogen ion. (Acetic acid is sometimes referred to by its systematic chemical name, ethanoic acid.)

Acids do not always dissociate completely when they are dissolved in water. The strength of an acid is determined by the extent to which it dissociated – in other words, by how much is present in a solution as the undissociated acid, and how much as ions. The acidity of a solution will depend on both the strength of the acid and its concentration (i.e. how much is present in the solution).

Hydrochloric acid is a strong acid: it is more or less completely dissociated in water. By contrast, acetic acid and carbon dioxide are relatively weak acids: they are only partially dissociated in water. A dilute solution of acetic acid (0.1 mol per L) is only 1.3 per cent dissociated at 25°C.

The opposite of acids are the alkalis or bases. These are compounds that dissolve in water to give positively charged ions (cations) and a negatively charged hydroxide ion (OH^-). An example of a strong base is sodium hydroxide (NaOH, caustic soda):

$$NaOH + H_2O \rightarrow Na^+ + OH^- + H_2O.$$

Like a strong acid, it is more or less completely dissociated in solution.

An example of a relatively weak base is ammonia (NH_3):

$$NH_3 + H_2O \rightleftharpoons NH_4{}^+ + OH^-.$$

In this case some ammonia (NH_3) remains in the solution, although some has gained a hydrogen ion from water to form the ammonium ion ($NH_4{}^+$).

If equal amounts of solutions of an acid and a base are mixed, the hydrogen ions of the acid solution react with the hydroxyl ions of the base, forming water:

$$H^+ + OH \rightarrow H_2O.$$

The result is a mixture of the positively charged ion of the base and the negatively charged ion of the acid. This is a salt. For example, mixing hydrochloric acid and sodium hydroxide results in the formation of sodium chloride (a mixture of Na^+ and Cl^- ions) – sodium chloride is ordinary table salt:

$$Na^+ + OH^- + H^+ + Cl^- \rightarrow Na^+ + Cl^- + H_2O$$

The reaction between hydrogen ions and hydroxide ions to form water proceeds with the production of a great deal of heat, and a concentrated solution may boil explosively. This is because, all other things being equal, H_2O is very much more stable than a mixture of H^+ and OH^- ions. In other words, the equilibrium $H^+ + OH^- \rightleftharpoons H_2O$ lies well over to the right-hand side.

3.4.1.1 *pH: a measure of acidity*

Only a minute proportion of pure water is ionized and present as hydrogen (H^+) and hydroxyl (OH^-) ions. The concentration of H^+ ions is only 10^{-7} mol per L, while there are 55 mol per L of H_2O. At neutrality, as in pure water, the concentration of OH^- ions equals that of H^+ ions. Both are 10^{-7} mol per L, and the product of multiplying the concentration of H^+ ions and that of OH^- ions = 10^{-14} – this is the ionic product of water.

The ionic product of water is a constant, and is always maintained at 10^{-14}; as a solution becomes more acidic (i.e. the concentration of H^+ ions increases), so the concentration of OH^- ions decreases, so that $[H^+] \times [OH^-] = 10^{-14}$. Conversely, as a solution becomes more alkaline (i.e. the concentration of OH^- ions increases), so the concentration of H^+ ions decreases so that $[H^+] \times [OH^-]$ still equals 10^{-14}.

The acidity or alkalinity of a solution can thus be expressed simply by considering the concentration of hydrogen ions present:

- at neutrality $[H^+] = 10^{-7}$ mol per L
- in an acid solution $[H^+] > 10^{-7}$ mol per L and $[OH^-] < 10^{-7}$ mol per L
- in an alkaline solution $[OH^-] > 10^{-7}$ mol per L and $[H^+] < 10^{-7}$ mol per L.

Although the concentration of hydrogen ions is sometimes used as a measure of acidity or alkalinity, it is a cumbersome system, and in order to give more easily manageable numbers, it is usual to use the negative logarithm of the hydrogen ion concentration. This is known as the pH of the solution (for potential hydrogen):

- at neutrality $[H^+] = 10^{-7}$ mol per L, therefore pH = 7
- in an acid solution $[H^+] > 10^{-7}$ mol per L, therefore pH < 7
- in an alkaline solution $[H^+] > 10^{-7}$ mol per L, therefore pH > 7.

The complete range of the pH scale is from 1 (which is very strongly acid) to 14 (which is very strongly alkaline). In biological systems there is usually a narrow range of pH around neutrality, from about 5 to 9, although it is noteworthy that the gastric juice is strongly acid, with a pH of about 1.5 to 2.

Using a logarithmic scale for pH disguises the fact that an apparently small change in pH represents a very large change in the concentration of H^+ ions, and hence a large change in acidity or alkalinity. A change of one pH unit represents a tenfold change in the concentration of H^+ ions. The apparently small change in plasma pH from the normal range of 7.35–7.45 down to 7.2 represents potentially life-threatening acidosis.

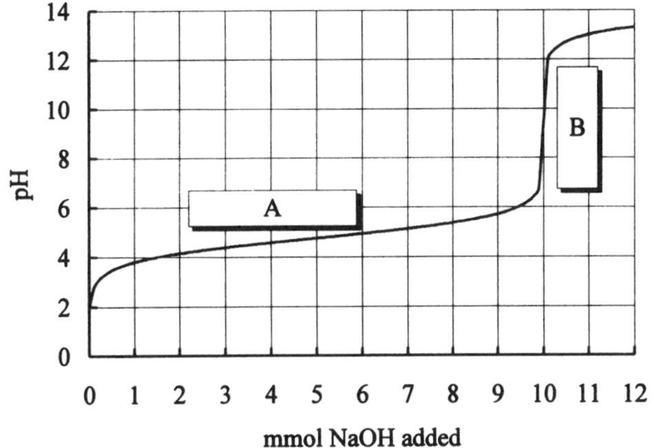

Figure 3.6 Titration of acetic acid with sodium hydroxide.

3.4.1.2 *Buffers and the maintenance of pH*

Since a small change in the pH of tissue fluids is vitally important, there is an obvious need for a chemical system that can take up spare H^+ ions when the pH begins to fall, and release H^+ ions as the pH begins to rise.

As discussed in §3.4.1, carbon dioxide is a weak acid and it undergoes partial dissociation when it dissolves in water:

$$CO_2 + H_2O \rightleftharpoons H^+ + HCO_3^-.$$

The position of the equilibrium (i.e. the proportion present as CO_2 as opposed to HCO_3^- and H^+ ions) depends on the relative concentrations of carbon dioxide and hydrogen ions. If the concentration of hydrogen ions rises, the equilibrium will shift to the left. Bicarbonate ions will break down to carbon dioxide and hydroxyl ions (OH^-), which then react with the hydrogen ions to form water. Conversely, if the concentration of hydrogen ions begins to fall, more of the carbon dioxide will react to form bicarbonate and hydrogen ions.

The equilibrium between carbon dioxide and bicarbonate thus acts to stabilize the concentration of hydrogen ions in a solution. Such a system is a buffer: it acts to absorb changes in hydrogen ion concentration and reduce their impact. It is only when the change in hydrogen ion concentration is greater than the capacity of the buffer system that there is a detectable change in pH.

The carbon dioxide/bicarbonate system is only one of several different buffer systems in the body, although it is one of the most important in terms of maintaining the pH of plasma. Proteins also have considerable buffering capacity, and other ions make a significant contribution.

Any weak acid or base can act as a buffer around the pH at which it undergoes ionization, stabilizing the pH as the concentration of H^+ ions changes, by changing between its ionized and un-ionized forms.

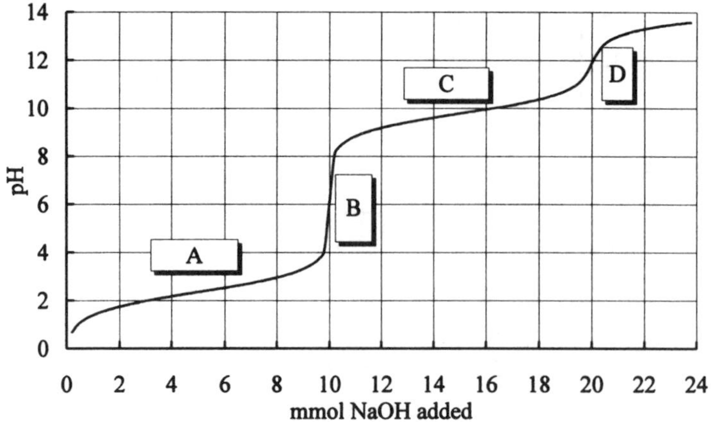

Figure 3.7 Titration of glycine hydrochloride with sodium hydroxide.

Figure 3.6 shows the effect on pH of adding increasing amounts of alkali to a solution containing 10 mmol of acetic acid. Initially, there is a sharp increase in pH, as the OH^- ions from the sodium hydroxide neutralize the H^+ ions of the acid. Then, in region A, there is a range over which addition of further sodium hydroxide has almost no effect on the pH of the solution. At pH 4.75 acetate is half-ionized; as the concentration of OH^- ions increases, so more of the acid ionizes, releasing H^+ ions, and so maintaining a more or less constant pH. Once the amount of sodium hydroxide added is almost equal to that of the acetic acid present (region B), all of the buffering capacity of the acid has been exhausted, and the pH of the solution increases rapidly as more of the strong alkali is added.

Figure 3.7 shows the effect of adding sodium hydroxide to a solution containing 10 mmol of the amino acid glycine ($H_2N—CH_2—COOH$), initially present as its hydrochloride salt. Glycine has both a weak acid group (—COOH, which can donate a hydrogen ion to form COO^-) and a weak basic group ($—NH_2$, which can accept a hydrogen ion to form $—NH_3{}^+$). In region A, at pH 2.35, the —COOH group is half-ionized, and it can therefore act as a buffer. When all of the —COOH groups have been neutralized by the sodium hydroxide (region B), the pH increases sharply as more alkali is added. In region C, at pH 9.78, the $—NH_2$ group is half-ionized, and it can act as a buffer around this pH. When all of the $—NH_3{}^+$ groups have been neutralized, there is again a sharp increase in pH as more alkali is added (region D).

3.5 Forces between molecules

Molecules interact with each other in three main ways: the formation of hydrogen bonds between molecules, van der Waals forces between molecules, and hydrophobic interactions. These interactions are responsible for the maintenance of the structures of such biologically important compounds as proteins (§6.4.2), nucleic acids (§10.2.1), and the lipid membranes of cells (§3.5.3.1).

3.5.1 Hydrogen bonding

Any compound in which one of the atoms sharing electrons in a bond exerts a greater attraction for the shared electrons than the other will have δ^- and δ^+ charges, as discussed for water in §3.3.1.

When an electronegative atom or group faces outwards from the overall molecule, there will be an exposed δ^- at the surface of the molecule. Similarly, if an electropositive atom or group faces outwards from the surface of the molecule, there will be an exposed δ^+ charge at the surface of the molecule.

These δ^+ and δ^- partial charges at the surface of molecules are capable of interacting with the oppositely charged poles of water molecules. This is the basis for the solubility of non-ionic compounds in water. Although there is no overall charge on the molecule, the partial charges allow considerable interaction with water molecules, and thus the molecules of the compound can readily be distributed through the water. Such water-soluble compounds are called hydrophilic (from the Greek for water-loving). Compounds that do not form such δ^+ and δ^- partial charges cannot interact with water. Such compounds, which are insoluble in water, are hydrophobic (from the Greek for water-hating).

In relatively large molecules, there may be some regions that develop partial δ^+ and δ^- charges, and therefore can interact with water (i.e. hydrophilic regions) and other regions which do not develop partial charges, and do not interact with water (hydrophobic regions). Compounds with both hydrophilic and hydrophobic regions in the molecule are sparingly soluble in water; the extent to which they dissolve depends on the relative sizes of the hydrophilic and hydrophobic regions.

Hydrophilic compounds in which δ^+ or δ^- partial charges can develop do not only interact with water molecules. They can also interact with other hydrophilic molecules, forming partial bonds (hydrogen bonds) between partial charges of opposite polarity. Hydrogen bonds between molecules are of critical importance in the structure and function of proteins (see §6.4.2) and nucleic acids (§10.2.1), and the binding of substrates to enzymes (§4.2), and hormones and neurotransmitters to receptors (§11.2). Although individual hydrogen bonds are weak, in large molecules the sum of many such weak bonds can result in very great structural stability.

3.5.2 van der Waals forces

Even when the different atoms in a chemical bond exert the same overall attraction on the shared electrons, so that there is no development of δ^+ and

δ^- partial charges, there are transient partial charges. This is because the electrons surrounding a nucleus are not static but move around the nucleus in their orbitals. In a covalent bond, the shared electrons are oscillating around both nuclei. At any instant, one atom will have a greater share in the electron than the other. This means that one atom will develop a minute negative charge, and the other an equally minute positive charge. This is only a transient separation of charge, and at another instant there may be either the opposite separation of charges, or an equal distribution of charge associated with both atoms. Nevertheless, for as long as a charge separation of this type exists, it provides the possibility of attraction to an opposite transient charge in a nearby molecule (or a nearby region of the same molecule in a large compound such as a protein).

Attractions between molecules based on transient minute inequality of the sharing of electrons of this type are called van der Waals forces, after their original discoverer. Individually, van der Waals forces are very much weaker than hydrogen bonds, and last for only an infinitesimally short time. Nevertheless, at any time there are a great many such temporary charge separations in a large molecule, and the sum of the van der Waals forces makes a considerable contribution to structure.

3.5.3 ***Hydrophobic interactions***

Not only can hydrophobic compounds not interact with water, they are repelled by the polar water molecules. If an oil (which is a hydrophobic compound) is shaken vigorously with water, it will mix in the water. However, it has not dissolved, but has merely been dispersed as a large number of very small droplets. The result is a milky-looking suspension of those droplets in water – an emulsion. The droplets are spherical, because this is the shape in which they have least need to interact with water. Gradually the emulsion begins to clear, and the oil forms larger and larger droplets. Eventually it separates from the water completely. This separation is again the result of repulsion between the slightly charged water molecules and the hydrophobic molecules. In order to minimize contact with water, the hydrophobic molecules associate with each other as much as possible.

In molecules that have both hydrophobic and hydrophilic regions, each region behaves as would be predicted. The hydrophilic regions of the molecule interact with water, whereas the hydrophobic regions are repelled by the water and interact with each other.

Fatty acids (see §6.3.1.1) are compounds with both hydrophobic and hydrophilic regions: they have a charged (and hence hydrophilic) group at one end of the molecule, and a chain of $-CH_2-$ groups, which is hydrophobic. The sodium salt of palmitic acid is $CH_3-(CH_2)_{16}-COO^- + Na^+$.

A fatty acid will dissolve in water, but, as the concentration increases, the hydrophobic tail regions group together, and the end result is a spherical

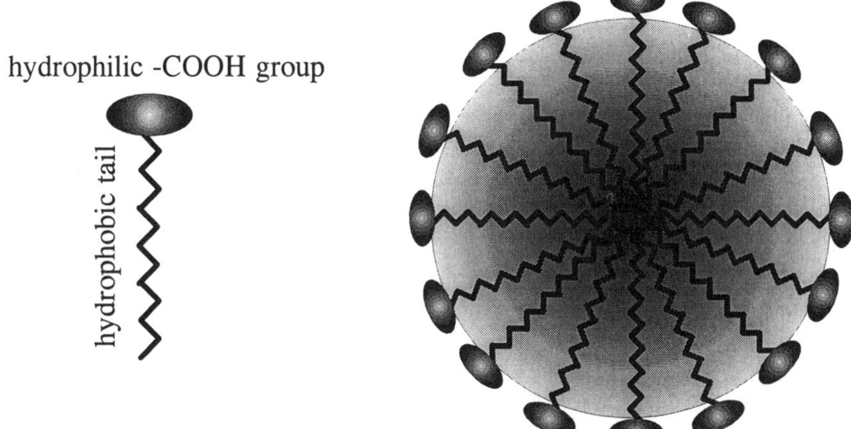

Figure 3.8 Fatty acids and the formation of lipid micelles.

globule called a micelle, as shown in Figure 3.8. The hydrophobic tails are inside and the hydrophilic groups face outwards, interacting with water. The sodium ions will interact with water and will be freely dispersed in the solution.

If oil and water are shaken together with sodium palmitate (or the salt of another fatty acid), the emulsion does not separate on standing. Both the oil and the hydrophobic tails of the fatty acid molecules have been repelled by the water and have formed mixed micelles. The hydrophilic charged groups of the fatty acid molecules stick out from the micelles and interact with water. Now the micelles do not come together to form larger droplets, because each one has an outer coat of hydrophilic groups which interact with water. This is a stable emulsion of oil in water.

This is the basis of the action of soaps and detergents; soap is a mixture of salts of fatty acids such as palmitate. Emulsification of dietary fats in the aqueous medium of the gut contents is essential for the digestion and absorption of fats (see §6.3.2). The bile salts secreted into the gut by the gall bladder and the fatty acids formed from the digestion of fats both act to stabilize the emulsion.

3.5.3.1 *The arrangement of lipids to form cell membranes*

As discussed in §6.3.1.2, phospholipids are molecules with both a hydrophobic tail (consisting of two fatty acid chains) and a highly hydrophilic head region. They can thus interact with both lipid and water in the same way as free fatty acids.

Phospholipids readily form a double layer (a lipid bilayer), with the hydrophobic chains of two layers of molecules interacting with each other in the centre of the bilayer. Both faces of the bilayer are made up of the hydrophilic groups, which interact with water. This is the basis of the structure of membranes around and within cells (see Figure 3.9). The lipid inner region of the membrane bilayer also contains cholesterol (see §6.3.1.3) and vitamin E (see §12.2.3), as well as other hydrophobic compounds.

Membranes also contain proteins. These may be located at the outer or inner face of the membrane, and some of the most important membrane proteins span the whole width of the membrane and interact with water at both surfaces. All membrane-associated proteins have hydrophobic regions, which interact with the lipids, and hydrophilic regions, which emerge from the lipid and interact with water. (See §6.4.2 for a discussion of protein structure and §11.2 for the role of membrane proteins in the responses to hormones.)

Membranes, both those within the cell and those surrounding the cell, are not rigid static structures, but have a considerable degree of fluidity. The proteins can move around in the lipid bilayer, and regions of membrane can form vesicles for the transport of compounds into and out of the cell. A region of cell membrane can invaginate, to form a depression in the cell surface. This deepens, and the space that communicates with the outside closes off, until a separate membrane-enclosed vesicle has been formed inside the cell. This is the process of **endocytosis**.

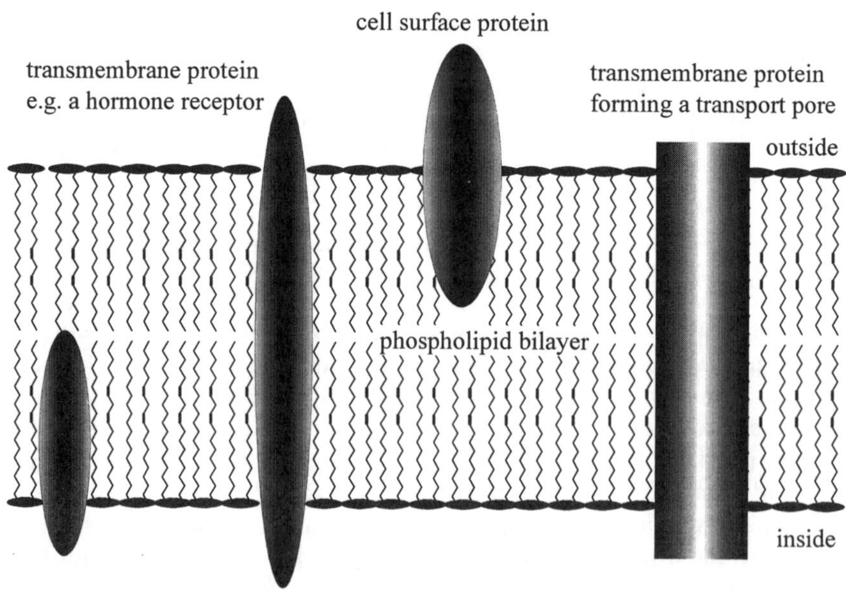

Figure 3.9 Arrangement of phospholipids to form a cell membrane (see also Figure 6.8).

The reverse process occurs in the secretion of proteins, hormones and neurotransmitters from the cell. The compounds to be exported are synthesized or accumulated in membrane-enclosed vesicles. These vesicles then migrate to the surface of the cell, where the membrane of the vesicle fuses with the cell membrane, leading to the formation of a pore in the membrane through which the contents of the vesicle can be exported into the extracellular fluid.

3.6 Component parts of biologically important molecules

Although there are 96 naturally occurring chemical elements, relatively few of them are important in biological systems. Indeed, most of the important compounds in biochemistry are composed of carbon, hydrogen, oxygen and nitrogen; sulphur and phosphorus also have important roles. Some other elements, shown in Table 3.1, are also important in biochemistry, and a few elements may be important because we are exposed to them and they may be poisonous (e.g. cadmium, lead and mercury).

The chemistry of biological systems is essentially the chemistry of carbon compounds; these are generally known as organic compounds because they were originally discovered in living (organic) matter. Simple carbonates and bicarbonates, and the whole host of compounds not involving carbon, are known as inorganic compounds. This chemical use of the word *organic* is quite different from that used to describe foods grown without the use of pesticides, fertilizers, and so on, which are sometimes known as organic foods. Chemically, they are exactly the same as conventional foods.

The inorganic compounds that are nutritionally important are often referred to as minerals because they are compounds that are (or can be) obtained by mining (see §12.3).

Just as the writing of chemical formulae is simplified by using abbreviations for the names of the elements, the structures of organic compounds can be simplified by omitting many of the carbon atoms and just drawing a skeleton of the structure of the molecule. Indeed, hydrogen atoms are not usually shown unless there is some reason to do so. Figure 3.10 shows how a variety of structures can be simplified and shown as skeletons.

When there is an atom other than carbon in the molecule it must be shown, since otherwise it would be assumed that there was a carbon atom there. For example, pyridine (see Figure 3.10) has a nitrogen atom incorporated into the ring – the other five positions of the ring are all carbon atoms.

Groups containing oxygen, nitrogen or sulphur in addition to carbon are attached to the hydrocarbon carbon 'skeleton' of biologically important molecules. It is these groups that provide the chemical reactivity of the compounds. They are hydrophilic groups and they interact with water.

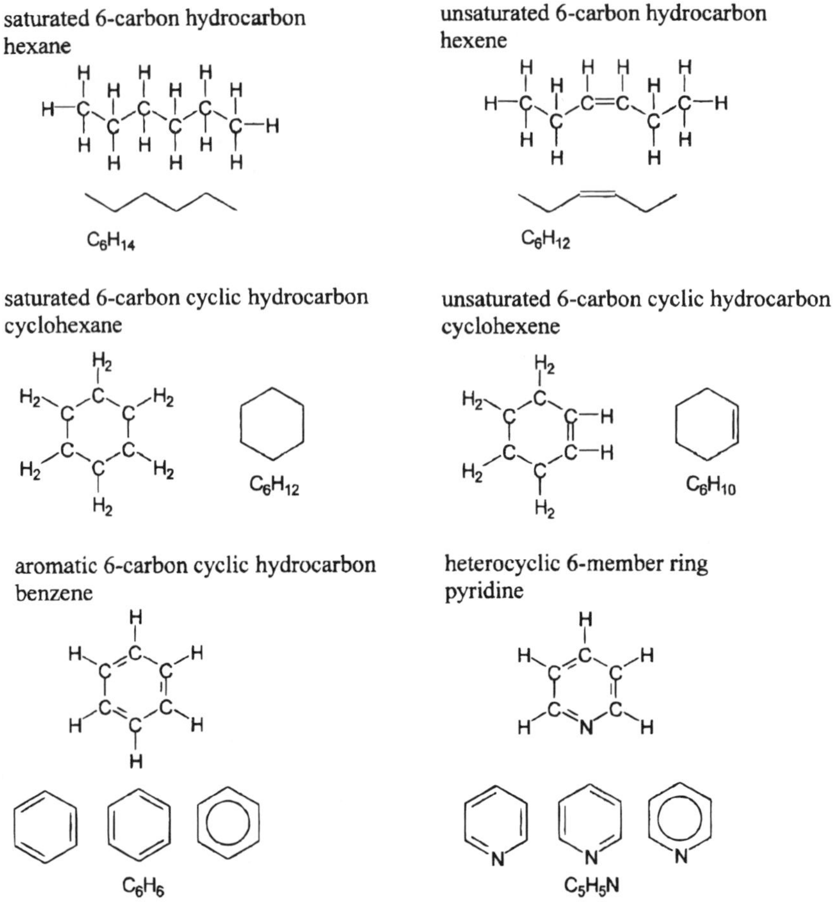

saturated 6-carbon hydrocarbon
hexane

C_6H_{14}

unsaturated 6-carbon hydrocarbon
hexene

C_6H_{12}

saturated 6-carbon cyclic hydrocarbon
cyclohexane

C_6H_{12}

unsaturated 6-carbon cyclic hydrocarbon
cyclohexene

C_6H_{10}

aromatic 6-carbon cyclic hydrocarbon
benzene

C_6H_6

heterocyclic 6-member ring
pyridine

C_5H_5N

Figure 3.10 Methods of representing molecular structures.

3.6.1 ***Hydrocarbons***

Hydrocarbons are compounds consisting of carbon and hydrogen only. They may consist of straight or branched chains of carbon atoms, or may form cyclic structures (rings), commonly consisting of five or six carbon atoms in biologically important compounds. Hydrocarbons do not have to be saturated with hydrogen; they may contain one or more carbon–carbon double bond (see the structures of hexane, hexene, cyclohexane and cyclohexene in Figure 3.10).

Simple hydrocarbons are not important in nutrition or biochemistry. However, many compounds contain relatively large regions which are hydrocarbon chains or rings. These cannot interact with water because they do not show charge separation in their covalent bonds, and so cannot form hydrogen bonds (see §3.5.1). Hydrocarbon regions of molecules are therefore hydrophobic.

3.6.1.1 *Aromatic compounds*

An important group of unsaturated hydrocarbons have a cyclic structure, with multiple double bonds in the ring. The simplest such compound is benzene. As shown in Figure 3.10, benzene is C_6H_6, and has three carbon–carbon double bonds in the 6-carbon ring. Although separate single and double bonds can be drawn, these could be in either of the arrangements shown in Figure 3.10, and can be considered to alternate rapidly between these two arrangements. It is conventional to draw the molecule with a circle in the middle of the hexagonal ring, to show the alternation of double and single bonds, and the fact that the single and double bonds cannot be localized to individual carbon atoms.

In compounds of this type, the electrons forming the covalent bonds are evenly shared between all the atoms in the ring, so that all the bonds in the ring are intermediate between single and double bonds. The ring itself is completely flat, with the delocalized electrons of the alternating single and double bonds forming electron-dense regions above and below the plane of the ring formed by the nuclei of the carbon atoms. Compounds of this type are called aromatic. This is a chemical term and it does not mean that all aromatic compounds have a smell or aroma, although the term was originally used because many of the aromatic oils from natural sources have this type of ring structure in their molecules.

In linear molecules, which have alternating single and double bonds in the carbon chain, the electrons that are shared to form the covalent bonds are delocalized, and shared between more than just two carbon atoms in almost the same way as occurs in aromatic compounds. Such compounds are not aromatic, but they share some chemical properties with aromatic compounds. A compound having alternating single and double bonds is said to have conjugated double bonds. They are important in the structure and function of compounds such as vitamin A and carotene (see §12.2.1).

3.6.2 **Heterocyclic compounds**

Carbon is not the only element that can be incorporated into ring structures. Oxygen or nitrogen, and sometimes also sulphur and other elements, may also be incorporated into carbon ring structures. Such compounds are called heterocyclic, from the Greek *heteros* meaning different, because they contain an atom other than carbon in the ring.

Heterocyclic compounds may be saturated or unsaturated, and indeed some are also aromatic. Nitrogen-containing heterocyclic rings are especially important in the purines and pyrimidines that make up the nucleic acids (see §10.2.1), as well as a variety of other important compounds.

3.6.3 Hydroxyl groups

A simple hydroxyl (—OH) group attached to a hydrocarbon chain forms an alcohol (see Figure 3.11). Some alcohols are important in nutrition and biochemistry, quite apart from ethanol (ethyl alcohol), which is the alcohol in alcoholic beverages (see §2.4.5 for notes on prudent levels of alcohol consumption).

Hydroxyl groups are important in carbohydrates (see §6.2.1) and in the glycerol that forms fats and oils by reaction with the fatty acids (see §6.3.1), as well as in other compounds.

A hydroxyl group attached to an aromatic ring can ionize relatively readily, giving up H^+ to form $—O^-$. Such aromatic hydroxyl compounds are called phenols; phenolic groups are important in compounds such as the amino acid tyrosine (see Figure 6.13), vitamin D (§12.2.2.2) and some of the steroid hormones (Figure 4.9), among others.

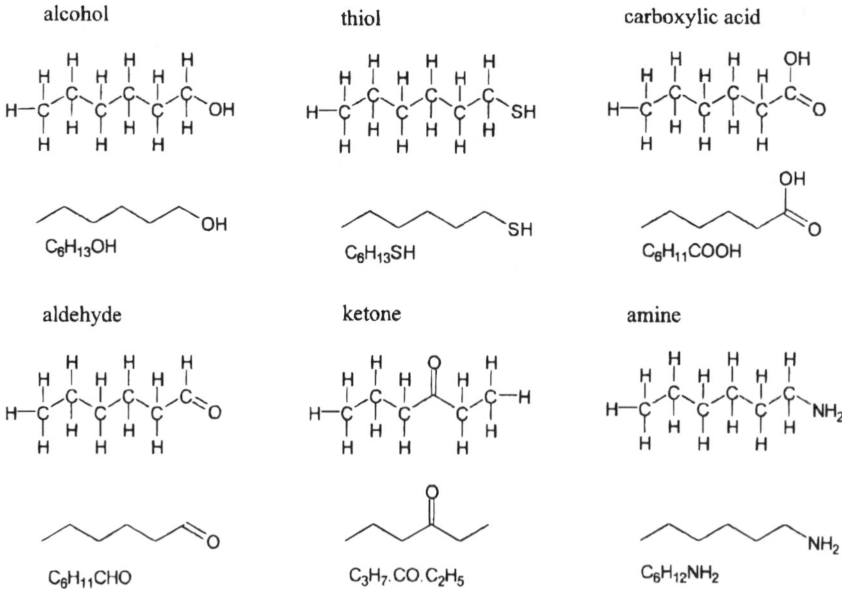

Figure 3.11 Biologically important functional groups in molecules.

3.6.4 *Sulphydryl groups*

In some ways, the sulphydryl group (-SH) is similar to the hydroxyl group. Compounds bearing a sulphydryl group are sometimes called thiols. The reactive part of coenzyme A (see §7.4.2.2) is a sulphydryl group.

Biologically, the most important feature of sulphydryl groups is that they readily undergo oxidation (see §5.3.1.2). For example, the -SH groups in two molecules of the amino acid cysteine can undergo oxidation, resulting in the formation of a new bond between the two sulphur atoms and joining the two cysteine molecules together to form the amino acid cystine. Oxidation of the sulphydryl groups of cysteine molecules in proteins, with the formation of cystine, plays an important role in the structure of proteins (see Figure 6.11).

3.6.5 *Carbonyl groups: aldehydes and ketones*

The carbonyl group (C=O) is important in two main groups of compounds:

- Aldehydes, in which one valency of the carbon of the carbonyl group is occupied by an aliphatic group (or sometimes an aromatic group), while the other is occupied by hydrogen.
- Ketones, in which two aliphatic groups are attached to the carbon which bears the carbonyl group.

Aldehydes and ketones arise from the oxidation of alcohols. For example, oxidation of ethyl alcohol (ethanol) results in the formation of acetaldehyde:

$$CH_3{-}CH_2{-}OH + \text{carrier} \rightleftharpoons CH_3{-}HC{=}O + \text{carrier}{-}H_2$$

The reaction is reversible, and reduction of an aldehyde results in the formation of the corresponding alcohol.

Carbonyl groups also occur in a variety of compounds that are strictly neither aldehydes nor ketones. Such a C=O group occurring in a molecule is sometimes called a keto group, although it is more correct to call it an oxo group. Keto-acids are intermediates in many of the metabolic pathways discussed in Chapter 7.

3.6.6 *Carboxylic acids*

The carbonyl group is important in a further class of compounds, the carboxylic acids. The acid group arises from the further oxidation of an aldehyde. Thus, oxidation of acetaldehyde results in the formation of acetic acid (ethanoic acid):

$$CH_3{-}HC{=}O + \text{acceptor} + H_2O \rightleftharpoons CH_3{-}COOH + \text{acceptor}{-}H_2.$$

Acetic acid (ethanoic acid, see §3.4.1) is the acid of vinegar. Although it can be synthesized chemically, much of the vinegar consumed is produced by fermentation of carbohydrates to form ethanol, followed by a further fermentation process to convert the alcohol to acetic acid.

In the reaction written above, the acid is shown as CH_3—COOH. This is a chemical shorthand way of writing the structure on a single line. As shown in Figure 3.11, the four valencies of the carbon atoms are occupied as follows:

- One carbon atom has three valencies occupied by hydrogen, forming a methyl group (CH_3-) and the fourth by bonding to carbon.
- The other carbon atom has one valency occupied by binding to the carbon of the methyl group, one to the oxygen of the hydroxyl group (-OH) and the other two to oxygen (a carbonyl group, C=O).

The hydrogen of the hydroxyl group of carboxylic acids can readily be lost, and as discussed in §3.4.1, acetic acid is a (relatively weak) acid. It dissociates in solution to form the acetate ion ($CH_3—COO^-$) and a hydrogen ion (H^+).

Almost all of the biologically important acids are carboxylic acids, including the fatty acids (see §6.3.1.1), the amino acids (§6.4.1) and compounds formed as intermediates in the metabolism of fats, carbohydrates and proteins.

3.6.6.1 *Esters*

Under appropriate conditions an alcohol and an acid can react together, with the elimination of water, forming an ester, as shown in Figure 3.12. The reaction is reversible, and esters can be cleaved to yield the acid and alcohol by the addition of water. The elimination of water to form an ester is a condensation reaction, whereas the reverse reaction, the cleavage of a bond by the addition of water, is hydrolysis.

Esters are important in biochemistry, especially in the formation of fats from fatty acids and the alcohol glycerol (which has three hydroxyl groups,

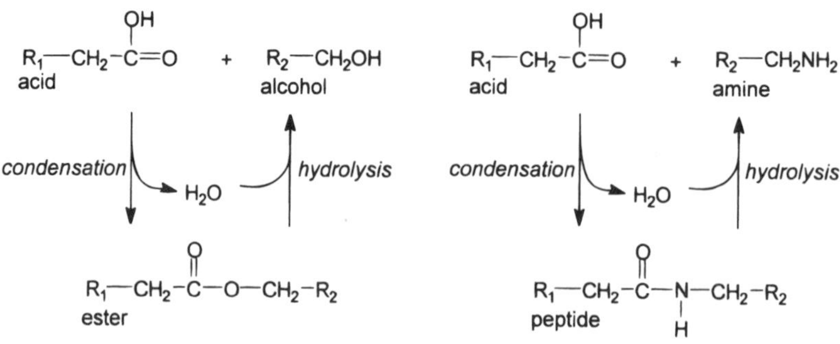

Figure 3.12 The formation and hydrolysis of ester and peptide bonds.

and can therefore form esters to three fatty acid molecules; see §6.3.1). Fatty acids can also form thio-esters to the sulphydryl group of a thiol, for example in the formation of acetyl CoA (see §7.4.2.2).

3.6.7 Amino groups and peptide bonds

The commonest nitrogen-containing group in metabolically important compounds is the amino group, $—NH_2$. Amino groups are found in the amino acids of proteins (see §6.4.1), and in the purines and pyrimidines of nucleic acids (see §10.2.1).

Amino groups can undergo a condensation reaction with a carboxylic acid similar to the formation of esters (see Figure 3.12). The elimination of water between an amino group and carboxylic acid results in the formation of a peptide bond, which is the basis of the structure of proteins (see §6.4.2). Again the reaction is reversible, and peptide bonds can be hydrolysed under appropriate conditions. The formation of peptide bonds is the basis of the formation of proteins from amino acids (see §10.3.2), and the hydrolysis of peptide bonds to release amino acids is the basis of the digestion of proteins (§6.4.3).

3.7 The naming of organic compounds

There are systematic chemical rules for the naming of organic compounds, based on the functional groups and the size and type of hydrocarbon structure of the compound. Such systematic names uniquely identify any given compound, in the same way as the structural formula does. However, they tend to be cumbersome, and many metabolically important compounds have more convenient, officially accepted, trivial names. In general, trivial names will be used in this book, rather than systematic names.

It is often necessary to be able to say which carbon atom of a compound has a reactive group attached. Here there is a simple rule. The carbon atoms are numbered from one end of the molecule. Carbon-1 is the one that carries the reactive group for which the compound is named. If the reactive group is an aldehyde or a carboxylic acid, then carbon-1 is the carbon of the carbonyl group.

There is also a slightly different system for numbering carbon atoms, using the letters of the Greek alphabet. The α-carbon is the one to which to the functional group for which the compound is named is attached. The next carbon is the β-carbon, and so on. Thus, in a fatty acid or aldehyde, the α-carbon is actually carbon-2, since the carbonyl group as a whole is the functional group. The carbon atom farthest from the α-carbon is sometimes called the ω-carbon: ω is the last letter of the Greek alphabet. (See §6.3.1.1, where this convention is used in the naming of unsaturated fatty acids.)

In cyclic compounds, the positions of the ring are numbered in such a way that the position to which the functional group for which the compound is named has the lowest number. In heterocyclic compounds, it is the non-carbon atom that is given the number 1, and the carbon atoms are numbered from that position.

3.7.1 *Isomerism: asymmetry and the shape of molecules*

Compounds that contain the same functional groups, but differently arranged in the molecule, are known as isomers. The simplest form of isomerism, positional isomerism, results from different arrangements of the functional groups on the carbon skeleton. For example, the amino acids leucine and isoleucine (see Figure 6.13) are positional isomers.

Positional isomers often have different chemical behaviour. Two further types of isomerism are important in biological systems; in these two cases the chemical behaviour of the isomers is more or less identical, but the molecules have different shapes, and therefore behave differently in metabolic reactions, where the shape of the molecule, as well as its chemical reactivity, is important.

3.7.1.1 Cis–trans *isomerism around double bonds*

Single bonds between carbon atoms permit free rotation of the various parts of the molecule. However, carbon–carbon double bonds do not. They impose rigidity on that part of the molecule. This means there are two different arrangements around a carbon–carbon double bond, as shown in Figure 3.13:

- Both parts of the chain may be on the same side of the double bond. This is the *cis*-configuration.
- The chain on one side of the double bond may be on the opposite side from the other. This is the *trans*-configuration.

This type of isomerism, where groups may be on the same side of a double bond (*cis*-) or opposite sides (*trans*-) is *cis–trans* isomerism. *Cis–trans* isomer-

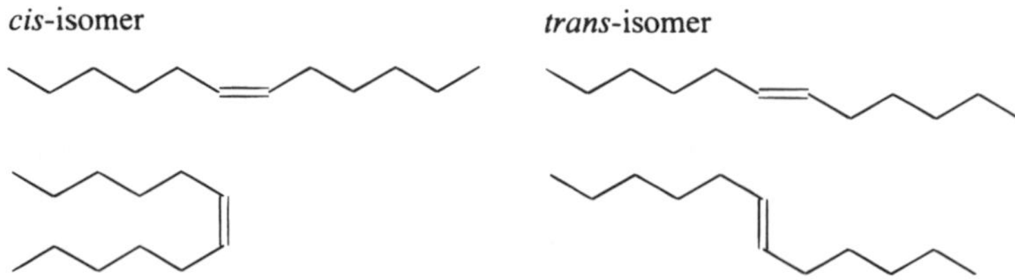

Figure 3.13 *Cis–trans* isomerism around a carbon–carbon double bond.

ism is extremely important in biochemistry, since the two isomers have very different shapes, and the overall shape of molecules is important in enzyme-catalysed reactions (see §4.2). For example, interconversion between the *cis*- and *trans*-isomers of retinol (vitamin A) is crucially important for its function in vision (§12.2.1.1). Although an increased consumption of polyunsaturated fats is considered desirable, this applies only to the *cis*-isomers; *trans*-unsaturated fatty acids are potentially deleterious to health and, as discussed in §2.4.2.1, it is considered that consumption should not increase.

3.7.1.2 *Asymmetric centres in molecules: DL-isomerism*

If four different groups are attached to a single carbon atom, their arrangement is important. As shown in Figure 3.14, there are two possible arrangements of four groups. These two arrangements are mirror images of each other, and cannot be superimposed on each other – in the same way as right and left hands or feet are mirror images of each other. In other words, the compounds are asymmetric. The carbon atom to which the four different groups are attached is a centre of asymmetry. The two forms of such compounds are conformational isomers. Chemically they react in the same way, but they have a different conformation or spatial arrangement of reactive groups in the molecule.

The two conformational isomers of the three-carbon sugar glyceraldehyde are shown in Figure 3.14. They are distinguished from each other by using the letters D (from the Greek *dextro* = right) and L (*laevo* = left). The assignment of conformation to other compounds is based on their relationship to D- or L-glyceraldehyde.

This system for assigning conformation is useful in biochemistry. Almost all of the metabolically important sugars have the D-conformation. Thus, in order to specify the (naturally occurring) isomer of glucose, it is called D-glucose

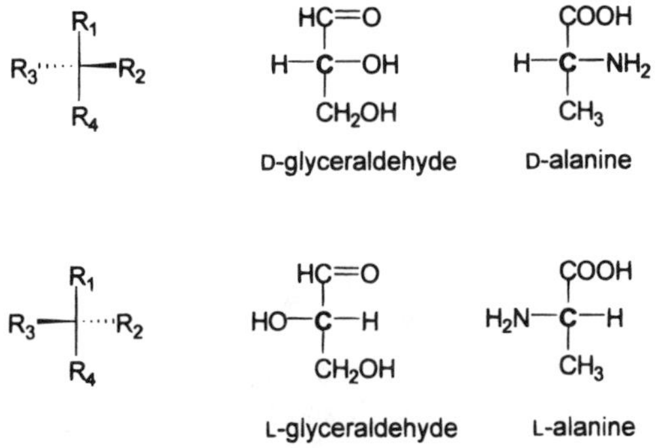

R_1, R_2, R_3, R_4

HC=O, H—C—OH, CH_2OH — D-glyceraldehyde

COOH, H—C—NH_2, CH_3 — D-alanine

HC=O, HO—C—H, CH_2OH — L-glyceraldehyde

COOH, H_2N—C—H, CH_3 — L-alanine

Figure 3.14 DL-Isomerism around an asymmetric carbon atom.

(sometimes referred to as dextrose). Similarly, almost all of the naturally occurring amino acids have the L-conformation. Small amounts of D-amino acids are ingested from bacterial proteins (see §10.3.1.1).

The opposite conformational isomer from the one that occurs naturally can have very different effects in the body. This is because it cannot bind to enzymes or receptors in the same way. For example, the metabolically important isomer of the amino acid tryptophan is the L-isomer. L-Tryptophan has a very strong, unpleasant bitter flavour. However, D-tryptophan has a pleasant sweet taste, some 40 times sweeter than sugar.

Chemical synthesis of compounds that have centres of asymmetry results in a mixture of equal amounts of the D- and L-isomers. This is the **racemic mixture**, and is shown by using the prefix DL- before the name of the compound. Frequently, D- and L-isomers of such synthesized compounds have to be separated before they can be used because the opposite isomer has undesirable effects. Increasingly, complex drugs are being synthesized by a mixture of chemical and biochemical (generally microbiological) techniques in order to achieve synthesis of only one isomer.

Although the system of naming asymmetric compounds by their relationship to the spatial arrangement of groups in glyceraldehyde has advantages for biochemistry, it does not follow the rigorous rules of chemical nomenclature. There is an alternative system, based on assignment of a strict hierarchy of chemically reactive groups around the asymmetric centre. Here the two possible stereoisomers are called *R* (from the Latin *rectus* = right) and *S* (*sinistra* = left).

This system of nomenclature does not give the same conformation for all of the naturally occurring amino acids and is relatively little used in biochemistry and nutrition. However, it is sometimes used, especially when considering complex molecules. For example, there are three asymmetric centres in the molecule of vitamin E (see §12.2.3). To distinguish between the possibilities, the conformation at each of these positions is given as *R* or *S*. The naturally occurring form of vitamin E is (*RRR*)-α-tocopherol (sometimes also called (all-*R*)-α-tocopherol).

3.8 Biologically important molecules

The biologically important types of compound can be divided into four main groups:

- *Carbohydrates*: Compounds containing carbon, hydrogen and oxygen, normally in the ratio $C_n:H_{2n}:O_n$. The structures of nutritionally important carbohydrates are discussed in §6.2.1.
- *Lipids*: Compounds mainly composed of carbon and hydrogen, for the most part in the ratio $C_n:H_{2n}$, but with small amounts of oxygen, and in some lipids (the phospholipids) also phosphorus and nitrogen. The structures of lipids are discussed in §6.3.1.

- *Amino acids* (and the proteins formed from them, which contain carbon, hydrogen, oxygen, nitrogen and small amounts of sulphur): The structures of amino acids and proteins are discussed in §6.4.1. The role of proteins that catalyse metabolic reactions (enzymes) is discussed in §4.2.
- *Nucleotides* (and the nucleic acids formed from them, which contain carbon, hydrogen, nitrogen and phosphorus): The structures of nucleotides are discussed in §5.1 and of the nucleic acids (DNA and RNA), which contain the genetic information of the cell, in §10.2.1.

In addition, there are a great many other compounds that do not fit into any of these categories; many of these are coenzymes (see §4.3.1) and hormones (§11.2 and §11.3), as well as intermediate compounds in the metabolism of carbohydrates, lipids, amino acids and nucleotides.

4

Chemical Reactions: Enzymes and Metabolic Pathways

All metabolic processes depend on reaction between molecules, with breaking of some covalent bonds and the formation of others, yielding compounds that are different from the starting materials. In order to understand nutrition and metabolism it is therefore essential to understand how chemical reactions occur, and how they are catalysed by enzymes.

4.1 Chemical reactions: breaking and making covalent bonds

Breaking covalent bonds (see §3.2.2) requires an input of energy in some form – normally as heat, but in some cases light or other radiation. This is the activation energy of the reaction. The process of breaking a bond requires activation of the electrons forming the bond – a temporary shift of one or more electrons from orbitals in which they have a stable configuration to other orbitals, further from the nucleus. Electrons that have been activated in this way now have unstable configurations, and the covalent bonds they had contributed to are broken. Electrons cannot remain in this unstable activated state for more than a fraction of a second. Sometimes they simply return to their original unexcited state, emitting the same energy as was taken up to excite them. Overall there is no change when this occurs.

More commonly, the excited electrons may adopt a different stable configuration by interacting with electrons associated with different atoms and molecules. The result is the formation of new covalent bonds, and hence the formation of new compounds. In this case, there are three possibilities (as shown in Figure 4.1):

- There may be an output of energy equal to the activation energy of the reaction, so that the energy level of the products is the same as that of the starting materials. Such a reaction is energetically neutral.
- There may be an output of energy greater than the activation of the reaction, so that the energy level of the products is lower than that of the starting materials. This is an exothermic reaction – it proceeds with the output of

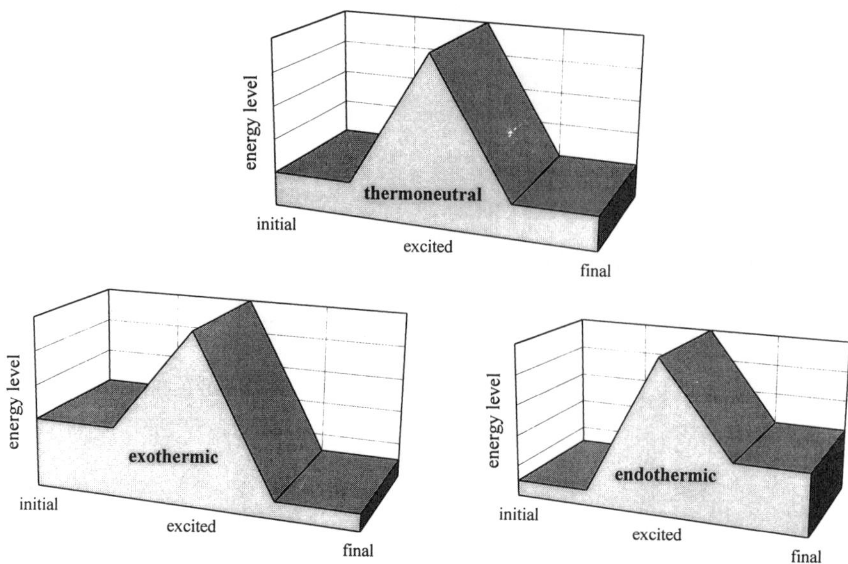

Figure 4.1 Changes in energy level in chemical reactions.

heat. An exothermic reaction will proceed spontaneously once the initial activation energy has been provided.

- There may be an output of energy less than the activation energy, so that the energy level of the products is higher than that of the starting materials. The solution will take up heat from its surroundings, and will have to be heated for the reaction to proceed. This is an endothermic reaction.

In general, reactions in which relatively large complex molecules are broken down to smaller molecules are exothermic, whereas reactions that involve the synthesis of larger molecules from smaller ones are endothermic.

4.1.1 *Equilibrium*

Some reactions, such as the burning of a hydrocarbon in air to form carbon dioxide and water, are highly exothermic, and the products of the reaction are widely dispersed. Such reactions proceed essentially in one direction only. However, most reactions do not proceed in only one direction. If two compounds, A and B, can react together to form X and Y, then X and Y can react to form A and B. The reactions can be written as:

$$A + B \rightarrow X + Y \quad (1)$$

$$X + Y \rightarrow A + B \quad (2)$$

Starting with only A and B in the solution, at first only reaction (1) will occur, forming X and Y. However, as X and Y accumulate, so they will undergo reaction (2), forming A and B. Similarly, starting with X and Y, at first only reaction (2) will occur, forming A and B. As A and B accumulate, so they will undergo reaction (1), forming X and Y.

In both cases, the final result will be a solution containing A, B, X and Y. The relative amounts of [A + B] and [X + Y] will be the same, regardless of whether the starting compounds (substrates) were A and B or X and Y. At this stage the rate of reaction (1) forming X and Y, and reaction (2) forming A and B, will be equal. This is equilibrium, and the reaction can be written as:

$$A + B \rightleftharpoons X + Y$$

If there is a large difference in energy level between [A + B] and [X + Y] – i.e. if the reaction is exothermic in one direction (and therefore endothermic in the other direction) – then the position of the equilibrium will reflect this. If reaction (1) above is exothermic, then at equilibrium there will be very little A and B remaining – most will have been converted to X and Y. Conversely, if reaction (1) is endothermic, then relatively little of the substrates will be converted to X and Y at equilibrium.

At equilibrium the ratio of [A + B]/[X + Y] is a constant for any given reaction, depending on the temperature. This means that a constant addition of substrates will disturb the equilibrium and increase the amount of product formed. Constant removal of products will similarly disturb the equilibrium and increase the rate at which substrate is removed.

4.1.2 ***Catalysts***

A catalyst is a compound that increases the rate at which a reaction comes to equilibrium, without itself being consumed in the reaction. This means that a relatively small amount of catalyst can act on a large number of molecules of reactants. Catalysts affect the rate at which equilibrium is achieved in three main ways:

- By providing a surface on which the molecules that are to undergo reaction can come together in higher concentration than would be possible in free solution, thus increasing the probability of them colliding and reacting. This binding may also align substrates in the correct orientation to undergo reaction.
- By providing a microenvironment for the reactants that is different from the solution as a whole.
- By participating in the reaction by withdrawing electrons from, or donating electrons to, covalent bonds. This enhances the breaking of bonds that is the essential prerequisite for chemical reaction, and lowers the activation energy of the reaction.

4.2 Enzymes

Enzymes are proteins that catalyse metabolic reactions. As discussed in §6.4.2, proteins are polymers of amino acids, linked in a linear sequence. Any protein adopts a characteristic pattern of folding, determined largely by the sequence of the different amino acids in its sequence. This folding of the protein chain results in reactive groups from a variety of amino acids, which might be widely separated in the linear sequence, coming together at the protein surface. This creates a site on the surface of the protein that has a defined shape and array of chemically reactive groups. This is the active site of the enzyme. It is the site that both binds the compounds which are to undergo reaction (the substrates) and catalyses the reaction.

The binding of substrates to enzymes involves interactions between the substrate and reactive groups of the amino acid side chains that make up the active site of the enzyme (see §6.4.1). This means that enzymes show a considerable degree of specificity for the substrates they bind. Normally, several different interactions must occur before the substrate can bind in the correct orientation to undergo reaction, and binding of the substrate often causes a change in the shape of the active site, bringing reactive groups closer to the substrate.

The specificity of enzymes is such that they distinguish between the D- and L-isomers (see §3.7.1.2) and between the *cis*- and *trans*-isomers (see §3.7.1.1) of the substrate, because the isomers have different shapes, although in non-enzymic chemical reactions the isomers may behave identically. The shape and conformation of the substrate are critically important for binding to an enzyme.

Enzymes are not simply passive surfaces that bind the substrates. The active site of the enzyme plays an important part in the reaction process. Various amino acid side chains of the enzyme molecule at the active site provide chemically reactive groups which can facilitate the making or breaking of specific chemical bonds in the substrate by donating or withdrawing electrons. In this way the enzyme can lower the activation energy of a chemical reaction (Figure 4.2). Rather than only an input of energy to excite the electrons in a bond, the enzyme achieves at least part of the excitation by interactions between the substrate and reactive groups at the active site.

Enzymes can also provide very distinctive microenvironments at the active site. An array of amino acids with hydrophobic side chains making up an active site will produce a non-aqueous environment in which water molecules are scarce, despite the fact that the solution as a whole is an aqueous solution. An array of amino acids with acidic side chains will produce, locally, a lower pH than in the solution as a whole, while an array of amino acids with basic side chains will produce, again only in the immediate area of the active site, a high pH.

The result of this is that an enzyme can achieve an increase in the rate at which a reaction attains equilibrium under much milder conditions than for a

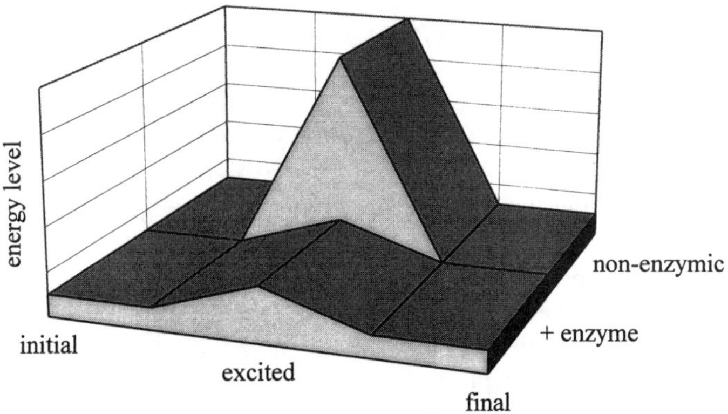

Figure 4.2 The effect of an enzyme on the activation energy of a reaction.

simple chemical catalyst. In order to hydrolyse a protein into its constituent amino acids in the laboratory, it is necessary to use concentrated acid as a catalyst and to heat the sample at 105°C overnight to provide the activation energy of the hydrolysis. As discussed in §6.4.3, this is the process of digestion of proteins, which occurs in the human gut under relatively mild acid or alkaline conditions, at 37°C, and is complete within a few hours of eating a meal.

The sequence of events in an enzyme-catalysed reaction can be written as:

$$E + S \rightleftharpoons E - S \rightleftharpoons E - P \rightleftharpoons E + P$$

Where E is the enzyme, S the substrate and P the product. The reaction occurs in three stages, all of which are reversible:

- Binding of the substrate to the enzyme, to form the enzyme-substrate complex:

  $$E + S \rightleftharpoons E - S$$

- Reaction of the enzyme-substrate complex to form the enzyme-product complex:

  $$E - S \rightleftharpoons E - P$$

- Breakdown of the enzyme-product complex, with release of the product:

  $$E - P \rightleftharpoons E + P$$

The fact that enzymes not only bind the substrates, but also participate in the reaction (although they emerge unchanged at the end of the reaction) means that, as well as conferring specificity for the substrates, an enzyme also confers specificity for the reaction that is followed. This means that if a substrate is capable of undergoing several reactions, its fate will be determined by which enzymes are present, and the relative activities of enzymes that compete with each other for the substrate.

4.2.1 *Factors affecting the activity of enzymes*

When an enzyme has been purified, it is possible to express the amount of enzyme in tissues as the number of moles of enzyme protein present. However, what is more important is not how much of the enzyme protein is present in the cell, but how much catalytic activity there is – how much substrate can be converted to product in a given time. Therefore, amounts of enzyme in tissues are usually expressed in terms of units of activity. The correct SI unit of catalysis is the katal, which equals 1 mol of substrate converted per second. However, enzyme activity is usually expressed as the number of micromoles of substrate converted (or of product formed) per minute. This is the standard unit of enzyme activity, determined under specified optimum conditions for that enzyme, at 30°C. This temperature is a compromise between mammalian biochemists, who work at body temperature (37°C for human beings) and microbiological biochemists, who normally work at 20°C.

4.2.1.1 *pH*

The binding of the substrate to the enzyme and the catalysis of the reaction both depend on interactions between the substrates and reactive groups in the amino acid side chains that make up the active site. This means that both the substrates and these various reactive groups have to be in the appropriate ionized form for binding and reaction to occur. The state of ionization depends on the pH of the medium. This means that an enzyme will have maximum activity at a specific pH. This is the optimum pH for that enzyme; obviously, it will be different for different enzymes. As the pH rises or falls away from the optimum, so the activity of the enzyme will decrease. Most enzymes have little or no activity 2–3 pH units away from their pH optimum. This is shown for two different enzymes, with different pH optima, in Figure 4.3.

There is very precise control over pH in the body. As discussed in §3.4.1.2, a relatively small change in the pH of blood plasma away from the normal value of 7.35–7.45 results in serious problems of acidosis (below 7.2) or alkalosis (above 7.6). Nevertheless, enzymes with pH optima very different from 7.4, and which may have no detectable activity at pH 7.4, are important in the body. This is because the pH within different subcellular compartments and organelles can be very different from the average pH of either the cell as a whole or of plasma.

4.2.1.2 *Temperature*

Chemical reactions proceed faster at higher temperatures, for two reasons:

- Molecules move faster at higher temperatures, and hence have a greater chance of colliding to undergo reaction.

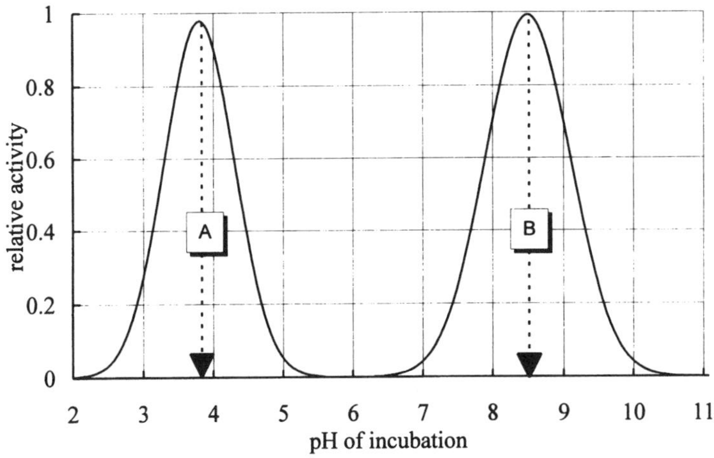

Figure 4.3 The effect of pH on the rate of an enzyme-catalysed reaction.

- At a higher temperature it is also easier for electrons to gain activation energy, and hence become excited into unstable orbitals to undergo reaction.

With enzyme-catalysed reactions, although the rate at which the reaction comes to equilibrium increases with temperature, there is a second effect of temperature: denaturation of the enzyme protein, leading to irreversible loss of activity. As the temperature increases, so the movement of parts of the protein molecules relative to each other increases, leading eventually to disruption of the hydrogen bonds (see §3.5.1) that maintain the folded structure of the protein. When this happens, the protein chain unfolds and ceases to be soluble, precipitating out from the solution. As the folding of the protein chain is lost, so the active site ceases to exist.

As shown in Figure 4.4, the temperature thus has two opposing effects on enzyme activity. At relatively low temperatures (up to about 50–55°C), increasing temperature results in an increase in the rate of reaction. However, as the temperature increases further, so denaturation of the enzyme protein becomes increasingly important, resulting in a rapid decrease in activity at higher temperatures. Both the increase in activity at lower temperatures and the denaturation at higher temperatures are characteristics of the enzyme concerned, depending on its structure.

The effect of temperature is not normally important in the body, since body temperature is normally maintained close to 37°C. However, some of the effects of fever (when body temperature may rise to 40°C) may be due to changes in the rates of enzyme reactions. Because enzymes respond differently

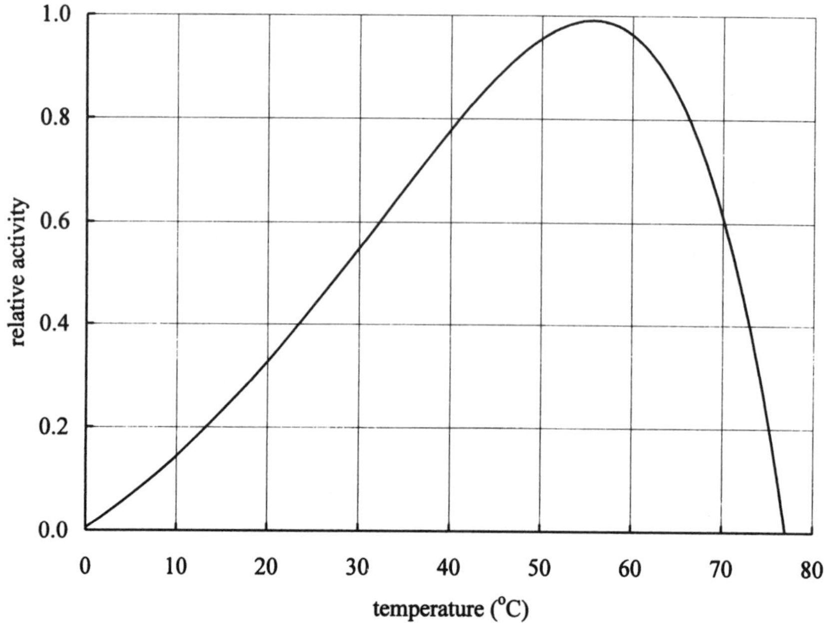

Figure 4.4 The effect of temperature on the rate of an enzyme-catalysed reaction.

to changes in temperature, there can be a considerable loss of the normal integration between different enzymic reactions and metabolic pathways.

4.2.1.3 *The concentration of substrate*

In a simple chemical reaction involving a single substrate, the rate at which product is formed increases in a linear fashion as the concentration of the substrate increases. At higher concentrations of substrate there is more substrate available to undergo the reaction, and therefore a greater probability of molecules undergoing reaction.

With enzyme-catalysed reactions, the change in the rate of formation of product with increasing concentration of substrate is not linear, but curved, as shown in Figure 4.5. At relatively low concentrations of substrate (region A in Figure 4.5), the catalytic site of the enzyme may be empty at times, until more substrate binds and undergoes reaction. Under these conditions, what limits the rate of formation of product is the time taken for another molecule of substrate to bind to the enzyme. Adding more substrate shortens this time, and so increases the rate of formation of product. A relatively small change in the concentration of substrate has a large effect on the rate at which product is formed in this region of the curve.

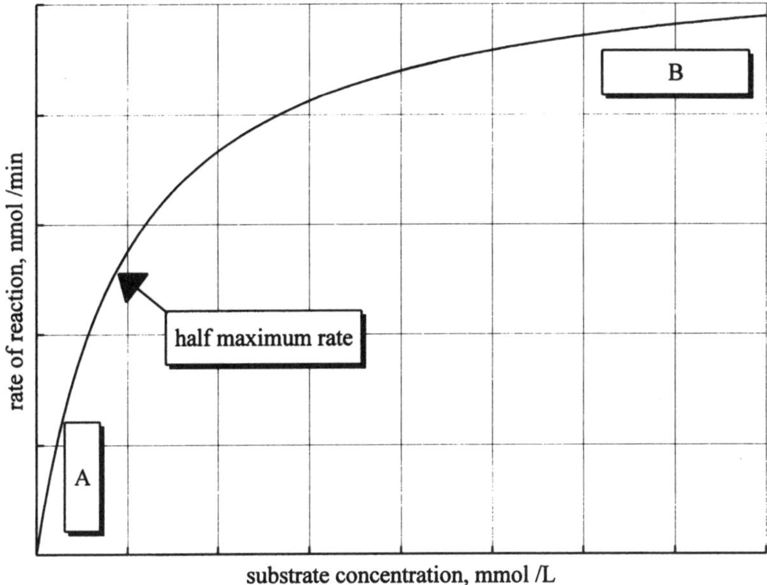

Figure 4.5 Substrate dependence of the rate of an enzyme-catalysed reaction.

At high concentrations of substrate (region B in Figure 4.5), as product leaves the catalytic site, another molecule of substrate binds. Under these conditions the enzyme is saturated with substrate; it is acting as fast as it can. The limiting factor in the formation of product is now that rate at which the enzyme can catalyse the reaction, and not the availability of substrate. The enzyme is acting at or near its maximum rate (or maximum velocity, usually abbreviated to V_{max}). Even a relatively large change in the concentration of substrate has little effect on the rate of formation of product in this region of the curve. Different enzymes have different values of V_{max} ; values of the order of 50–5000 mol of substrate converted per mole of enzyme per minute are common.

From a graph of the rate of formation of product versus the concentration of substrate (Figure 4.5), it is easy to estimate the maximum rate of reaction that an enzyme can achieve (V_{max}) when it is saturated with substrate. However, it is not possible to determine from this graph the concentration of substrate required to achieve saturation, because the enzyme gradually approaches its maximum rate of reaction as the concentration of substrate increases.

It is easy to find the concentration of substrate at which the enzyme has achieved half its maximum rate of reaction. The concentration of substrate to achieve half V_{max} is called the Michaelis constant of the enzyme (abbreviated to

K_m), to commemorate Michaelis, who, together with Menten, first formulated a mathematical model of the dependence of the rate of enzymic reactions on the concentration of substrate.

The K_m of an enzyme is not affected by the amount of the enzyme protein that is present. It is an (inverse) index of the ease with which an enzyme can bind substrate. An enzyme with a high K_m has a relatively poor ability to bind its substrate compared with an enzyme with a lower K_m. The higher the value of K_m, the greater is the concentration of substrate required to achieve half saturation of the enzyme.

In general, enzymes with a low K_m compared with the normal concentration of substrate in the cell are likely to be acting at or near their maximum rate, and hence to have a more or less constant rate of reaction, despite (modest) changes in the concentration of substrate. By contrast, an enzyme with a high K_m compared with the normal concentration of substrate in the cell will show a large change in the rate of reaction, with relatively small changes in the concentration of substrate.

If two enzymes in a cell can both act on the same substrate, catalysing different reactions, the enzyme with the lower K_m will be able to bind more substrate, and therefore its reaction will be favoured at relatively low concentrations of substrate.

Cooperative (allosteric) enzymes Not all enzymes show the simple hyperbolic dependence of rate of reaction on substrate concentration shown in Figure 4.5. Some enzymes consist of several separate protein chains, each with an active site. In many such enzymes, the binding of substrate to one active site causes changes in the conformation not only of that active site, but of the whole multi-subunit array. This change in conformation affects the other active sites, altering the ease with which substrate can bind to the other active sites. This is cooperativity – the different subunits of the complete enzyme cooperate with each other. Because there is a change in the conformation (or shape) of the enzyme molecule, the phenomenon is also called allostericity (from the Greek for *different shape*), and such enzymes are called allosteric enzymes.

Figure 4.6 shows the change in rate of reaction with increasing concentration of substrate for an enzyme which displays substrate cooperativity. At low concentrations of substrate, the enzyme has little activity. As one of the binding sites is occupied, this causes a conformational change in the enzyme, and so increases the ease with which the other sites can bind substrate. Therefore, there is a steep increase in the rate of reaction with increasing concentration of substrate. Of course, as all the sites become saturated, so the rate of reaction cannot increase any further with increasing concentration of substrate; the enzyme achieves its maximum rate of reaction.

Enzymes that display substrate cooperativity are often important in controlling the overall rate of metabolic pathways. Their rate of reaction is extremely sensitive to the concentration of substrate. Furthermore, this sensitivity can readily be modified by a variety of compounds that bind to specific

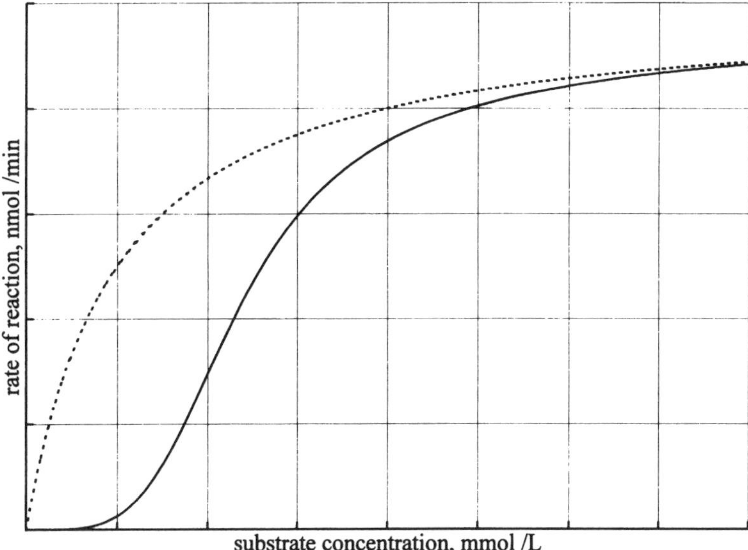

Figure 4.6 Substrate dependence of the rate of an enzyme-catalysed reaction for an enzyme showing cooperative binding (see also Figure 11.2).

regulator sites on the enzyme and affect its conformation, so affecting the conformation of all of the active sites of the multi-subunit complex. As discussed in §11.1, end-products and precursors of metabolic pathways often act in this way to modify the activity of regulatory enzymes.

4.2.1.4 *Inhibitors*

As discussed in §11.1, some metabolic intermediates can act as inhibitors of specific enzymes, reducing their activity, and so regulating metabolic pathways. Many of the drugs used to treat various diseases are inhibitors of enzymes. Some act by inhibiting the activity of the patient's enzyme, so altering metabolic regulation; others act by preferentially inhibiting key enzymes in the bacteria or other microorganisms that are causing disease.

Compounds that act as inhibitors of enzymes may either act reversibly, so that the inhibition gradually wears off as the inhibitor is metabolized, or irreversibly, causing chemical modification of the enzyme protein, so that the effect of the inhibitor is prolonged, and only diminishes gradually as the enzyme protein is broken down and replaced (see §10.1). Obviously, it is important when designing drugs to know whether they act as reversible or irreversible inhibitors. An irreversible inhibitor may need to be administered only every few days; however, it is more difficult to adjust the dose of an irreversible inhibitor to match the patient's needs, because of the long duration of action. By contrast, it is easy to adjust the dose of a reversible inhibitor to produce the desired effect, but such a compound may have to be taken several times a day, depending on the rate at which it is metabolized in, and excreted from, the body.

Irreversible inhibitors are chemical analogues of the substrate and they bind to the enzyme in the same way as does the substrate, then undergo part of the reaction sequence of the normal reaction. However, at some stage they form a covalent bond to a reactive group in the active site, resulting in inactivation of the enzyme. Such inhibitors are sometimes called mechanism-dependent inhibitors, or suicide inhibitors, because they cause the enzyme to commit suicide.

There are two main classes of reversible inhibition of enzymes: competitive and non-competitive. Which type of inhibitor will be more appropriate for a given drug depends on the effect that is desired.

Competitive inhibition A competitive inhibitor is a compound that binds to the active site of the enzyme in place of the substrate. Commonly, but not always, such compounds are chemical analogues of the substrate. Although a competitive inhibitor binds to the active site, it does not undergo reaction, or if it does, not to yield the product that would have been obtained by reaction of the normal substrate.

A competitive inhibitor reduces the rate of reaction because, at any time, some molecules of the enzyme have bound the inhibitor, and therefore are not free to bind the substrate. However, the binding of the inhibitor to the enzyme is reversible, and therefore there is competition between the substrate and the inhibitor for the enzyme.

If the concentration of substrate is increased, it will compete more effectively with the inhibitor for the active site of the enzyme. This means that at high concentrations of substrate the enzyme will achieve the same maximum rate of reaction (V_{max}) in the presence or absence of inhibitor. It is simply that in the presence of inhibitor the enzyme requires a higher concentration of substrate to achieve saturation; in other words, the K_m of the enzyme is higher in the presence of a competitive inhibitor.

The effect of a drug that is a competitive inhibitor is that the rate at which product is formed is unchanged, but there is an increase in the concentration of the substrate of the inhibited enzyme in the cell. This means that a competitive inhibitor is appropriate for use as a drug where the aim is to increase the available pool of substrate (perhaps so as to allow an alternative reaction to proceed), but inappropriate if the aim is to reduce the amount of product formed. As the inhibitor acts, so it will cause an increase in the concentration of substrate in the cell, and eventually this will rise high enough for the enzyme to reach a more or less normal rate of reaction.

Non-competitive inhibition Compounds that are non-competitive inhibitors bind to the enzyme–substrate complex, rather than to the enzyme itself. The enzyme–substrate–inhibitor complex only breaks down to enzyme + product + inhibitor slowly, so the effect of a non-competitive inhibitor is to slow down the rate at which the enzyme catalyses the formation of product.

Because there is no competition between the inhibitor and the substrate for binding to the enzyme, increasing the concentration of substrate has no effect on the activity of the enzyme in the presence of a non-competitive inhibitor. The K_m of the enzyme is unaffected by a non-competitive inhibitor, but the V_{max} is reduced.

A non-competitive inhibitor would be the choice for use as a drug when the aim is either to increase the concentration of substrate in the cell or to reduce the rate at which the product is formed, since, unlike a competitive inhibitor, the accumulation of substrate has no effect on the extent of inhibition.

4.3 Coenzymes and prosthetic groups

Although enzymes are proteins, many contain small non-protein molecules as an integral part of their structure. These may be organic compounds, which are known as coenzymes, or they may be metal ions. In either case, they are essential to the function of the enzyme, and the enzyme has no activity in the absence of the metal ion or coenzyme.

Coenzymes may be relatively loosely bound to the enzyme, so that they can be lost or exchanged between different enzymes, or they may be very tightly bound. When a coenzyme is covalently bound to the protein, as a result of a chemical reaction between the coenzyme and the enzyme protein, it is sometimes called a prosthetic group. Like the enzyme itself, the coenzyme or prosthetic group participates in the reaction, but at the end emerges unchanged. Sometimes the coenzyme is chemically modified in one reaction, then restored to its original state by reaction with a second enzyme.

Many of the coenzymes are derived from vitamins; despite their importance, they cannot be made in the body, but must be provided in the diet. Table 4.1 shows the major coenzymes, the vitamins they are derived from, and their principal metabolic functions.

4.3.1 *Coenzymes and metals in oxidation and reduction reactions*

In its simplest form, oxidation is the combination of a molecule with oxygen. Thus, if carbon is burnt in air, it is oxidized to carbon dioxide: $C + O_2 \rightarrow CO_2$. Similarly, if a carbohydrate such as glucose ($C_6H_{12}O_6$) is burnt in air, it is oxidized to carbon dioxide and water:

$$C_6H_1O_6 + 6 \times O_2 \rightarrow 6 \times CO_2 + 6 \times H_2O.$$

Oxidation reactions need not always involve the addition of oxygen to the compound being oxidized. Oxidation can also be considered as a process of removing electrons from a molecule. Thus, the conversion of the iron Fe^{2+} ion

Table 4.1 The major coenzymes

	Full name	Source	Functions
CoA	Coenzyme A	Pantothenic acid	Acyl transfer reactions
FAD	Flavin adenine dinucleotide	Vitamin B_2	Oxidation reactions
FMN	Flavin mononucleotide	Vitamin B_2	Oxidation reactions
NAD	Nicotinamide adenine dinucleotide	Niacin	Oxidation and reduction reactions
NADP	Nicotinamide adenine dinucleotide phosphate	Niacin	Oxidation and reduction reations
PLP	Pyridoxal phosphate	Vitamin B_6	Amino acid metabolism

There are a number of other coenzymes, which are discussed as they are relevant to specific metabolic pathways. In addition to those shown in this table, most of the other vitamins also function as coenzymes; see §12.2.

to Fe^{3+} is also an oxidation, although in this case there is no direct involvement of oxygen.

In many reactions, the removal of electrons in an oxidation reaction does not result in the formation of a positive ion – hydrogen ions (H^+) are removed together with the electrons. This means that the removal of hydrogen from a compound is also oxidation. For example, a hydrocarbon such as ethane (C_2H_6) is oxidized to ethene (C_2H_4) by removing two hydrogen atoms onto a carrier:

$$CH_3{-}CH_3 + \text{carrier} \rightleftharpoons CH_2{=}CH_2 + \text{carrier}{-}H_2\,.$$

Reduction is the reverse of oxidation; the addition of hydrogen or electrons, or the removal of oxygen, are all reduction reactions. In the reaction above, ethane was oxidized to ethene at the expense of a carrier, which was reduced in the process. The addition of hydrogen to the carrier is a reduction reaction. Similarly, the addition of electrons to a molecule is a reduction, so just as the conversion of Fe^{2+} to Fe^{3+} is an oxidation reaction, the reverse reaction, the conversion of Fe^{3+} to Fe^{2+}, is a reduction.

Most of the reactions involved in the generation of metabolically useful energy involve the oxidation of metabolic fuels, whereas many of the biosynthetic reactions involved in the formation of metabolic fuel reserves and the synthesis of body components are reductions.

In some metabolic oxidation and reduction reactions, the hydrogen acceptor or donor is an integral part of the molecule of the enzyme that catalyses the reaction (e.g. riboflavin, see §4.3.1.2). In other cases the hydrogen acceptor or donor acts as a substrate of the enzyme (e.g. the nicotinamide nucleotide coenzymes; see §4.3.1.3).

4.3.1.1 *Metal ions*

The electron acceptor or donor may be a metal ion which can have two different stable electron configurations. Commonly iron (which can form Fe^{2+} or

Fe^{3+} ions) and copper (which can form Cu^{+} or Cu^{2+} ions) are involved. In some enzymes the metal ion is bound to the enzyme, in others it is incorporated in an organic molecule, which in turn is attached to the enzyme. For example, haem is an organic compound containing iron, which is the coenzyme for a variety of enzymes collectively known as the cytochromes (see §5.3.1.2). Haem is also the prosthetic group of haemoglobin, the protein in red blood cells that binds and transports oxygen between the lungs and other tissues, and myoglobin in muscle. However, in haemoglobin and myoglobin the iron of haem does not undergo oxidation; it binds oxygen but does not react with it.

4.3.1.2 *Riboflavin and flavoproteins*

Vitamin B_2 (riboflavin, see §12.2.6) is important in many oxidation and reduction reactions. A few enzymes contain riboflavin itself, whereas others contain a riboflavin derivative: either riboflavin phosphate (sometimes called flavin mononucleotide) or flavin adenine dinucleotide (FAD, see Figure 12.10). When an enzyme contains riboflavin, it is usually covalently bound at the active site. Although riboflavin phosphate and FAD are not normally covalently bound to the enzyme, they are tightly bound, and can be regarded as

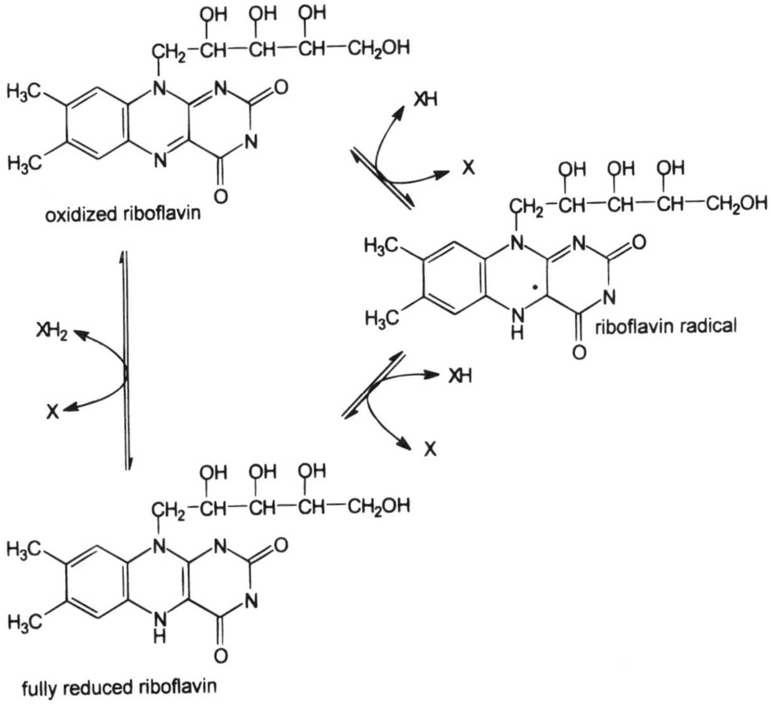

Figure 4.7 Oxidation and reduction of the riboflavin coenzymes (see also Figure 12.10).

prosthetic groups. The resultant enzymes with attached riboflavin are collectively known as flavoproteins.

As shown in Figure 4.7, the riboflavin part of flavoproteins can undergo two reduction reactions. It can accept one hydrogen, to form the flavin radical (generally written as flavin-H˙), followed by a second hydrogen forming fully reduced flavin-H_2.

Some reactions involve transfer of a single hydrogen to a flavin, forming flavin-H˙, which is then recycled in a separate reaction. Sometimes two molecules of flavin each accept one hydrogen atom from the substrate to be oxidized. Other reactions involve the sequential transfer of two hydrogens onto the flavin, forming first the flavin-H˙ radical, then fully reduced flavin-H_2.

As discussed in §2.5.1, the reoxidation of reduced flavins in enzymes that react with oxygen is a major source of potentially damaging oxygen radicals.

4.3.1.3 The nicotinamide nucleotide coenzymes: NAD and NADP

The vitamin niacin (see §12.2.7) is important for the formation of two closely related compounds, the nicotinamide nucleotide coenzymes. These are nicotinamide adenine dinucleotide (NAD) and nicotinamide adenine dinucleotide phosphate (NADP). As shown in Figure 4.8, they differ only in that NADP has an additional phosphate group attached to the ribose. The whole of the

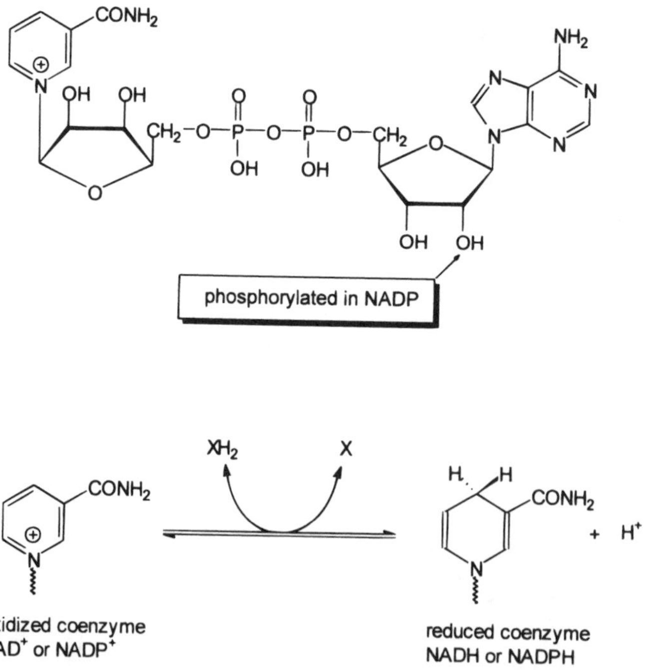

Figure 4.8 Oxidation and reduction of the nicotinamide nucleotide coenzymes, NAD and NADP (see also Figure 12.11).

coenzyme molecule is essential for binding to enzymes, and most enzymes can bind and use only one of these two coenzymes, despite the overall similarity in their structures.

The functionally important part of the nicotinamide nucleotide coenzymes is the nicotinamide ring, which undergoes a two electron reduction. In the oxidized coenzymes there is a positive charge associated with the nitrogen atom in the nicotinamide ring, and the oxidized forms of the coenzymes are usually shown as NAD^+ and $NADP^+$. Reduction involves the transfer of two electrons and two hydrogen ions (H^+) from the substrate to the coenzyme. One electron neutralizes the positive charge on the nitrogen atom. The other, with its associated H^+ ion, is incorporated into the ring as a second hydrogen at carbon-4. In the oxidized coenzyme there was one hydrogen at carbon-4, but this is not shown when the ring is drawn. In the reduced coenzymes both hydrogens are shown, with a dotted bond to one hydrogen and a bold bond to the other, to show that the ring as a whole is flat, with one hydrogen at carbon-4 above the plane of the ring and the other below.

The second H^+ ion removed from the substrate remains associated with the coenzyme. This means that the reaction can be shown as:

$$X{-}H_2 + NAD^+ \leftrightharpoons X + NADH + H^+,$$

where $X{-}H_2$ is the substrate and X is the product (the oxidized form of the substrate).

Note that the reaction is reversible, and NADH can act as a reducing agent:

$$X + NADH + H^+ \leftrightharpoons X{-}H_2 + NAD^+$$

where X is now the substrate and $X{-}H_2$ is the product (the reduced form of the substrate).

The usual notation is that NAD and NADP are used when the oxidation state is not relevant, and NAD(P) when either NAD or NADP is being discussed. The oxidized coenzymes are shown as $NAD(P)^+$, and the reduced forms as NAD(P)H.

Unlike flavins and metal coenzymes, the nicotinamide nucleotide coenzymes do not remain bound to the enzyme, but act as substrates, binding to the enzyme, undergoing reduction and then leaving. The reduced coenzyme is then reoxidized either by reaction with another enzyme, for which it acts as a hydrogen donor, or by way of the mitochondrial electron transport chain (see §5.3.1.2). Cells contain only a small amount of NAD(P) (of the order of 400 nmol per g in liver), which is rapidly cycled between the oxidized and reduced forms by different enzymes.

In general, NAD^+ is the coenzyme for oxidation reactions, with most of the resultant NADH being reoxidized by the mitochondrial electron transport chain, whereas NADPH is the main coenzyme for reduction reactions (e.g. the synthesis of fatty acids; see §7.6.1). Much of the NADPH that is required for

Table 4.2 Classification of enzyme-catalysed reactions

Oxidoreductases	Oxidation and reduction reactions:	
	dehydrogenases	addition or removal of H
	oxidases	two-electron transfer to O_2 forming H_2O_2
		two-electron transfer to $\frac{1}{2}O_2$ forming H_2O
	oxygenases	incorporate O_2 into product
	hydroxylases	incorporate $\frac{1}{2}O_2$ into product as -OH and form H_2O
	peroxidases	use as H_2O_2 as oxygen donor, forming H_2O
Transferases	Transfer a chemical group from one substrate to the other	
	kinases	transfer phosphate from ATP onto substrate
Hydrolases	Hydrolysis of C–O, C–N, O–P and C–S bonds (e.g. esterases, proteases, phosphatases, deamidases)	
Lyases	Addition across a carbon–carbon double bond: (e.g. dehydratases, hydratases, decarboxylases)	
Isomerases	Intramolecular rearrangements	
Ligases (synthetases)	Formation of bonds between two substrates: frequently linked to utilization of ATP, with intermediate formationof phosphorylated enzyme or substrate	

fatty acid synthesis is produced by the pentose phosphate pathway of carbohydrate metabolism (see §7.4.1.1).

4.4 The classification and naming of enzymes

There is a formal system of enzyme nomenclature, in which each enzyme has a number, and the various enzymes are classified according to the type of reaction catalysed and the substrates, products and coenzymes of the reaction. This is used in research publications, when there is a need to identify an enzyme unambiguously, but for general use there is a less formal system of naming enzymes. Almost all enzyme names end in *-ase*, and many are derived simply from the name of the substrate acted on, with the suffix *-ase*. In some cases, the type of reaction catalysed is also included.

Altogether there are some 5000 enzymes in human tissues. However, they can be classified into only six groups, depending on the types of chemical reaction they catalyse:

- oxidation and reduction reactions
- transfer of a reactive group from one substrate onto another
- hydrolysis of bonds

- addition across carbon–carbon double bonds
- rearrangement of groups within a single molecule of substrate
- formation of bonds between two substrates, frequently linked to the hydrolysis of ATP → ADP + phosphate.

This classification of enzymes is expanded in Table 4.2, to give some examples of the types of reactions catalysed.

4.5 Metabolic pathways

A simple reaction, such as the oxidation of ethanol (alcohol) to carbon dioxide and water, can proceed in a single step – for example, simply by setting fire to the alcohol in air. The reaction is exothermic, and the oxidation of ethanol to carbon dioxide and water yields an output of 29 kJ per g.

When alcohol is metabolized in the body, although the overall reaction is the same, it does not proceed in a single step, but as a series of linked reactions, each resulting in a small change in the substrate. As shown in Figure 4.9, the metabolic oxidation of ethanol involves 11 enzyme-catalysed reactions, as well as the mitochondrial electron transport chain (see §5.3.1.2). The energy yield is still 29 kJ per g, since the starting material (ethanol) and the end-products (carbon dioxide and water) are the same, and hence the change in energy level is the same overall, regardless of the route taken. Such a sequence of linked enzyme-catalysed reactions is a metabolic pathway.

Metabolic pathways can be divided into three broad groups:

- Catabolic pathways, involved in the breakdown of relatively large molecules, and oxidation, ultimately to carbon dioxide and water. These are the main energy-yielding metabolic pathways.
- Anabolic pathways, involved in the synthesis of compounds from simpler precursors. These are the main energy-requiring metabolic pathways. Many are reduction reactions, and many involve condensation reactions. Similar reactions are also involved in the metabolism of drugs and other foreign compounds, and hormones and neurotransmitters, to yield products that are excreted in the urine or bile.
- Central pathways, involved in interconversions of substrates, that can be regarded as being both catabolic and anabolic. The principal such pathway is the citric acid cycle (see §7.4.2.3).

4.5.1 Linear and branched pathways

The simplest type of metabolic pathway is a single sequence of reactions in which the starting material is converted to the end-product with no possibility of alternative reactions or branches in the pathway.

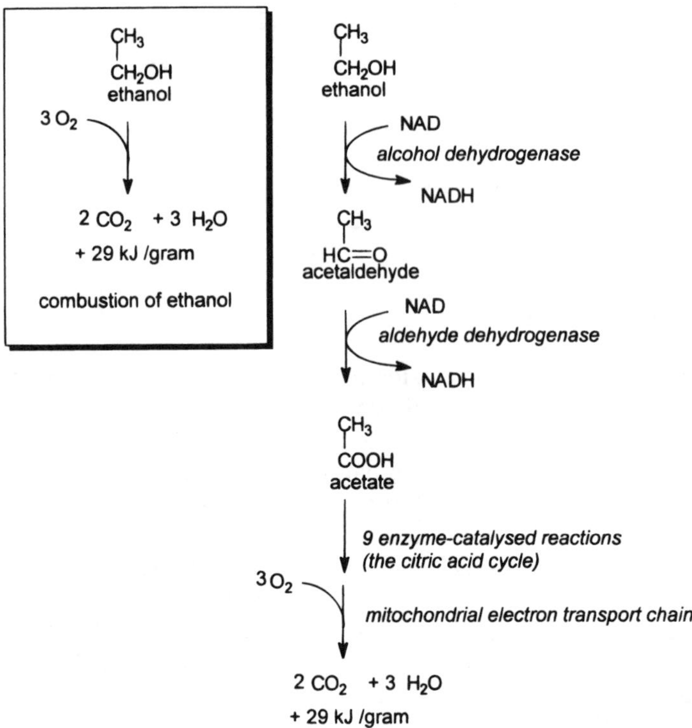

Figure 4.9 A simple metabolic pathway: the oxidation of ethanol to carbon dioxide and water.

Simple linear pathways are rare, since many of the intermediate compounds in metabolism can be used in a variety of different pathways, depending on the body's need for various end-products. Many metabolic pathways involve branch points, where an intermediate may proceed down one branch or another. The fate of an intermediate at a branch point will depend on the relative activities of the two enzymes that are competing for the same substrate. Enzymes catalysing reactions at branch points are usually subject to regulation (see §11.1), so as to direct substrates through one branch or the other, depending on the body's requirements at the time.

4.5.2 Looped reaction sequences

Sometimes a complete metabolic pathway involves repeating a series of similar reactions several times over. Thus, the synthesis of fatty acids (see §7.6.1) involves the repeated addition of two-carbon units until the final chain length (commonly 14, 16 or 18 carbon units) has been achieved. The addition of each two-carbon unit involves four separate reaction steps, which are repeated each time. Similarly, the oxidation of fatty acids (see §7.5.2) proceeds by the sequential removal of two-carbon units. Again the removal of each two-carbon unit involves a repeated sequence of reactions.

4.5.3 Cyclic pathways

The third type of metabolic pathway is cyclic: the end-product is the same compound as the starting material. Thus, in the synthesis of urea (see §10.3.1.4), the molecule of urea is built up in a series of stages as part of a larger carrier molecule. At the end of the reaction sequence, the urea is released by hydrolysis, resulting in the formation of the starting material to undergo a further cycle of reaction. Similarly, in the citric acid cycle (see §7.4.2.3) the four-carbon compound oxaloacetate can be considered to be the beginning of the pathway. It reacts with the two-carbon compound acetate to form a six-carbon compound, citrate. Two carbon atoms are lost as carbon dioxide in the reaction sequence, so that at the end oxaloacetate is reformed.

The intermediates in a cyclic pathway can be considered to be catalysts in that they participate in the reaction sequence, but at the end they emerge unchanged.

A note on metabolic pathways

A metabolic pathway is no more than a map showing the steps by which one compound is converted to another. Along the way are points of interest: key steps that allow for the regulation and integration of different pathways; enzymes that may be targets for drugs or poisons; enzymes that are affected by disease, etc.

There is no more point in 'learning' a metabolic pathway than there is 'learning' a road map. What is important is to be able to read the pathways like a map, to see how metabolic intermediates are related to each other, how changes in one system affect other systems, and which are the points of interest.

5

The Role of ATP in Metabolism

The coenzyme adenosine triphosphate (ATP) acts as the central link between energy-yielding metabolic pathways and energy expenditure on physical and chemical work. The oxidation of metabolic fuels is linked to the phosphorylation of adenosine diphosphate (ADP) to adenosine triphosphate (ATP); the expenditure of metabolic energy for the synthesis of body constituents, transport of compounds across cell membranes and the contraction of muscle results overall in the hydrolysis of ATP to yield ADP and phosphate ions. The total body content of ATP plus ADP is under 350 mmol, but the amount of ATP synthesized and used each day is about 100 mol – an amount equal to the total body weight.

Under normal conditions, the processes shown in Figure 5.1 are tightly coupled, so that the oxidation of metabolic fuels is controlled by the availability of ADP, which in turn is controlled by the rate at which ATP is being utilized in performing physical and chemical work. Work output, or energy expenditure, thus controls the rate at which metabolic fuels are oxidized, and hence the amount of food that must be eaten to meet energy requirements. As discussed in §7.3.1, metabolic fuels in excess of immediate requirements are stored as reserves of glycogen in muscle and liver, and fat in adipose tissue.

5.1 The adenosine nucleotides

Nucleotides consist of a purine or pyrimidine base linked to the 5-carbon sugar ribose. The base plus sugar is a nucleoside; in a nucleotide the sugar is phosphorylated. Nucleotides may be mono-, di- or triphosphates. In addition to the functions discussed here, purine and pyrimidine nucleotides are important in RNA (see §10.2.2) and DNA (§10.2.1), where the sugar is deoxyribose rather than ribose.

The nucleotides formed from the purine adenine, adenosine monophosphate (AMP), adenosine diphosphate (ADP) and adenosine triphosphate

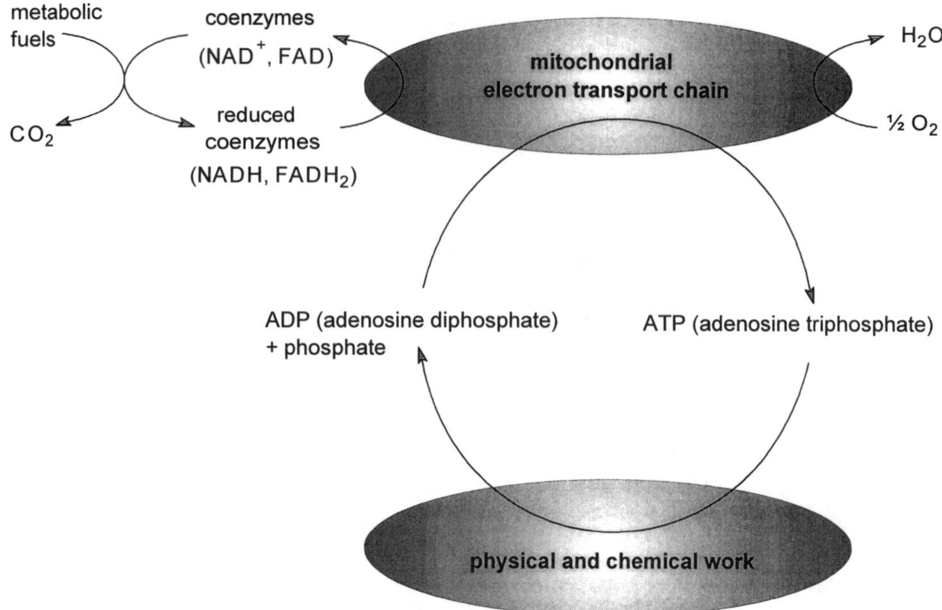

Figure 5.1 The role of ATP in metabolism: obligatory linkage between the oxidation of metabolic fuels and the performance of physical and chemical work.

(ATP), are shown in Figure 5.2. Similar nucleotides are also formed from the purine guanine (the guanosine nucleotides) and the pyrimidine uracil (the uridine nucleotides). See also §11.2.2 for a discussion of the role of cyclic AMP in metabolic regulation and hormone action.

In the nucleic acids (DNA and RNA, see §10.2.1 and §10.2.2) it is the purine or pyrimidine that is important, carrying the genetic information. However, in the link between energy-yielding metabolism and the performance of physical and chemical work, what is important is the phosphorylation of the ribose. Although most reactions are linked to adenosine triphosphate, a few are linked to guanosine triphosphate (GTP; see, for example, §7.4.2.3 and §7.7) or uridine triphosphate (UTP, see §7.6.2).

5.2 Functions of ATP

In all of the reactions in which ATP is utilized, what is observed overall is hydrolysis of ATP to ADP and phosphate. However, as discussed below, although this is the overall reaction, simple hydrolysis of ATP does not achieve any useful result; it is the intermediate steps in the reaction of ATP $+ H_2O \rightarrow ADP +$ phosphate that are important.

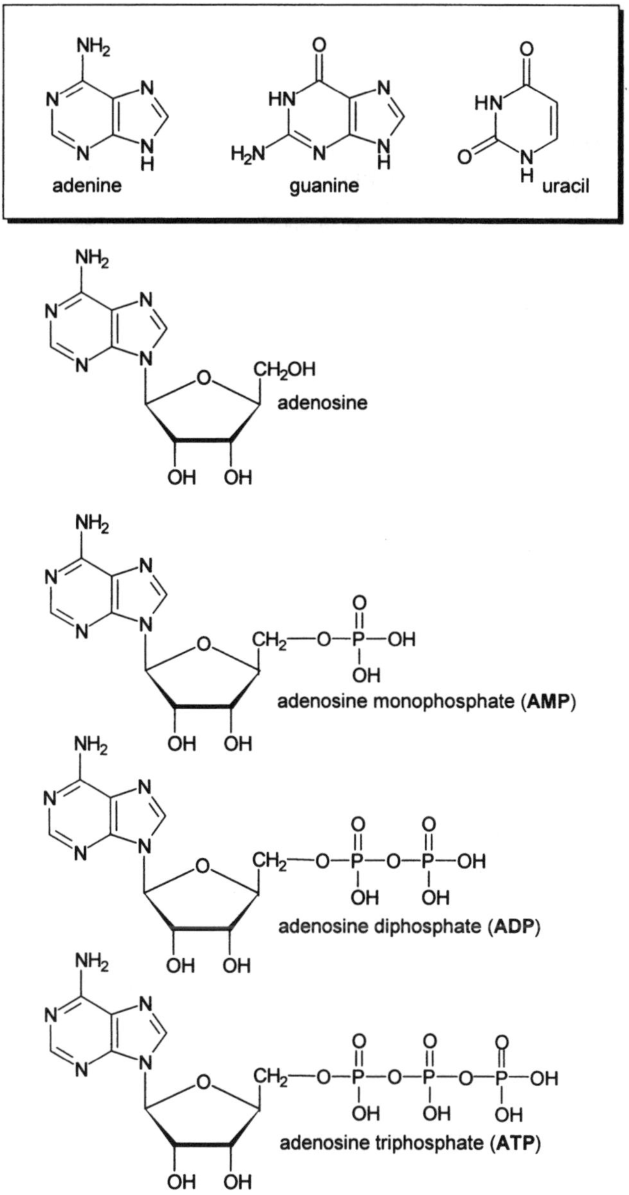

Figure 5.2 The adenine nucleotides, and (inset) the purines adenine and guanine, and the pyrimidine uracil.

a) Phosphorylation of the enzyme

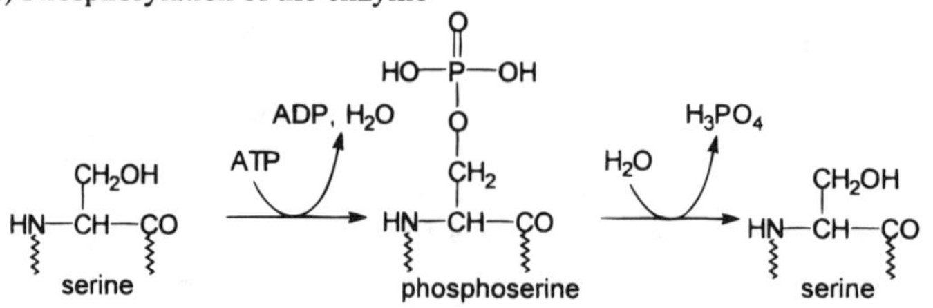

serine → (ATP → ADP, H_2O) → phosphoserine → (H_2O → H_3PO_4) → serine

b) Phosphorylation of the substrate

glutamate → (NH_4^+, ATP → ADP, Pi; *overall reaction*) → glutamine

glutamate → (ATP → ADP) → γ-glutamyl phosphate → (NH_4^+ → H_3PO_4) → glutamine

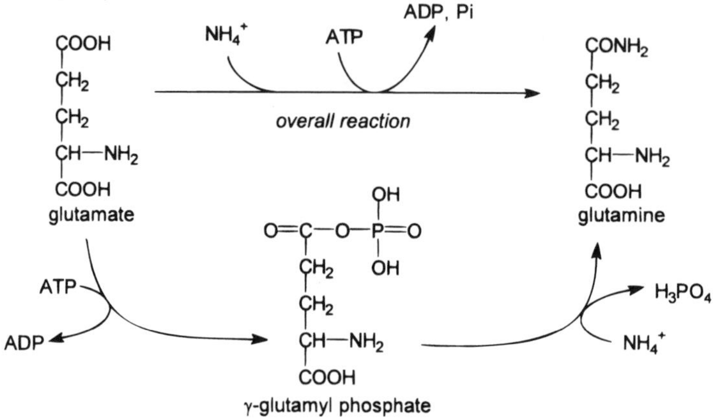

c) Adenylation of the substrate

methionine → (ATP → H_3PO_4 + pyrophosphate; *methionine adenosyltransferase*) → *S*-adenosylmethionine → (X → X—CH_3) → adenosine + homocysteine

pyrophosphate → (H_2O; *pyrophosphatase*) → 2 x H_3PO_4

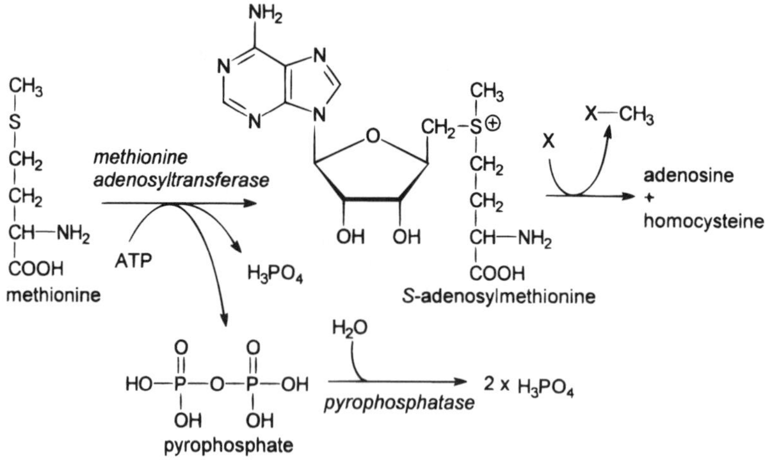

Figure 5.3 The role of ATP in endothermic enzyme-catalysed reactions.

5.2.1 *The role of ATP in endothermic reactions*

As discussed in §4.1, the equilibrium of an endothermic reaction A + B ⇌ C + D lies well to the left unless there is an input of energy, usually as heat. The hydrolysis of ATP is exothermic, and the equilibrium of the reaction ATP + H_2O ⇌ ADP + phosphate lies well to the right. Linkage between the two reactions could thus ensure that the (unfavoured) endothermic reaction could proceed together with overall hydrolysis of ATP → ADP + phosphate.

Such linkage between two apparently unrelated reactions can easily be achieved in enzyme-catalysed reactions; there are three possible mechanisms:

- Phosphorylation of the hydroxyl group of a serine, threonine or tyrosine residue in the enzyme (see Figure 5.3a), thus altering the chemical nature of its catalytic site. As discussed in §11.2, such phosphorylation of the enzyme is also important in regulating metabolic pathways, especially in response to hormone action.
- Phosphorylation of one of the substrates; as shown in Figure 5.3b, the synthesis of glutamine from glutamate and ammonia involves the formation of a phosphorylated intermediate.
- Transfer of the adenosyl group of ATP onto one of the substrates, as shown in Figure 5.3c for the activation of the methyl group of the amino acid methionine for methyl-transfer reactions.

Not only is the hydrolysis of ATP → ADP and phosphate an exothermic reaction, but the concentration of ATP in cells is always very much higher than that of ADP (the ratio of ATP to ADP is about 500 : 1), so again ensuring that the reaction will indeed proceed in the direction of ATP hydrolysis. Furthermore, the concentration of ADP in cells is maintained extremely low by rephosphorylation to ATP, linked to the oxidation of metabolic fuels (see §5.3). Again this serves to ensure that the equilibrium of the reaction ATP + H_2O → ADP + phosphate lies well to the right.

In some cases, there is a further mechanism to ensure that the equilibrium of an ATP-linked reaction is kept well to the right, to such an extent that the reaction is essentially irreversible. As shown in Figure 5.4, such reactions result in the hydrolysis of ATP to AMP and pyrophosphate. There is an active pyrophosphatase in cells, which catalyses the hydrolysis of pyrophosphate to yield two phosphates, so removing one of the products of the reaction, and ensuring that it is essentially irreversible.

5.2.2 *Transport of materials across cell membranes*

Compounds that are lipid soluble will diffuse freely across cell membranes, since they can dissolve in the lipid of the membrane (see Figure 3.9): this is passive diffusion. Hydrophilic compounds require a transport protein in order

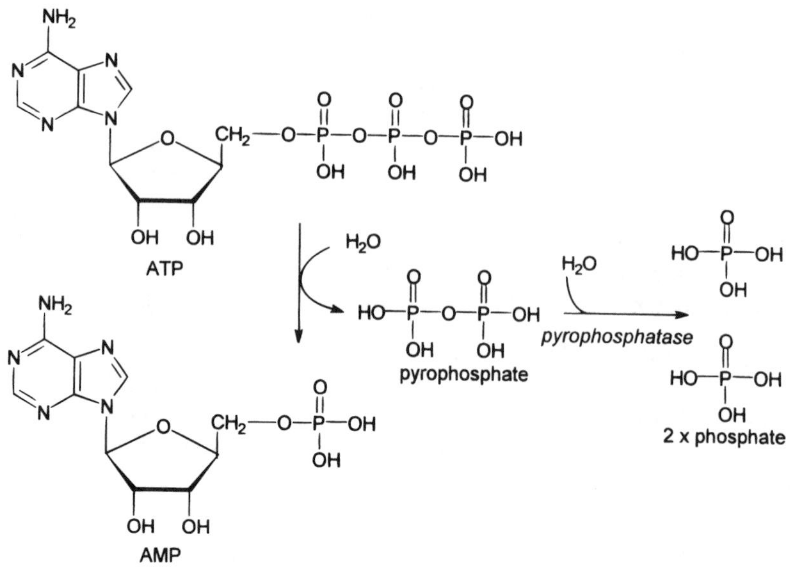

Figure 5.4 The hydrolysis of ATP to AMP and pyrophosphate.

to cross the lipid membrane – this is facilitated diffusion. Neither passive nor facilitated diffusion alone can lead to a greater concentration of the material being transported inside the cell than that present outside.

Concentrative uptake of the material being transported may be achieved in three main ways: protein binding, metabolic trapping and active transport. These last two mechanisms are both ATP-dependent.

5.2.2.1 *Protein binding for concentrative uptake*

For a hydrophilic compound that enters a cell by facilitated diffusion, a net increase in concentration inside the cell can be achieved by binding the material to a protein that has a higher affinity for the compound than does the membrane carrier. It is only material in free solution that equilibrates across the membrane, not that which is protein bound. Such binding proteins are important, for example, in the intestinal absorption of calcium (see §12.3.1.1) and iron (§6.6).

For hydrophobic compounds that enter the cell by passive diffusion, the situation is slightly more complex. Hydrophobic compounds cannot dissolve in plasma to any significant extent, but are transported bound to more or less specific transport proteins. For example, serum albumin binds a great many drugs and also free fatty acids (see §7.5). There are also highly specific binding proteins in plasma, such as the retinol binding protein that transports vitamin A (see §12.2.1.3), and cortisol and sex hormone binding globins that transport steroid hormones. The lipid-soluble compounds being transported will dissolve in cell membranes, but the cells will accumulate them significantly only if there is also an intracellular binding protein that has a higher affinity than does the plasma binding protein, such as the steroid hormone receptor proteins in target cells (see §11.3).

5.2.2.2 Metabolic trapping

Glucose enters liver cells freely by carrier-mediated diffusion (although uptake into other tissues is by active transport). Once inside the cell, glucose is phosphorylated to glucose 6–phosphate, a reaction catalysed by the enzyme hexokinase, using ATP as the phosphate donor (see §7.4.1). Glucose 6–phosphate does not cross cell membranes, and therefore there is a net accumulation of [glucose plus glucose 6–phosphate] inside the cell, at the expense of 1 mol of ATP utilized per mole of glucose trapped in this way. Vitamins B_6 (see §12.2.8) and B_2 (riboflavin, see §12.2.6) are similarly accumulated inside cells by phosphorylation at the expense of ATP.

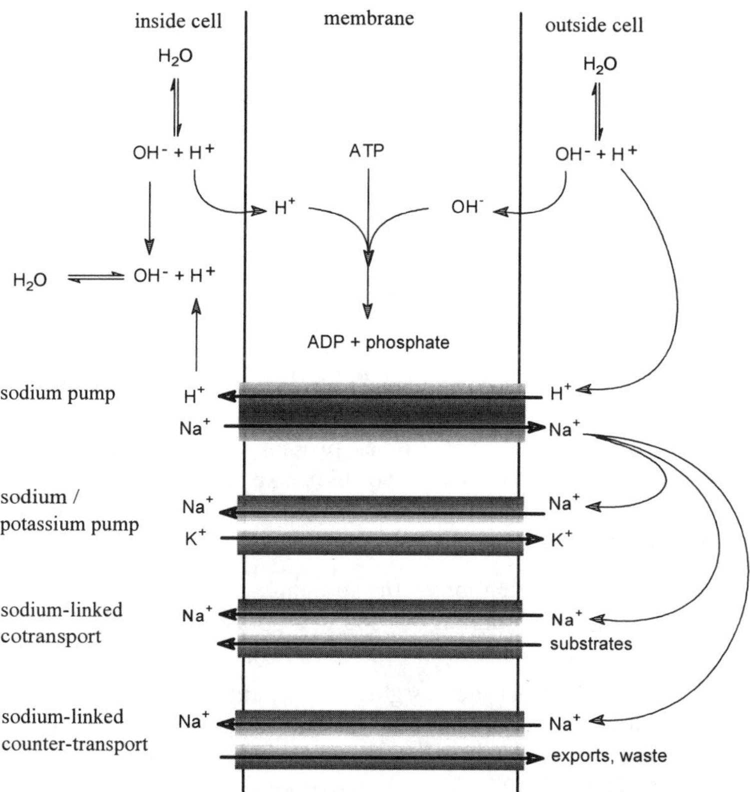

Figure 5.5 The role of ATP in membrane transport: ATPase and the sodium pump.

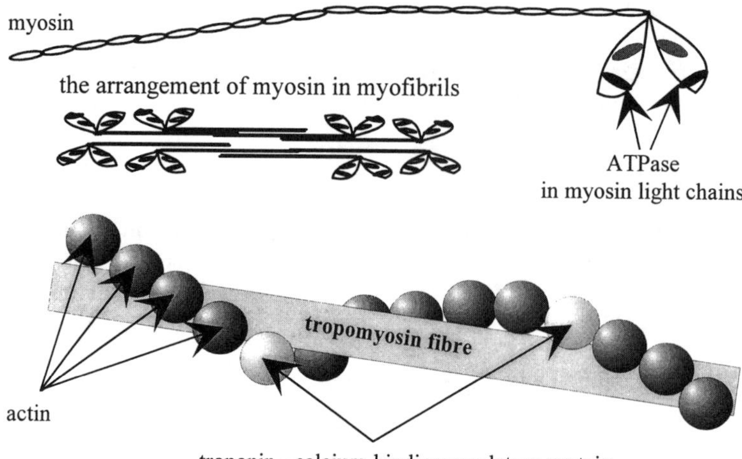

Figure 5.6 Actin and myosin, the major proteins of muscle.

5.2.2.3 *Ion pumps and active transport*

There is active pumping of ions across cell membranes, so that there is a higher concentration of potassium ions (K^+) inside cells than in the extracellular fluid, and a higher concentration of sodium ions (Na^+) outside cells than inside. This is accompanied by the hydrolysis of ATP $\rightarrow$ ADP + phosphate. The key to understanding the role of ATP in ion pumps lies in the fact that the hydrolysis is effected not by H_2O, but by H^+ and OH^- ions.

As shown in Figure 5.5, the ATPase which catalyses the hydrolysis of ATP $\rightarrow$ ADP + phosphate is within the membrane, and takes an H^+ ion from inside the cell and an OH^- ion from the extracellular fluid. The resultant surplus protons in the extracellular fluid then enter the cell on a carrier protein, and react with the surplus hydroxyl ions within the cell, so discharging the pH gradient. The carrier protein that transports the protons across the cell membrane only does so in exchange for sodium ions, so maintaining approximate electrical neutrality across the membrane. The sodium ions in turn re-enter the cell in one of three ways:

- In exchange for potassium ions – the sodium–potassium pump. This is especially important in maintaining the sodium–potassium gradient across nerve cells that is the basis of electrical conductivity of nerves.
- Together with substrates such as glucose and amino acids, thus providing a mechanism for net accumulation of these substrates, driven by the sodium gradient, which in turn has been created by the proton gradient produced by the hydrolysis of ATP. This is the process of active transport; it is a cotransport mechanism since the sodium ions and substrates travel in the same direction across the cell membrane.

- In exchange for compounds being exported or excreted from the cell. This is again active transport, in this case a counter-transport mechanism, since the sodium ions and the compounds being transported move in opposite directions across the membrane.

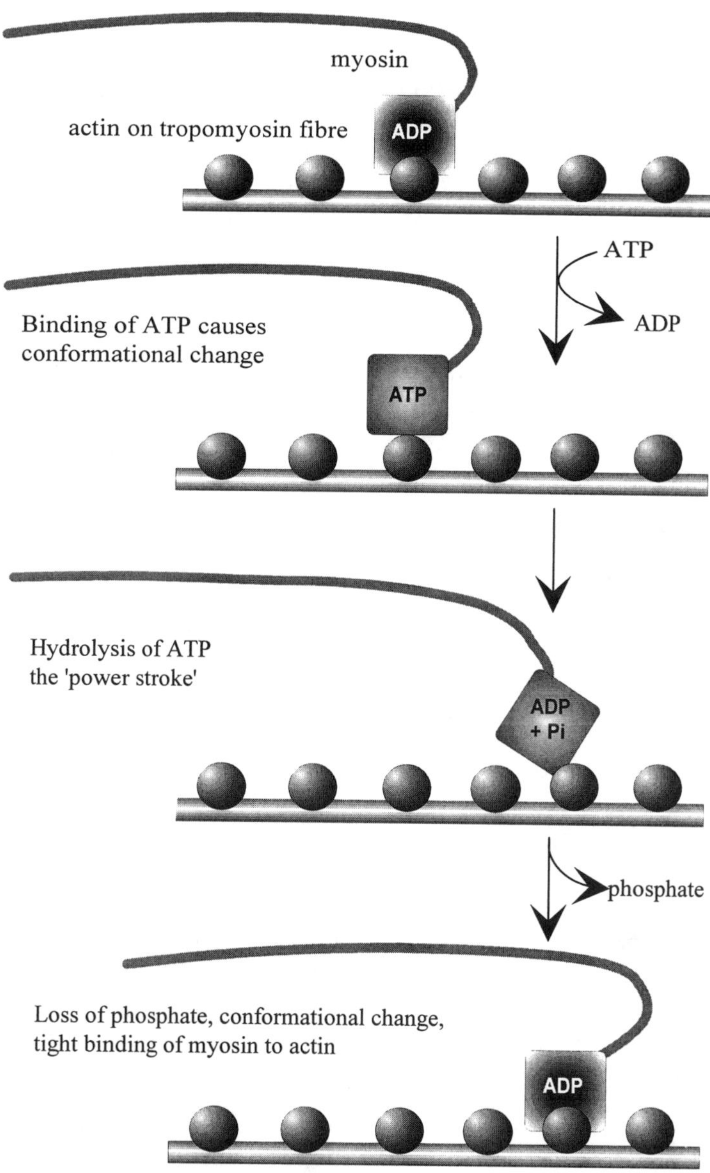

Figure 5.7 The role of ATP in muscle contraction.

5.2.3 *The role of ATP in muscle contraction*

The important proteins of muscle are actin and myosin. As shown in Figure 5.6, myosin is a filamentous protein, consisting of several subunits, and with ATPase activity in the head region. In myofibrils, myosin molecules are arranged in clusters with the tail regions overlapping. Actin is a smaller, globular protein, and actin molecules are arranged around a fibrous protein, tropomyosin, so creating a chain of actin molecules, interspersed with molecules of a calcium-binding regulatory protein, troponin.

In resting muscle, each myosin head unit binds ADP and is bound to an actin molecule, as shown in Figure 5.7. The binding of ATP to myosin displaces the bound ADP and causes a conformation change in the molecule, so that, while it remains associated with the actin molecule, it is no longer tightly bound. Hydrolysis of the bound ATP to ADP and phosphate causes a further conformational change in the myosin molecule, this time affecting the tail region, so that the head region becomes associated with an actin molecule farther along. This is the power stroke which causes the actin and myosin filaments to slide over one another. When the phosphate is released, the head region of myosin undergoes the reverse conformational change, so that it now becomes tightly bound to the new actin molecule, and is ready to undergo a further cycle of ATP binding, hydrolysis and movement.

5.3 The phosphorylation of ADP to ATP

A few metabolic reactions involve direct transfer of phosphate from a phosphorylated substrate onto ADP, forming ATP. Two such reactions are shown in Figure 5.8; both are reactions in the glycolytic pathway of glucose metabolism (see §7.4.1). Such reactions are of relatively minor importance in ensuring

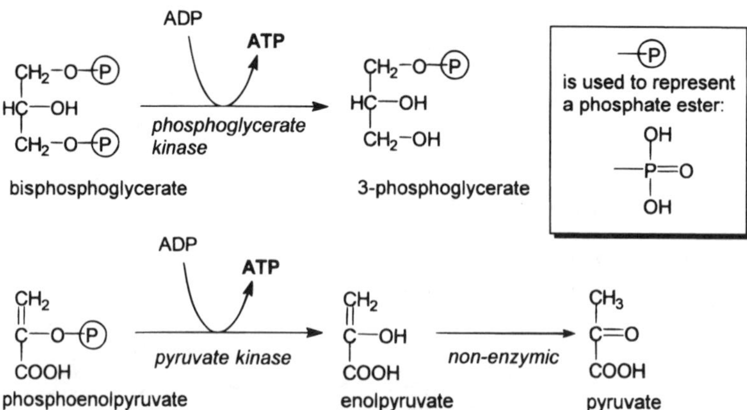

Figure 5.8 Substrate-level phosphorylation of ADP to ATP.

a supply of ATP (although they become important in muscle under conditions of maximum exertion); under normal conditions almost all of the phosphorylation of ADP to ATP occurs in the mitochondria, by the process of oxidative phosphorylation.

5.3.1 *Oxidative phosphorylation: the phosphorylation of ADP to ATP linked to the oxidation of metabolic fuels*

With the exception of glycolysis (see §7.4.1), most of the reactions in the oxidation of metabolic fuels occur inside the mitochondria and lead to the reduction of nicotinamide nucleotide and flavin coenzymes (see §4.3.1.2 and §4.3.1.3). The reduced coenzymes are then reoxidized. Within the inner membrane of the mitochondrion (see §5.3.1.1) there is a series of coenzymes that are able to undergo reduction and oxidation. The first coenzyme in the chain is reduced by reaction with NADH, and is then reoxidized by reducing the next coenzyme. In turn, each coenzyme in the chain is reduced by the preceding coenzyme, and then reoxidized by reducing the next one. The final step is the oxidation of a reduced coenzyme by oxygen, resulting in the formation of water.

This stepwise oxidation of NADH and reduction of oxygen to water is linked to the phosphorylation of ADP → ATP, and this linkage is obligatory under normal conditions. Three moles of ATP are formed for each mole of NADH that is oxidized. Flavoproteins reduce an intermediate coenzyme in the chain, and 2 mol of ADP are phosphorylated to ATP for each mole of reduced flavoprotein that is oxidized.

5.3.1.1 *The mitochondrion*

Both the number and size of mitochondria vary in different cells – for example, a liver cell contains some 800 mitochondria, a renal tubule cell some 300 and a sperm about 20. As shown in Figure 5.9, mitochondria are intracellular organelles, with a double membrane structure. The outer membrane is permeable to a great many substrates; the inner membrane provides a barrier to regulate the uptake of substrates and output of products (see, for example, the regulation of acyl CoA uptake into the mitochondrion in §7.5.1). The inner membrane is highly folded, forming cristae.

The five compartments of the mitochondrion have a range of specialized functions:

- The outer membrane contains the enzymes that are responsible for the elongation of fatty acids synthesized in the cytosol (see §7.6.1), the enzymes for triacylglycerol synthesis from fatty acids (§7.6.1.2) and phospholipases that catalyse the hydrolysis of phospholipids (§6.3.1.2):

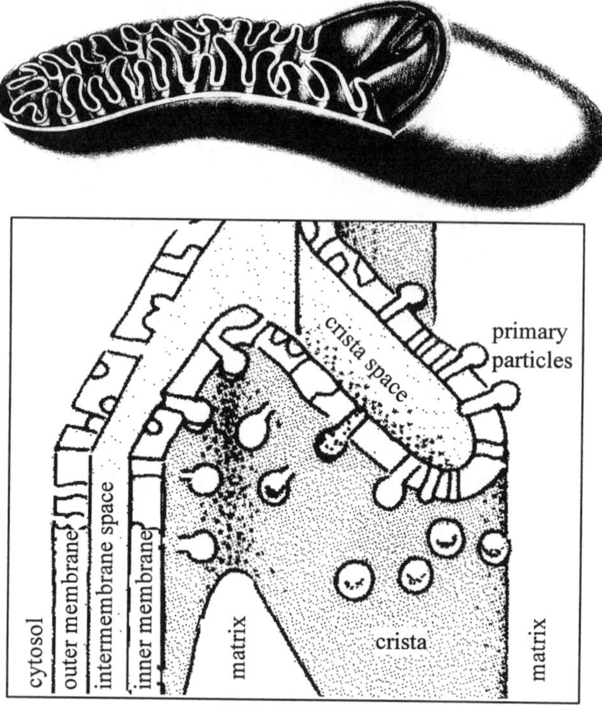

Figure 5.9 The mitochondrion.

- The intermembrane space contains enzymes involved in nucleotide metabolism, transamination of amino acids (see §10.3.1.2) and a variety of kinases.
- The inner membrane regulates the uptake of substrates into the matrix.
- The membrane of the cristae contains the coenzymes associated with electron transport, the oxidation of reduced coenzymes, and the reduction of oxygen to water. The primary particles on the inner surface of the cristae contain the enzymes that catalyse the phosphorylation of ADP to ATP.
- The mitochondrial matrix contains the enzymes concerned with the oxidation of fatty acids (see §7.5.2), the citric acid cycle (§7.4.2.3), a variety of other oxidases and dehydrogenases, the enzymes for mitochondrial replication and the DNA that codes for some of the mitochondrial proteins.

The overall process of oxidation of reduced coenzymes, reduction of oxygen to water, and phosphorylation of ADP to ATP requires intact mitochondria, or intact sealed vesicles of mitochondrial inner membrane prepared by disruption of mitochondria; it will not occur with solubilized preparations from mitochondria, nor with open fragments of mitochondrial inner membrane.

5.3.1.2 *The mitochondrial electron transport chain*

The mitochondrial electron transport chain is a series of enzymes and coenzymes in the inner membrane, each of which is reduced by the preceding coenzyme, and in turn reduces the next, until finally the protons and electrons that have entered the chain from either NADH or reduced flavin reduce oxygen to water. The sequence of the electron carriers shown in Figure 5.10 has been determined in two ways:

- By consideration of their electrochemical redox potentials, which permits determination of which carrier is likely to reduce another, and which is likely to be reduced. There is a gradual fall in redox potential between the enzyme that oxidizes NADH and that which reduces oxygen to water.
- By incubation of mitochondria with substrates, in the absence of oxygen, when all of the carriers become reduced, then introducing a limited amount of oxygen, and following the sequence in which the carriers become oxidized. The oxidation state of the carriers is determined by following changes in their absorption spectra.

Studies with inhibitors of specific electron carriers, and with artificial substrates that oxidize or reduce one specific carrier, permit analysis of the electron transport chain into four complexes of electron carriers:

- Complex I catalyses the oxidation of NADH and the reduction of ubiquinone, and is associated with the phosphorylation of 1 mol of ADP to ATP per mole of NADH oxidized.

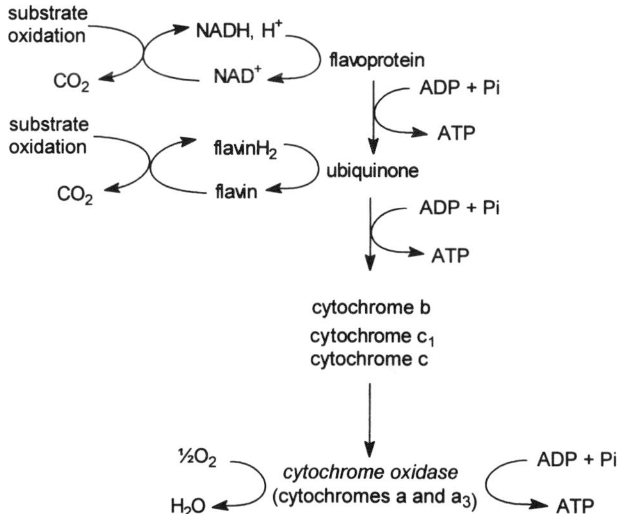

Figure 5.10 Overview of the mitochondrial electron transport chain.

- Complex II catalyses the oxidation of reduced flavins and the reduction of ubiquinone. This complex is not associated with phosphorylation of ADP to ATP.
- Complex III catalyses the oxidation of reduced ubiquinone and the reduction of cytochrome c, and is associated with the phosphorylation of 1 mol of ADP to ATP per mole of reduced ubiquinone oxidized.
- Complex IV catalyses the oxidation of reduced cytochrome c and the reduction of oxygen to water, and is associated with the phosphorylation of 1 mol of ADP to ATP per mole of reduced cytochrome c oxidized.

In order to understand how the transfer of electrons through the electron transport chain can be linked to the phosphorylation of ADP to ATP, it is necessary to consider the chemistry of the various electron carriers. They can be classified into two groups (see §4.3.1):

- Hydrogen carriers, which undergo reduction and oxidation reactions involving both protons and electrons; these are NAD, flavins and ubiquinone. NAD undergoes a two-electron oxidation/reduction reaction (see Figure 4.8), whereas both the flavins (Figure 4.7) and ubiquinone (Figure 5.11) undergo two single electron reactions to form a half-reduced radical, then the fully reduced coenzyme. Flavins can also undergo a two-electron reaction in a single step.

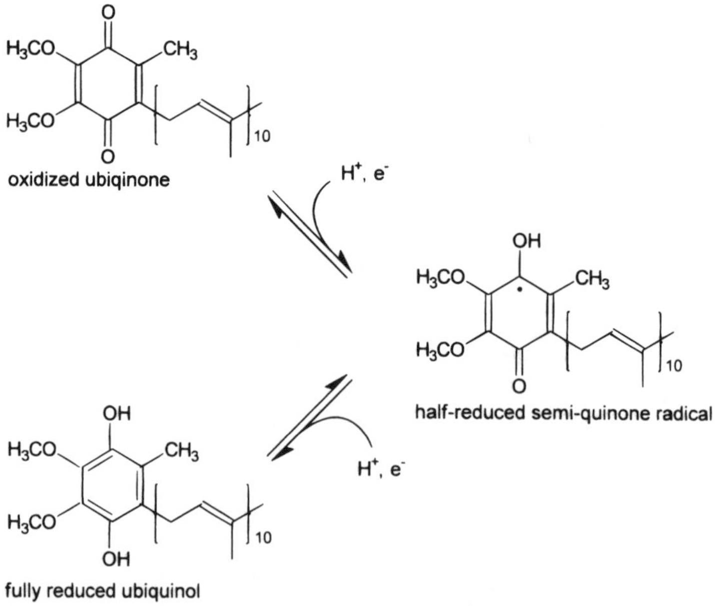

Figure 5.11 The oxidation and reduction of ubiquinone (coenzyme Q).

- Electron carriers, which contain a metal ion (iron in most, but both iron and copper in cytochrome oxidase) and undergo oxidation and reduction by electron transfer alone. These are the cytochromes, in which the iron is present in a haem molecule, and non-haem iron proteins, sometimes called iron–sulphur proteins, because the iron is bound to the protein through the sulphur of the amino acid cysteine. These are shown in Figure 5.12. All of the electron carriers undergo a single electron reaction, in which one iron atom at a time is reduced or oxidized.

The hydrogen and electron carriers of the electron transport chain are arranged in sequence in the crista membrane, as shown in Figure 5.13. Some carriers are entirely within the membrane; others are located on the inner or outer face of the membrane.

There are two steps in which a hydrogen carrier reduces an electron carrier: the reaction between the flavin and non-haem iron protein in complex I, and the reaction between ubiquinol and cytochrome b plus a non-haem iron protein in complex II. The reaction between non-haem iron protein and ubiquinone in complex I is the reverse – a hydrogen carrier is reduced by an electron carrier. When a hydrogen carrier reduces an electron carrier, there is a proton that is not transferred onto the electron carrier, but is extruded from the membrane into the intermembrane space, as shown in Figure 5.14.

When an electron carrier reduces a hydrogen carrier, there is a need for a proton to accompany the electron that is transferred. This is acquired from the mitochondrial matrix, thus shifting the equilibrium between H_2O and $H^+ + OH^-$, resulting in an accumulation of hydroxyl ions in the matrix.

5.3.1.3 *Phosphorylation of ADP linked to electron transport*

The result of alternation between hydrogen carriers and electron carriers in the electron transport chain is a separation of protons and hydroxyl ions across the mitochondrial membrane, with an accumulation of protons in the

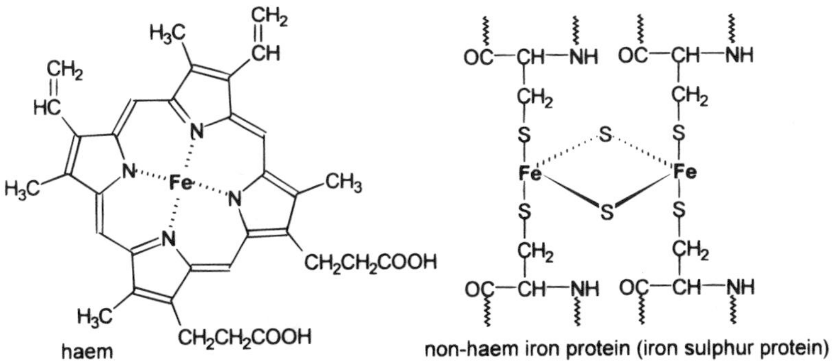

haem

non-haem iron protein (iron sulphur protein)

Figure 5.12 Haem and non-haem iron proteins (iron sulphur proteins).

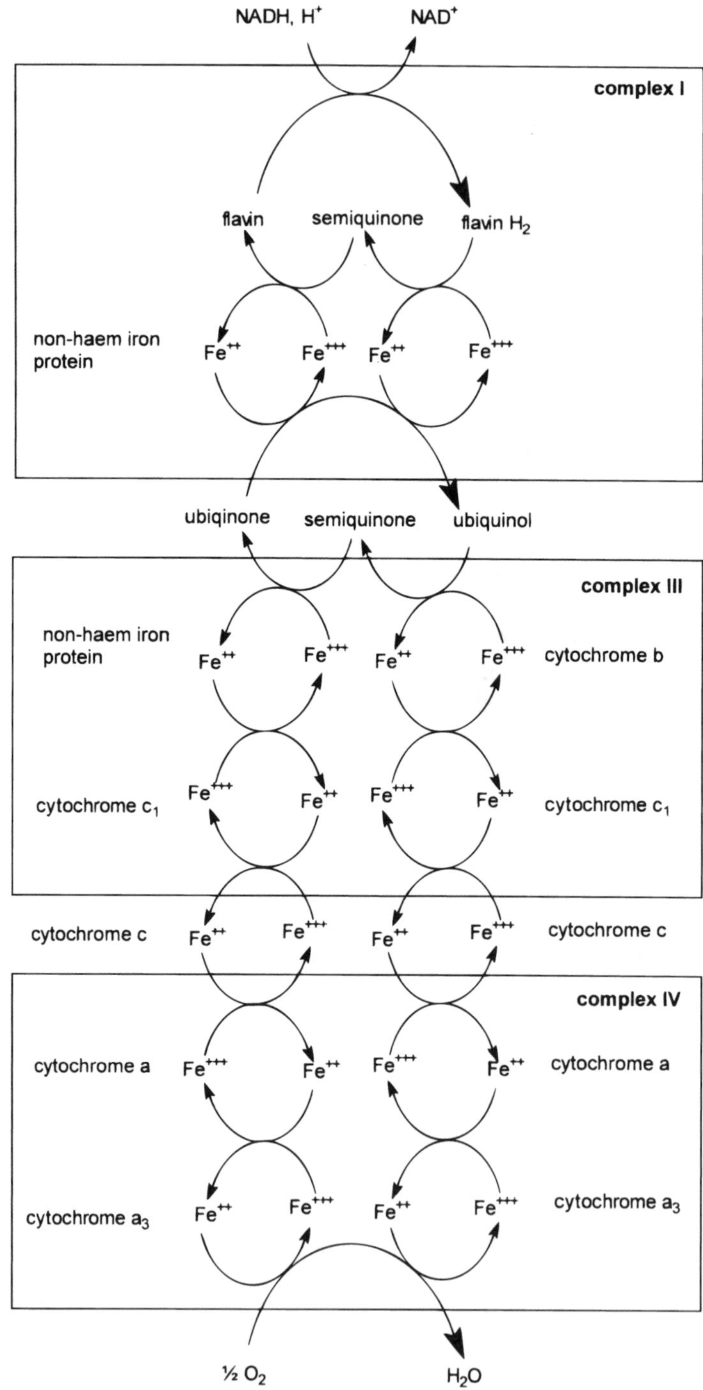

Figure 5.13 The mitochondrial electron transport chain.

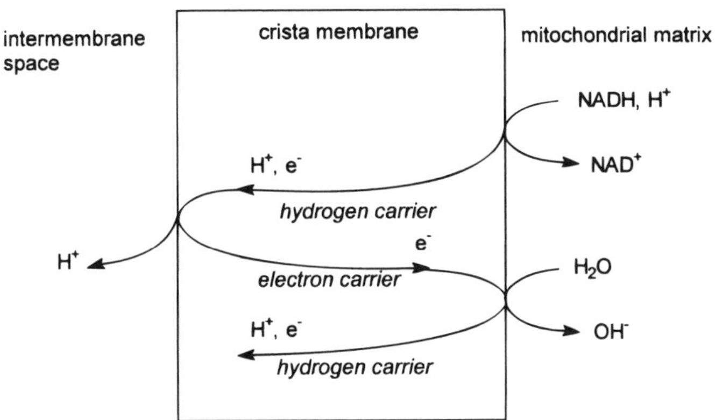

Figure 5.14 Interaction between hydrogen carriers and electron carriers in the mitochondrial electron transport chain; formation of the transmembrane proton gradient.

intermembrane space, and an accumulation of hydroxyl ions in the matrix (i.e. creation of a pH gradient across the inner membrane).

The reaction between ADP and phosphate to form ATP is a condensation reaction: ADP + phosphate → ATP + H_2O. Just as the hydrolysis of ATP involves protons and hydroxyl ions, rather than un-ionized water (see §5.2.2.3), so the condensation reaction involves the removal of a proton from one substrate and a hydroxyl ion from the other, so that although water is one of the ultimate products of the reaction, the immediate products are $H^+ + OH^-$, as shown in Figure 5.15. The protons and hydroxyl ions leave the enzyme from separate sites.

The condensation between ADP and phosphate is endothermic, and under normal conditions would not proceed to any significant extent. However, as discussed in §4.1.1, the equilibrium of a chemical reaction can be shifted by removal of one of more of the products. This is what occurs in mitochondrial ATP synthesis. The proton gradient across the mitochondrial inner membrane produced during electron transport is in the reverse direction to that which is produced by ATP synthase, and thus serves to remove the protons and hydroxyl ions produced in ATP synthesis.

The enzyme that catalyses the reaction, ATP synthase, occurs in the primary particles on the inner face of the crista membrane, which as shown in Figure 5.9, are attached to the membrane by a stalk that spans the membrane. As shown in Figure 5.15, this stalk provides a channel through which the protons ejected from the membrane during electron transport re-enter the mitochondrion and react with the hydroxyl ions produced in the condensation of ADP and phosphate, forming H_2O. The protons formed in the condensation reaction enter the mitochondrial matrix and react with the excess hydroxyl ions accumulated in the matrix during electron transport, again forming H_2O.

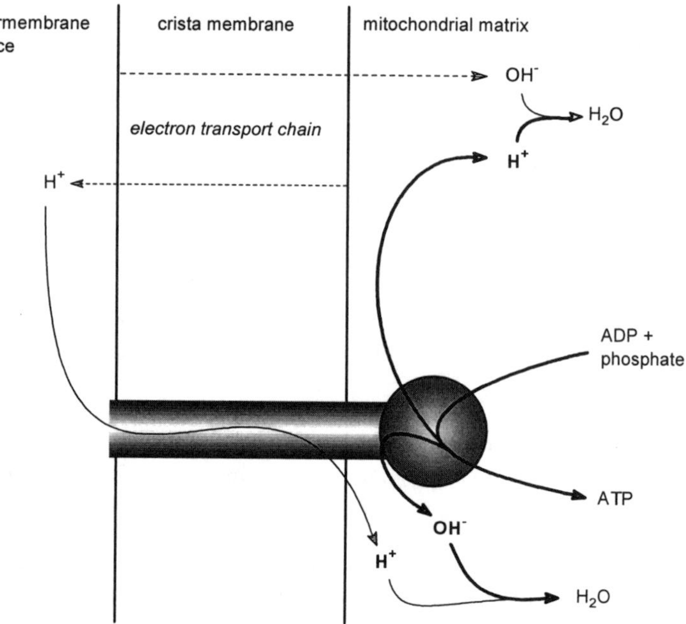

Figure 5.15 The reaction of the mitochondrial ATP synthase; utilization of the transmembrane proton gradient.

5.3.1.4 *The coupling of electron transport, oxidative phosphorylation and fuel oxidation*

The two processes of the oxidation of NADH or reduced flavins and the phosphorylation of ADP to ATP are normally tightly coupled. ADP phosphorylation cannot occur in mitochondria unless there is creation of the gradient of H^+ ions across the membrane as a result of the oxidation of NADH or reduced flavins.

Equally, if there is little or no ADP available, the oxidation of NADH and reduced flavins is inhibited because the H^+ gradient builds up and inhibits the transport reactions. This means that NADH and reduced flavoproteins are only oxidized when there is ADP available.

In turn, metabolic fuels can only be oxidized when NAD^+ and oxidized flavoproteins are available. Therefore, if there is little or no ADP available in the mitochondria (i.e. it has all been phosphorylated to ATP), there will be an accumulation of reduced coenzymes, and hence a slowing down of the rate of oxidation of metabolic fuels. In other words, metabolic fuels are oxidized only when there is a need for the phosphorylation of ADP to ATP. This means that metabolic fuels are oxidized only when ATP has been hydrolysed to ADP and phosphate by linkage to synthetic reactions, transport of compounds across cell membranes or muscle contraction.

It is possible to break this tight coupling between electron transport and ADP phosphorylation by adding compounds that render the mitochondrial membrane freely permeable to H^+ ions. In the presence of such compounds, the H^+ ions transported out do not accumulate, but are transported into the mitochondrial matrix, where they react with the OH^- ions, forming water. Under these conditions ADP is not phosphorylated to ATP, and the oxidation of NADH and reduced flavins can continue unimpeded.

The result of this uncoupling of electron transport from the phosphorylation of ADP is that a great deal of substrate is oxidized, with little production of ATP, although heat is produced. This is one of the physiological mechanisms for heat production to maintain body temperature without performing physical work: non-shivering thermogenesis. The process is especially important in infants, but also occurs to a limited extent in adults. Brown adipose tissue in various parts of the body (which is distinct from the white adipose tissue that is the main reserve of metabolic fuel) contains a protein called thermogenin. Under appropriate conditions this protein transports protons across the mitochondrial inner membrane, and so uncouples the processes of electron transport and phosphorylation of ADP to a limited extent, permitting oxidation of substrates and heat production without control by the availability of ADP.

6

Digestion and Absorption

The major components of the diet are starches, sugars, fats and proteins. These have to be hydrolysed to their constituent smaller molecules for absorption and metabolism. Starches and sugars are absorbed as monosaccharides; fats may either be absorbed intact or as free fatty acids and glycerol; proteins are absorbed as their constituent amino acids and small peptides.

The fat-soluble vitamins (A, D, E and K) are absorbed dissolved in dietary lipids; there are active transport systems (see §5.2.2.3) in the small intestinal mucosa for the absorption of the water-soluble vitamins. The absorption of vitamin B_{12} (see §6.5) requires a specific binding protein that is secreted in the gastric juice in order to bind to the mucosal transport system.

Minerals generally enter the intestinal mucosal cells by carrier-mediated diffusion (see §5.2.2.1) and are accumulated inside the cell by binding to specific binding proteins. They are then transferred into the bloodstream by active transport mechanisms at the serosal side of the epithelial cells, commonly again onto specific binding proteins in plasma. The absorption of calcium is discussed in §12.3.1.1, and that of iron in §6.6.

6.1 The gastrointestinal tract

The gastrointestinal tract is shown in Figure 6.1. The major functions of each region are:

1 Mouth
   (i) starch hydrolysis catalysed by amylase, secreted by the salivary glands
   (ii) fat hydrolysis catalysed by lingual lipase, secreted by the tongue
   (iii) absorption of small amounts of vitamin C and a variety of non-nutrients (including nicotine)

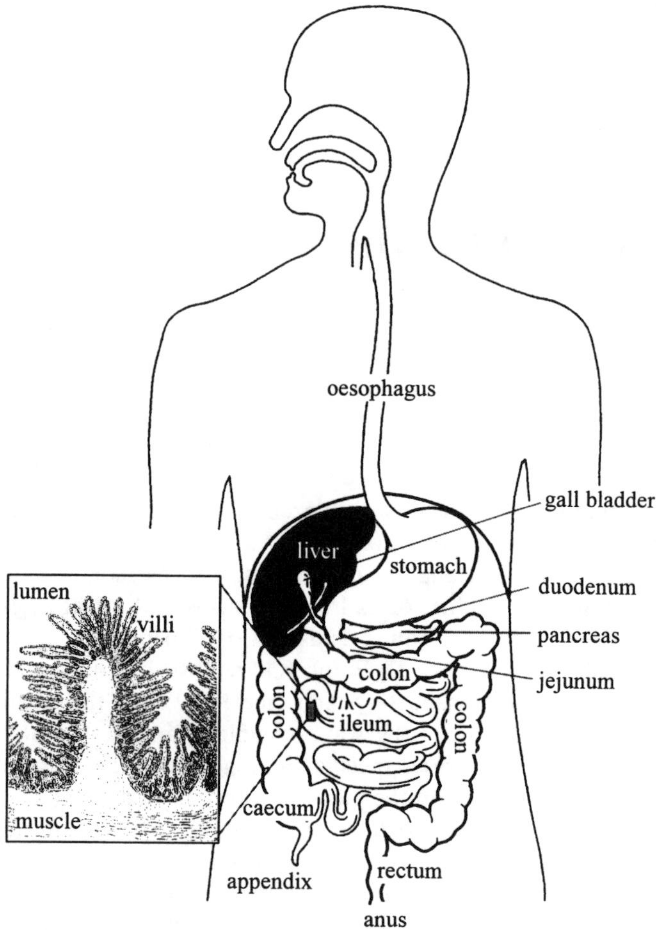

Figure 6.1 The gastrointestinal tract and (inset) the microscopic appearance of the small intestinal mucosa.

2 Stomach
- (i) gastric acid is important in the denaturation of dietary proteins (see §6.4.2) and the release of vitamin B_{12} (§6.5), iron and other minerals from protein binding
- (ii) protein hydrolysis catalysed by pepsin
- (iii) fat hydrolysis catalysed by lipase
- (iv) secretion of intrinsic factor for the absorption of vitamin B_{12} (see §6.5)

3 Small intestine (duodenum, jejunum and ileum)
- (i) starch hydrolysis catalysed by amylase secreted by the pancreas
- (ii) hydrolysis of disaccharides within the brush border of the intestinal mucosa

(iii) fat hydrolysis catalysed by lipase secreted by the pancreas
(iv) protein hydrolysis catalysed by a variety of exo- and endopeptidases (see §6.4.3) secreted by the pancreas and small intestinal mucosa
(v) hydrolysis of di- and tripeptides within the brush border of the intestinal mucosa
(vi) absorption of the products of digestion

4 Large intestine (caecum and colon)
(i) absorption of water (failure of water absorption, as in diarrhoea, can lead to serious dehydration)
(ii) bacterial metabolism of undigested carbohydrates and shed intestinal mucosal cells
(iii) absorption of some of the products of bacterial metabolism

5 Rectum
(i) storage of undigested gut contents prior to evacuation as faeces

Throughout the gastrointestinal tract, and especially in the small intestine, the surface area of the mucosa is considerably greater than would appear from its superficial appearance. As shown in the inset in Figure 6.1, the intestinal mucosa is folded longitudinally into the lumen. The surface of these folds is covered with villi; finger-like projections into the lumen, some 0.5–1.5 mm long. There are some 20–40 villi per mm^2, giving a total absorptive surface area of some 300 m^2 in the small intestine.

There is rapid turnover of the cells of the intestinal mucosa; epithelial cells proliferate in the crypts, alongside the cells that secrete digestive enzymes, and migrate to the tip of the villus, where they are shed into the lumen. The average life of an intestinal mucosal epithelial cell is about 48 hours. As discussed in §6.6, this rapid turnover of epithelial cells is important in controlling the absorption of iron, and possibly other minerals.

The rapid turnover of intestinal mucosal cells is also important for protection of the intestine against the digestive enzymes secreted into the lumen. Further protection is afforded by the secretion of mucus, a solution of proteins that are resistant to enzymic hydrolysis, which coats the intestinal mucosa. The secretion of intestinal mucus explains a considerable part of an adult's continuing requirement for dietary protein (see §10.1).

6.2 Digestion and absorption of carbohydrates

Carbohydrates are compounds of carbon, hydrogen and oxygen in the ratio $C_n:H_{2n}:O_n$. The basic unit of the carbohydrates is the sugar molecule or monosaccharide. Note that sugar is used here in a chemical sense, and includes a variety of simple carbohydrates, which are collectively known as sugars. Ordinary table sugar (cane sugar or beet sugar) is correctly known as sucrose; as discussed in §6.2.1.2, it is a disaccharide. It is just one of many different sugars.

6.2.1 The classification of carbohydrates

Dietary carbohydrates can be considered in two main groups: sugars and polysaccharides; as shown in Figure 6.2, the polysaccharides can be further subdivided into starches and non-starch polysaccharides.

The simplest type of sugar is a monosaccharide – a single sugar unit (see §6.2.1.1). Monosaccharides normally consist of between three and seven carbon atoms (and the corresponding number of hydrogen and oxygen atoms). A few larger monosaccharides also occur, although they are not important in nutrition and metabolism.

Disaccharides (see §6.2.1.2) are formed by condensation between two monosaccharides to form a glycoside bond. The reverse reaction, cleavage of the glycoside bond to release the individual monosaccharides, is a hydrolysis.

Oligosaccharides consist of three or four monosaccharide units (trisaccharides and tetrasaccharides) and occasionally more, linked by glycoside bonds. Nutritionally they are not particularly important, and indeed they are generally not digested, although they may be fermented by intestinal bacteria and make a significant contribution to the production of intestinal gas.

Nutritionally, it is useful to consider sugars (both monosaccharides and disaccharides) in two groups:

- Intrinsic sugars that are contained within plant cell walls in foods.
- Sugars that are in free solution in foods, and therefore provide a substrate for oral bacteria, leading to the formation of dental plaque and caries. These are known as extrinsic sugars; as discussed in §2.4.3.1, it is considered desir-

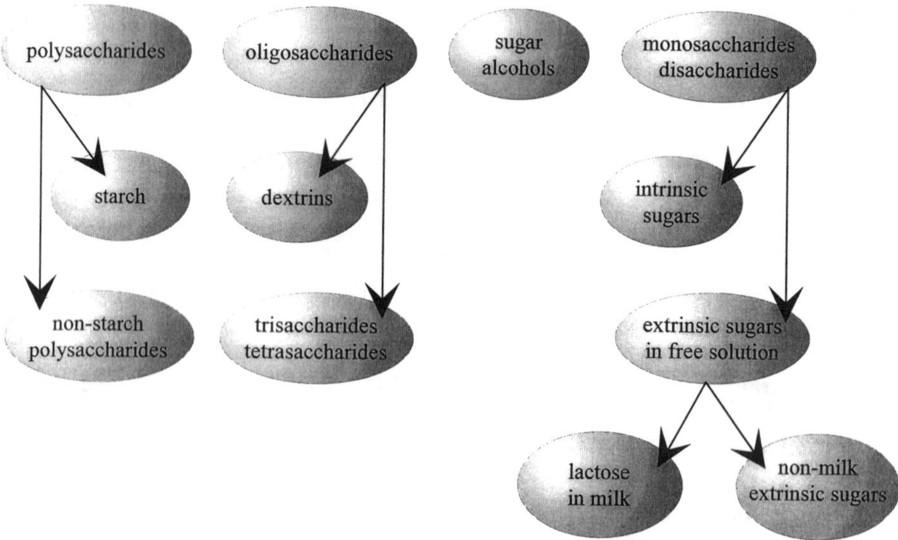

Figure 6.2 Nutritional classification of carbohydrates.

able to reduce the consumption of extrinsic sugars, because of their role in dental decay and also the ease with which excessive amounts of sweet foods can be consumed, thus leading to obesity (see §8.2) and possibly also increasing the risks of developing diabetes mellitus (§11.5).

A complication in the classification of sugars as intrinsic (which are considered desirable in the diet) and extrinsic (which are considered undesirable) is that lactose (see §6.2.1.2) is in free solution in milk, and hence is an extrinsic sugar. However, lactose is not a cause of dental decay, and milk is an important source of calcium (see §12.3.1), protein (see Chapter 10) and vitamin B_2 (§12.2.6). It is not considered desirable to reduce intakes of milk, which is the only significant source of lactose, and extrinsic sugars are further subdivided into milk sugar and non-milk extrinsic sugars.

Polysaccharides are polymers of many hundreds of monosaccharide units, again linked by glycoside bonds. The most important are starch and glycogen (see §6.2.1.4), both of which are polymers of the monosaccharide glucose. There are also other polysaccharides, composed of different monosaccharides or of glucose units linked differently from the linkages in starch and glycogen. Collectively these are known as non-starch polysaccharides. They are generally not digested, but have important roles in nutrition (see §6.2.1.5).

6.2.1.1 *Monosaccharides*

The classes of monosaccharides are named by the number of carbon atoms in the ring, using the Greek names for the numbers, with the ending *-ose* to show that they are sugars (the names of all sugars end in *-ose*):

- three-carbon monosaccharides are trioses
- four-carbon monosaccharides are tetroses
- five-carbon monosaccharides are pentoses
- six-carbon monosaccharides are hexoses
- seven-carbon monosaccharides are heptoses

In general, trioses, tetroses and heptoses are important as intermediate compounds in the metabolism of pentoses and hexoses, which are the nutritionally important sugars.

The pentoses and hexoses can exist as straight-chain compounds or can form heterocyclic rings (Figure 6.3). By convention, the ring of sugars is drawn with the bonds of one side thicker than the other. This is to show that the rings are planar, and can be considered to lie at right angles to the plane of the paper. The boldly drawn part of the molecule is then coming out of the paper, while the lightly drawn part is going behind the paper. The hydroxyl groups lie above or below the plane of the ring, in the plane of the paper. Each carbon has a hydrogen atom attached as well as a hydroxyl group. For convenience in drawing the structures of sugars, this hydrogen is generally omitted when the structures are drawn as rings.

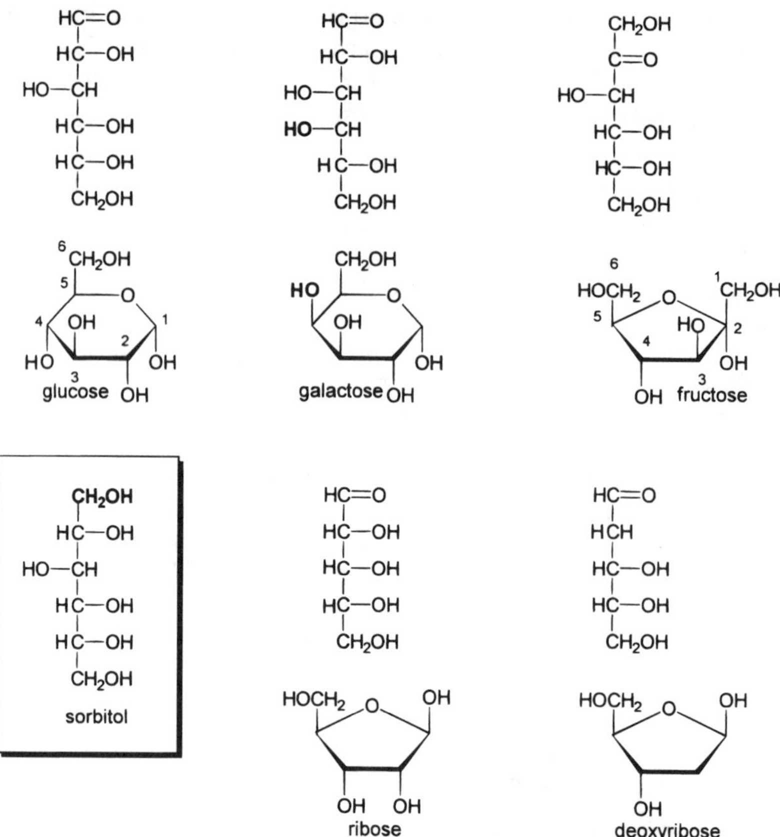

Figure 6.3 Nutritionally important monosaccharides: hexose and pentose sugars and (inset) the sugar alcohol sorbitol, showing the numbering of the carbon atoms of glucose and fructose.

The nutritionally important hexoses are glucose, galactose and fructose. Glucose and galactose differ from each other only in the arrangement of one hydroxyl group above or below the plane of the ring. Fructose differs from glucose and galactose in that it has a C=O (keto) group at carbon 2, whereas the other two have an H-C=O (aldehyde) group at carbon 1.

There are two important pentose sugars, ribose and deoxyribose. Deoxyribose is unusual, in that it has lost one of its hydroxyl groups. The main role of ribose and deoxyribose is in the nucleotides (see §5.1) and the nucleic acids, RNA in which the sugar is ribose (see §10.2.2) and DNA, in which the sugar is deoxyribose (§10.2.1).

Sugar alcohols are formed by the reduction of the aldehyde group of a monosaccharide to a hydroxyl (—OH) group. The most important of these is sorbitol, formed by the reduction of glucose. It is only slowly absorbed from the intestinal tract and metabolized, so that it has very much less effect on the concentration of glucose in the bloodstream than do other carbohydrates. Because of this, it is widely used in preparation of foods suitable for use by diabetics, since it tastes sweet and can replace sucrose and other sugars in food manufacture. However, sorbitol is metabolized as a metabolic fuel, with an energy yield approximately equal to that of glucose, so that it is not suitable for the replacement of carbohydrates in weight-reducing diets.

Xylitol is the sugar alcohol formed by reduction of the five-carbon sugar xylose, an isomer of ribose. It is of interest because unlike other sugars, which promote dental carries (see §2.4.3.1), xylitol has an anticariogenic action. The reasons for this are not well understood, but sucking sweets made from xylitol results in a significant reduction in the incidence of caries; such sweets are sometimes called 'tooth-friendly' because of this.

6.2.1.2 *Disaccharides*

The four common disaccharides are shown in Figure 6.4 – they are:

- Sucrose, cane or beet sugar, which is a dimer of glucose and fructose.
- Lactose, the sugar of milk, which is a dimer of glucose and galactose.
- Maltose, the sugar originally isolated from malt, which is a dimer of glucose.
- Isomaltose, which is also a dimer of glucose, but linked from carbon-1 of one glucose to carbon-6 of the other.

Both maltose and isomaltose arise from the digestion of starch.

6.2.1.3 *Reducing and non-reducing sugars*

Chemically, the aldehyde group of glucose is a reducing agent. That is, it reacts to reduce another compound, itself being oxidized to an acid group (—COOH) in the process. This forms the basis of a simple test for glucose in urine. In alkaline conditions, glucose reacts with copper ions, reducing them to copper oxide, and itself being oxidized. The original solution of copper ions has a blue colour; the copper oxide forms a yellow-brown precipitate.

This reaction is not specific for glucose. Other sugars with a free aldehyde group at carbon-1 are also reducing agents, and can undergo the same reaction. This lack of specificity can cause problems when a positive result of such a test is interpreted as meaning the presence of glucose. Some monosaccharides (including vitamin C, see §12.2.13), some pentose sugars that occur in foods and several disaccharides (including maltose and lactose, but not sucrose) will also react with copper ions and give a positive result. Although copper reagents are sometimes used to measure urine glucose in monitoring diabetic control (see §11.5), there are more specific tests using the enzyme glucose oxidase, which measure only glucose.

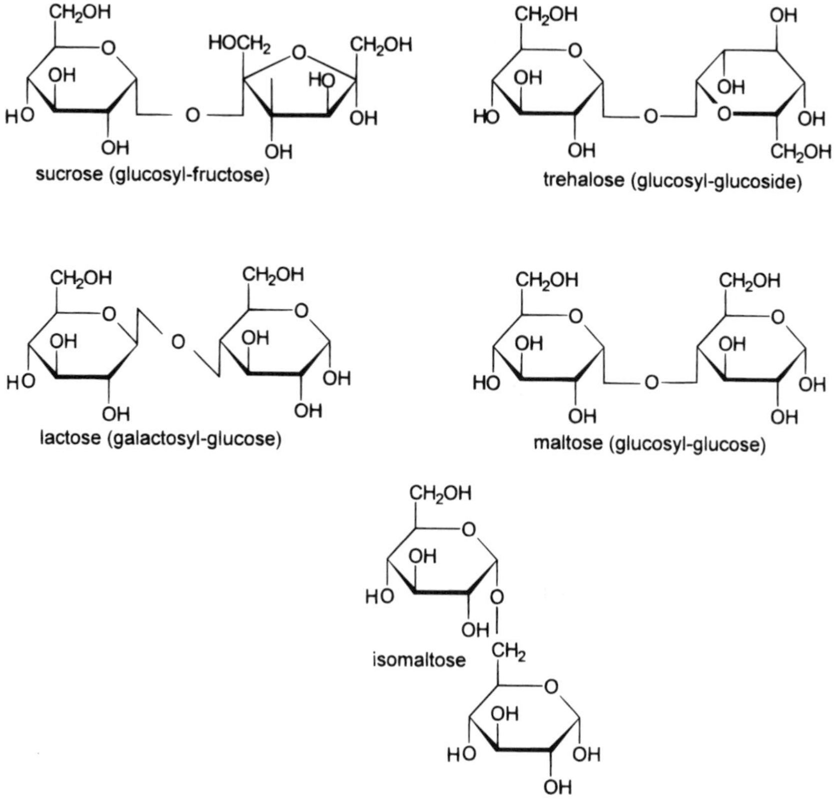

sucrose (glucosyl-fructose)

trehalose (glucosyl-glucoside)

lactose (galactosyl-glucose)

maltose (glucosyl-glucose)

isomaltose

Figure 6.4 Nutritionally important disaccharides.

It is important to realize that the term *reducing sugars* reflects a chemical reaction of the sugars: the ability to reduce a suitable acceptor such as copper ions. It has nothing to do with weight reduction and slimming, although some people erroneously believe that reducing sugars somehow help one to reduce excessive weight. This is not correct; the energy yield from reducing sugars and non-reducing sugars is exactly the same, and excess of either will contribute to obesity.

6.2.1.4 *Polysaccharides: starches and glycogen*

Starch is a polymer of glucose containing a large, but variable, number of glucose units. It is thus impossible to quote a relative molecular mass for starch, or to discuss amounts of starch in terms of moles. It can, however, be hydrolysed to glucose, and the results expressed as moles of glucose.

The simplest type of starch is amylose, a straight chain of glucose molecules, with glycoside links between carbon-1 of one glucose unit and carbon-4 of the next. Some types of starch have a branched structure, where every so often one glucose molecule has glycoside links to three others instead of just two. The branch is formed by linkage between carbon-1 of one glucose unit and carbon-6 of the next (Figure 6.5). This is amylopectin.

Starches are the storage carbohydrates of plants, and the relative amounts of amylose and amylopectin differ in starches from different sources, as indeed does the size of the overall starch molecule. On average, about 20–25 per cent of starch in foods is the straight chain polymer amylose, and the remaining 75–80 per cent is amylopectin.

Glycogen is the storage carbohydrate of mammalian muscle and liver. It is synthesized from glucose in the fed state (see §7.6.2), and its constituent glucose units are used as a metabolic fuel in the fasting state. Glycogen is a branched polymer, with essentially the same structure as amylopectin.

6.2.1.5 *Non-starch polysaccharides (dietary fibre)*

There are other polysaccharides in foods. Collectively they are known as non-starch polysaccharides, the major components of dietary fibre (see §2.4.3.2). Non-starch polysaccharides are not digested by human enzymes, although all can be fermented to some extent by intestinal bacteria, and the products of bacterial fermentation may be absorbed and metabolized as metabolic fuels. The major non-starch polysaccharides are:

- Cellulose, a polymer of glucose in which the configuration of the glycoside bond between the glucose units is in the opposite configuration ($\beta 1 \rightarrow 4$) from that in starch ($\alpha 1 \rightarrow 4$), and cannot be hydrolysed by human enzymes.
- Hemicelluloses, branched polymers of pentose (five-carbon) and hexose (six-carbon) sugars.
- Inulin, a polymer of fructose, which is the storage carbohydrate of Jerusalem artichoke and some other root vegetables.
- Pectin, a complex polymer of a variety of monosaccharides, including some methylated sugars.

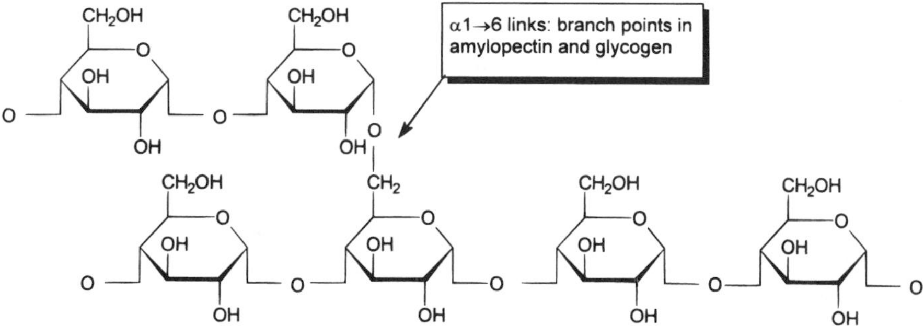

Figure 6.5 The structures of starch and glycogen.

- Plant gums, such as gum arabic, tragacanth, acacia, carob and guar gums – complex polymers of mixed monosaccharides.
- Mucilages such as alginates, agar and carrageen; complex polymers of mixed monosaccharides found in seaweeds and other algae.

Cellulose, hemicelluloses and inulin are insoluble non-starch polysaccharides; pectin and the plant gums and mucilages are soluble non-starch polysaccharides. The other major constituent of dietary fibre, lignin, is not a carbohydrate at all, but a complex polymer of a variety of aromatic alcohols.

6.2.2 *Carbohydrate digestion and absorption*

The digestion of carbohydrates is by hydrolysis of the glycoside bonds between monosaccharide units to liberate small oligosaccharides, then free mono- and disaccharides.

6.2.2.1 Starch digestion

The enzymes that catalyse the hydrolysis of starch are amylases, which are secreted both in the saliva and the pancreatic juice (salivary amylase is sometimes known by its old name of ptyalin). The digestion of starch begins when food is chewed, and continues for a time in the stomach. However, the gastric juice is very acid (about pH 1.5–2), and amylase is inactive at this pH; as the food bolus is mixed with gastric juice, so starch digestion ceases. When the food leaves the stomach and enters the small intestine, it is neutralized by the alkaline pancreatic juice (pH 8.8) and bile (pH 8). Amylase secreted by the pancreas continues the digestion of starch begun by salivary amylase. The products of amylase action are free glucose, maltose and isomaltose (from the branch points in amylopectin).

It might be thought that the increase in blood glucose (the glycaemic index) after consumption of starch would be the same as that from an equivalent amount of glucose. However, when the glycaemic index of starch is determined, it is significantly lower than that of glucose or any of the disaccharides. This is because not all of the dietary starch is hydrolysed by amylase. A proportion of the starch in foods is still enclosed in plant cell walls, which are mainly composed of cellulose. Cellulose is not digested by human enzymes, and therefore this starch is protected against digestion. Uncooked starch is resistant to amylase action, because it is present as small insoluble granules. The process of cooking swells the starch granules, resulting in a gel on which amylase can act. However, as cooked starch cools, a proportion undergoes crystallization to a form that is again resistant to amylase action – this is part of the process of staling of starchy foods. Some of this resistant starch is metabolized by bacteria in the colon, and a proportion of the products of bacterial metabolism, including fatty acids, may be absorbed and metabolized.

6.2.2.2 *Digestion of disaccharides*

The enzymes that catalyse the hydrolysis of disaccharides (the disaccharidases) are located on the brush border of the intestinal mucosal cells; the resultant monosaccharides return to the lumen of the small intestine, and are absorbed together with dietary monosaccharides and glucose arising from the digestion of starch (see §6.2.2.1):

- Maltase catalyses the hydrolysis of maltose to two molecules of glucose.
- Isomaltase (which occurs as a bifunctional enzyme with sucrase) catalyses the hydrolysis of isomaltose to two molecules of glucose.
- Lactase catalyses the hydrolysis of lactose to glucose and galactose.
- Trehalase catalyses the hydrolysis of trehalose to two molecules of glucose.
- Sucrase catalyses the hydrolysis of sucrose to glucose and fructose.

Deficiency of the enzyme lactase is common. Indeed, it is only in people of European origin that lactase persists after childhood. In most other people, and in some Europeans, lactase is gradually lost through adolescence; this is called alactasia. In the absence of lactase, lactose cannot be absorbed. It remains in the intestinal lumen, where it is a substrate for bacterial fermentation to lactate (see §7.4.1), resulting in a considerable increase in the osmotic pressure of the gut contents, since 1 mol of lactose yields 4 mol of lactate. In addition, bacterial fermentation produces carbon dioxide, methane and hydrogen, and the result of consuming a moderate amount of lactose is an explosive watery diarrhoea and severe abdominal pain. Even the relatively small amounts of lactose in milk may upset people with a complete deficiency of lactase. Such people can normally tolerate yogurt and other fermented milk products, since much of the lactose has been converted to lactic acid. Fortunately for people who suffer from alactasia, milk is the only significant source of lactose in the diet, so it is relatively easy to avoid consuming lactose.

Rarely, people may lack sucrase or maltase. This may either be a genetic lack of the enzyme, or an acquired loss as a result of intestinal infection. They are intolerant of sucrose or maltose, and suffer in the same way as alactasic subjects given lactose. It is relatively easy to avoid maltose, since there are few sources of it in the diet; the small amount formed in the digestion of starch does not seem to cause any significant problems. People who lack sucrase have a more serious problem, since as well as the obvious sugar in cakes and biscuits, jams, and so on, many manufactured foods contain added sucrose.

6.2.2.3 *The absorption of monosaccharides*

As shown in Figure 6.6, there are two separate mechanisms for the absorption of monosaccharides in the small intestine. Glucose and galactose are absorbed

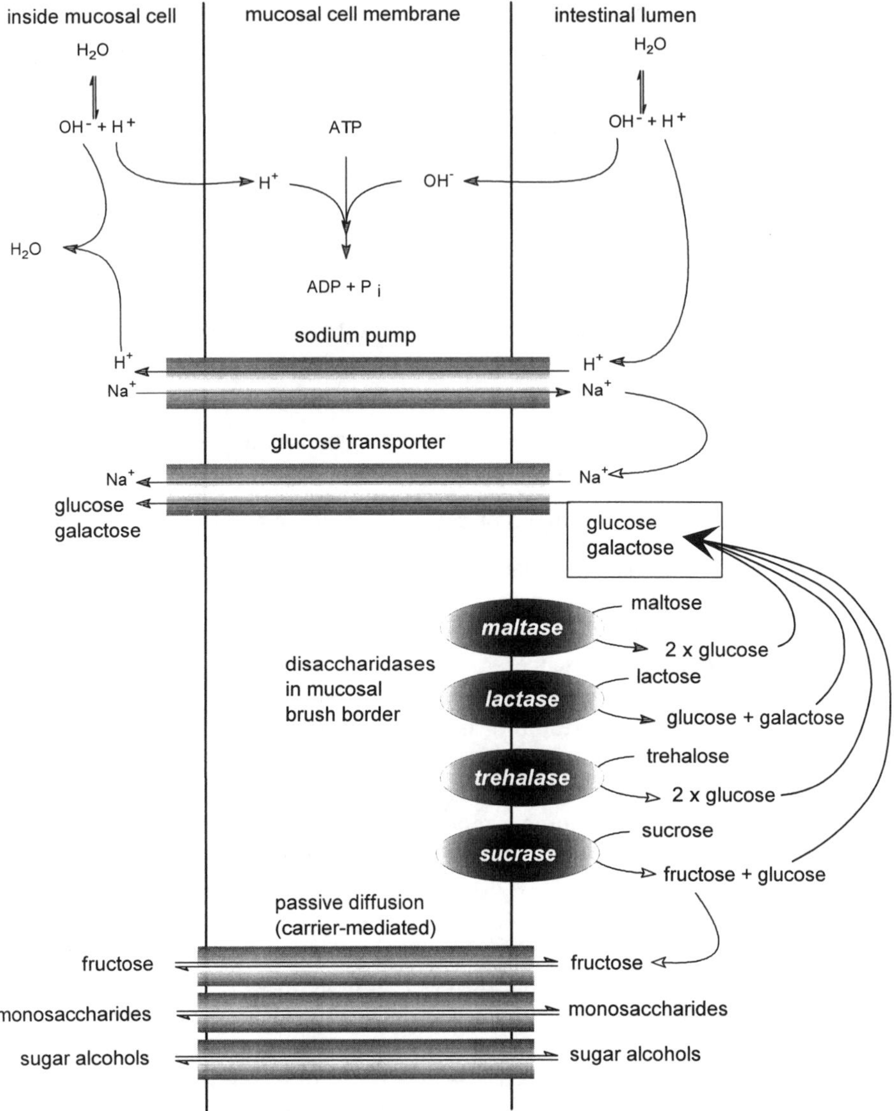

Figure 6.6 Intestinal digestion and absorption of sugars.

by a sodium-dependent active process. As discussed in §5.2.2.3, the hydrolysis of ATP within the mucosal cell membrane results in a proton gradient across the membrane; the protons re-enter the cell in exchange for sodium ions, and the sodium ions then re-enter the cell together with glucose or galactose. These two monosaccharides are carried by the same transport protein, and compete with each other for intestinal absorption.

Other monosaccharides are absorbed by passive carrier-mediated diffusion; there are at least three distinct carrier proteins, one for fructose, one for other monosaccharides and one for sugar alcohols. Because the absorption of these sugars is passive, fructose and sugar alcohols are only absorbed to a limited extent, and after a moderately high intake a significant amount will avoid absorption and remain in the intestinal lumen, acting as a substrate for colon bacteria and, like unabsorbed disaccharides in people with disaccharidase deficiency, causing abdominal pain and diarrhoea.

6.3 Digestion and absorption of fats

The major fats in the diet are triacylglycerols and, to a lesser extent, phospholipids. These are hydrophobic molecules, and have to be emulsified to very fine droplets (micelles, see §3.5.3) before they can be absorbed. This emulsification is achieved by partial hydrolysis to yield free fatty acids, and also by the action of the bile salts.

6.3.1 *The classification of dietary lipids*

Four groups of metabolically important compounds can be considered under the heading of lipids:

- Triacylglycerols (sometimes also known as triglycerides); these are the common oils and fats of the diet, which provide between 30 and 50 per cent of average energy intake (the difference between oils and fats is that oils are liquid at room temperature, whereas fats are solid).
- Phospholipids, which are chemically similar to triacylglycerols, but with a phosphate group in the molecule.
- Steroids, including cholesterol and extremely small amounts of steroid hormones (see §11.3); chemically these are completely different from triacylglycerols and phospholipids.
- A variety of other compounds, including vitamin A and carotenes (see §12.2.1), vitamin D (§12.2.2), vitamin E (§12.2.3) and vitamin K (§12.2.4).

Triacylglycerols have the general structure shown in Figure 6.7: they consist of a molecule of the three-carbon sugar alcohol glycerol esterified to three fatty acid molecules (acyl groups). The three fatty acids esterified to any one glycerol molecule will rarely all be the same. Triacylglycerols provide a major tissue reserve of metabolic fuel, within specialized tissue known as adipose tissue. Cells of adipose tissue contain only a relatively small amount of cytoplasm; 80 per cent of the cell is triacylglycerol. As discussed in §7.6.1, fatty

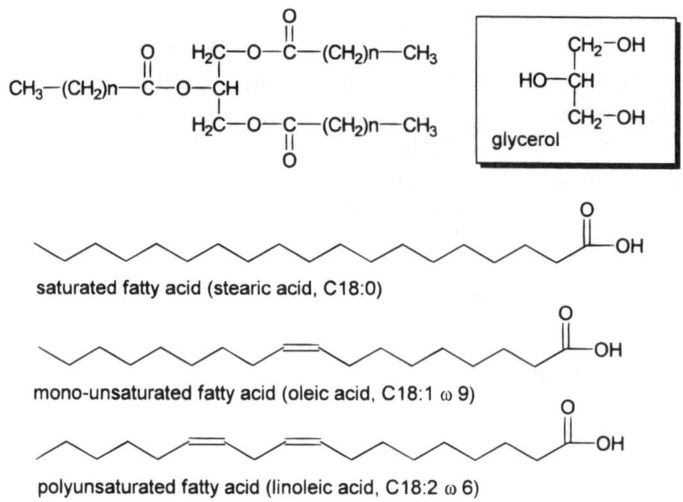

Figure 6.7 The structure of triacylglycerols and examples of saturated, mono-unsaturated and polyunsaturated fatty acids.

acids and triacylglycerols are synthesized, and added to adipose tissue reserves, after a meal. They are hydrolysed and the resultant free fatty acids and glycerol are released for use as metabolic fuels in the fasting state.

6.3.1.1 *Fatty acids*

There are various different fatty acids, differing in both the length of the carbon chain and whether or not they have one or more double bonds ($-CH{=}CH-$) in the chain. Those with no double bonds are saturated fatty acids – the carbon chain is completely saturated with hydrogen. Those with double bonds are unsaturated fatty acids – the carbon chain is not completely saturated with hydrogen (see §3.2.2.1). Fatty acids with one double bond are known as mono-unsaturated; those with two or more double bonds are known as polyunsaturated.

Although it is the fatty acids that are saturated or unsaturated, it is common to discuss saturated and unsaturated fats. Although this is not really correct, it is a useful shorthand, reflecting the fact that fats from different sources have a greater or lesser proportion of saturated and unsaturated fatty acids in their triacylglycerols (see Table 2.6).

As shown in Table 6.1, there are three different ways of naming the fatty acids:

- Many have trivial names, often derived from the source from which they were originally isolated. Thus, oleic acid was first isolated from olive oil, stearic acid from beef tallow, palmitic acid from palm oil, linoleic and linolenic acids from linseed oil, and so on.

Table 6.1 Fatty acid nomenclature

Fatty acid	C atoms	Double bonds Number	Double bonds First	Shorthand
Saturated				
Butyric	4	0	—	C4:0
Caproic	6	0	—	C6:0
Caprylic	8	0	—	C8:0
Capric	10	0	—	C10:0
Lauric	12	0	—	C12:0
Myristic	14	0	—	C14:0
Palmitic	16	0	—	C16:0
Stearic	18	0	—	C18:0
Arachidic	20	0	—	C20:0
Behenic	22	0	—	C22:0
Lignoceric	24	0	—	C24:0
Mono-unsaturated				
Palmitoleic	16	1	6	C16:1 ω6
Oleic	18	1	9	C18:1 ω9
Cetoleic	22	1	11	C22:1 ω11
Nervonic	24	1	9	C24:1 ω9
Polyunsaturated				
Linoleic	18	2	6	C18:2 ω6
α-Linolenic	18	3	3	C18:3 ω3
γ-Linolenic	18	3	6	C18:3 ω6
Arachidonic	20	4	6	C20:4 ω6
Eicosapentaenoic	20	5	3	C20:5 ω3
Docosatetraenoic	22	4	6	C22:4 ω6
Docosapentaenoic	22	5	3	C22:5 ω3
Docosapentaenoic	22	5	6	C22:5 ω6
Docosahexaenoic	22	6	3	C22:6 ω3

- All have systematic chemical names, based on the number of carbon atoms in the chain and the number and position of double bonds (if any).
- There is a shorthand notation to show the number of carbon atoms in the molecule, followed by a colon and the number of double bonds. The position of the first double bond from the methyl group of the fatty acid is shown by n- or ω- (the ω-carbon is the farthest from the α-carbon, which is the one to which the –COOH group is attached; see §3.7).

In the nutritionally important unsaturated fatty acids, the carbon–carbon double bonds are in the *cis*-configuration (see §3.7.1.1). The *trans*-isomers of unsaturated fatty acids do occur in foods to some extent, but they do not have the desirable biological actions of the *cis*-isomers, and indeed there is some evidence that *trans*-fatty acids may have adverse effects. As discussed in

§2.4.2.1, it is recommended that the consumption of *trans*-unsaturated fatty acids should not increase above the present average 2 per cent of energy intake.

Polyunsaturated fatty acids have two main functions in the body: in cell membranes (see §3.5.3.1) and as precursors for the synthesis of a group of compounds that includes prostaglandins, prostacyclins and thromboxanes. These function as local hormones, being secreted by cells into the extracellular fluid, and acting on nearby cells. Prostaglandins and the other compounds derived from polyunsaturated fatty acids are important in the regulation of the normal adhesiveness of blood cells, inflammation reactions, and so on.

The polyunsaturated fatty acids can be interconverted to a limited extent in the body, but there is a requirement for a dietary intake of linoleic acid (C18:2 ω6) and linolenic acid (C18:3 ω3), since these two, which can each be considered to be the parent of a family of related fatty acids, cannot be synthesized in the body. An intake of polyunsaturated fatty acids greater than the amount to meet physiological requirements confers benefits in terms of lowering the plasma concentration of cholesterol and reducing the risk of atherosclerosis and ischaemic heart disease. The requirement is less than 1 per cent of energy intake, but it is recommended that 6 per cent of energy intake should come from polyunsaturated fatty acids.

6.3.1.2 *Phospholipids*

Phospholipids are, as their name suggests, lipids that also contain the element phosphorus, as a phosphate group. As shown in Figure 6.8, they consist of glycerol esterified to two fatty acid molecules, one of which (esterified to carbon-2 of glycerol) is a polyunsaturated fatty acid. The third hydroxyl group of glycerol is not esterified to a fatty acid as in triacylglycerols, but to phos-

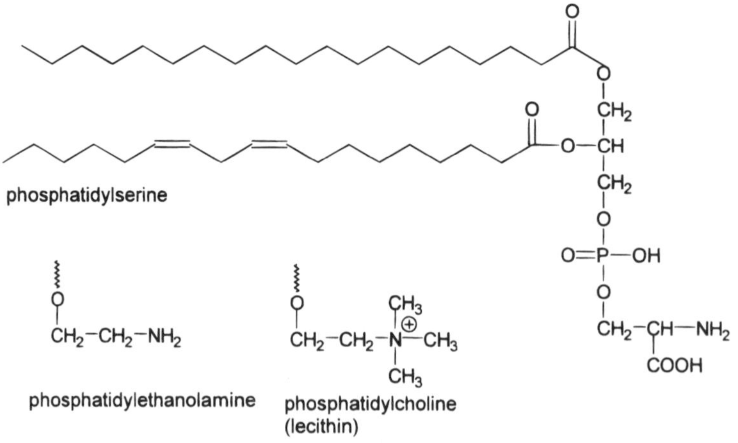

Figure 6.8 The structure of phospholipids (see also Figure 11.7).

phate. The phosphate in turn is esterified to one of a variety of compounds, including the amino acid serine (see §6.4.1), ethanolamine (which is formed from serine), choline (which is formed from ethanolamine), inositol or one of a variety of other compounds.

A phospholipid lacking the group esterified to the phosphate is known as a phosphatidic acid, and the complete phospholipids are called phosphatidyl serine, phosphatidyl ethanolamine, phosphatidyl choline (also called lecithin), phosphatidyl inositol, and so on.

In addition to its role in the structure of cell membranes (see §3.5.3.1), phosphatidyl inositol has a specialized role in membranes, acting to release inositol trisphosphate and diacylglycerol as intracellular second messengers to hormones (see §11.2.3).

6.3.1.3 *Cholesterol and the steroids*

As can be seen from Figure 6.9, steroids are chemically different from triacylglycerols or phospholipids. However, steroids are also hydrophobic molecules and they share some chemical and physical properties with other lipids. The parent compound of all the steroids in the body is cholesterol; different steroids are then formed by replacing one or more of the hydrogens with

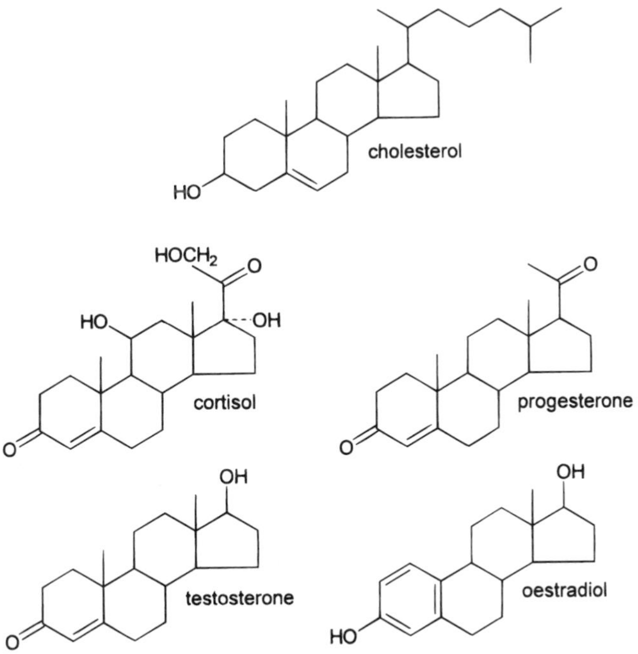

Figure 6.9 Cholesterol and the steroid hormones.

hydroxyl groups or oxo groups, and in some cases by shortening the side chain.

Apart from cholesterol, which has a major role in membrane structure and the synthesis of bile salts (see §6.3.2.1), the steroids are hormones – compounds synthesized in one tissue, then released into the circulation to act on a variety of other tissues (see §11.3). Vitamin D (§12.2.2) is a derivative of cholesterol, and can also be considered to be a steroid hormone.

The cholesterol required for membrane synthesis, and the very much smaller amount required for the synthesis of steroid hormones, may either be synthesized in the body or provided by the diet; average intakes are of the order of 500 mg (1.3 mmol) per day.

A raised concentration of cholesterol in plasma is a risk factor for atherosclerosis and ischaemic heart disease; concentrations of cholesterol above 5.2 mmol per L are associated with increased risk, and between 4–4.5 mmol per L with least risk. There is little evidence that for most healthy people the dietary intake of cholesterol has any significant effect on the plasma concentration of cholesterol. Various factors, including the total intake of dietary fat and the relative amounts of saturated and unsaturated fatty acids, can affect the amount of cholesterol formed in the liver. Saturated fatty acids generally increase the rate of cholesterol synthesis and unsaturated fatty acids reduce it. This is the basis for the recommendation that fat should provide 30 per cent of energy intake, with only 10 per cent from saturated fatty acids (see §2.4.2).

In general, if the dietary intake of preformed cholesterol is relatively high, then synthesis in the liver will be reduced. It is only in people with genetic defects of the control of cholesterol synthesis (familial hyperlipidaemia) that the dietary intake of cholesterol has any significant effect on plasma cholesterol. However, the main sources of preformed cholesterol in the diet are the same animal fats that are the main sources of saturated fatty acids (which tend to increase cholesterol synthesis). A lower intake of these foods will reduce the intake of preformed cholesterol and, more importantly, will reduce the synthesis of cholesterol in the body.

6.3.2 ***Digestion and absorption of triacylglycerols***

The digestion of triacylglycerols begins with lipase secreted by the tongue and continues in the stomach, where gastric lipase is secreted. As shown in Figure 6.10, hydrolysis of the fatty acids esterified to carbons 1 and 3 of the triacylglycerol results in the liberation of free fatty acids and 2-mono-acylglycerol. These are both hydrophobic and hydrophilic molecules, and, as discussed in §3.5.3, will therefore emulsify the lipid into increasingly small droplets. Triacylglycerol hydrolysis continues in the small intestine, catalysed by pancreatic lipase. Monoacylglycerols are hydrolysed to glycerol and free fatty acids by pancreatic esterase in the intestinal lumen and intracellular lipase within intestinal mucosal cells.

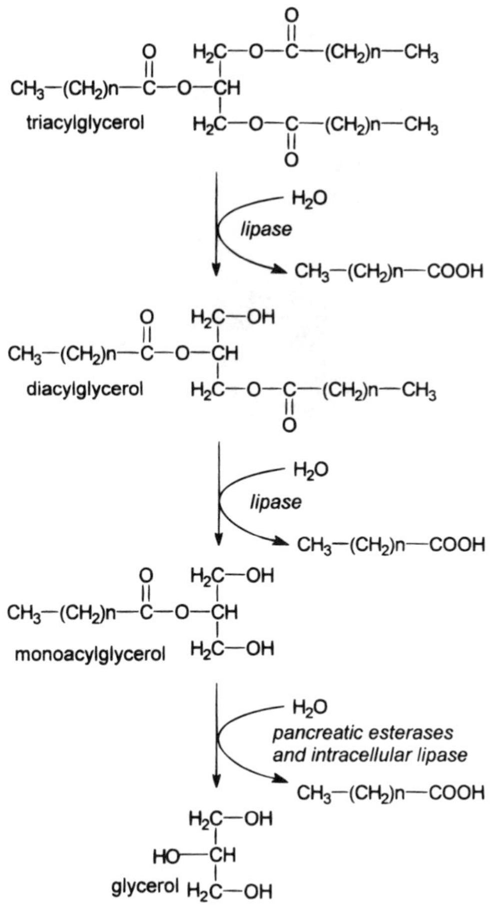

triacylglycerol

H_2O — *lipase* → $CH_3-(CH_2)n-COOH$

diacylglycerol

H_2O — *lipase* → $CH_3-(CH_2)n-COOH$

monoacylglycerol

H_2O — *pancreatic esterases and intracellular lipase* → $CH_3-(CH_2)n-COOH$

glycerol

Figure 6.10 Hydrolysis of triacylglycerol by lipase.

6.3.2.1 *Bile salts*

The final emulsification of dietary lipids into micelles that are small enough to be absorbed across the intestinal mucosa is achieved by the action of the bile salts. The bile salts are synthesized from cholesterol in the liver and are secreted, together with phospholipids and cholesterol, by the gall bladder. As shown in Figure 6.11, some 2 g of cholesterol and 30 g of bile salts are secreted by the gall bladder each day, almost all of which is re-absorbed, so that the total faecal output of steroids and bile salts is 1–2 g per day.

The primary bile salts (those synthesized in the liver) are conjugates of chenodeoxycholic acid and cholic acid with taurine or glycine (see Figure 6.12). Intestinal bacteria catalyse deconjugation and further metabolism to yield the secondary bile salts, lithocholic and deoxycholic acids. These are also

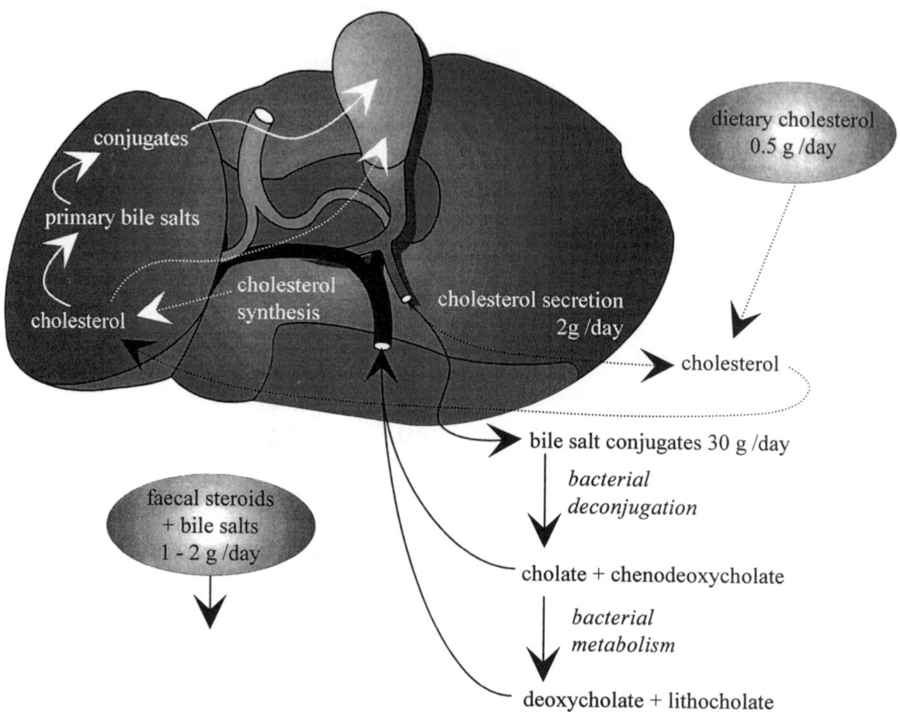

Figure 6.11 Enterohepatic circulation of cholesterol and the bile salts.

absorbed from the gut, and are reconjugated in the liver and secreted in the bile.

Both cholesterol and the bile salts can be bound physically by non-starch polysaccharide in the gut lumen, so that they cannot be re-absorbed. This is the basis of the cholesterol-lowering effect of moderately high intakes of dietary fibre (see §2.4.3.2) – if the bile salts are not re-absorbed and re-utilized, then there will be further synthesis from cholesterol in the liver.

Under normal conditions, the concentration of cholesterol in bile, relative to that of bile salts and phospholipids, is such that cholesterol is at or near its limit of solubility. It requires only a relatively small increase in the concentration of cholesterol in bile for it to crystallize out, resulting in the formation of gallstones. Obesity (see §8.2.2) and high fat diets (especially diets high in saturated fat, which increase the synthesis of cholesterol in the liver) are associated with a considerably increased incidence of gallstones.

6.3.2.2 *Lipid absorption and chylomicron formation*

The finely emulsified lipid micelles, containing intact triacylglycerol, monoacylglycerol, phospholipids, free fatty acids, and the fat-soluble vitamins A, D, E and K, as well as carotene (see Chapter 12), are absorbed across the intesti-

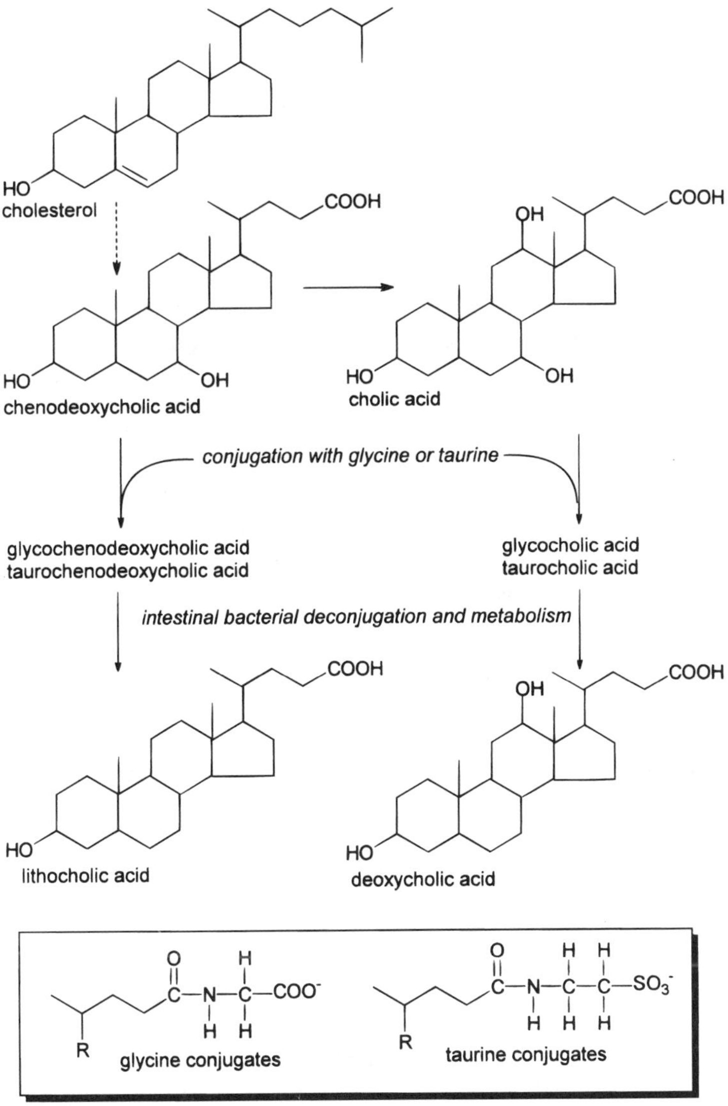

Figure 6.12 Metabolism of the bile salts.

nal wall into the mucosal cells. Here they are re-esterified to form triacylglycerols and are packaged together with proteins synthesized in the mucosal cells to form chylomicrons. Unlike the products of carbohydrate and protein digestion, which are absorbed into the veins draining the small intestine, and hence enter the body via the hepatic portal vein, chylomicrons leave the mucosal cell via the lymphatic system and enter the bloodstream at the thoracic duct. This means that, although the liver has a major function in regulating the amounts of carbohydrate and amino acids entering the peripheral circulation, the products of fat absorption are available to extrahepatic tissues in a more or less unregulated manner before they come to the liver.

6.4 Digestion and absorption of proteins

Proteins are large polymers. Unlike starch and glycogen, which are polymers of only a single type of monomer unit (glucose), proteins consist of a variety of amino acids. There is an almost infinite variety of proteins, composed of different numbers of the different amino acids (50–1000 amino acids in a single protein molecule) in different order. There are some 50 000 different proteins and polypeptides in the human body. Each protein has a specific sequence of amino acids.

Small proteins have a relative molecular mass of about $50–100 \times 10^3$, whereas some of the large complex proteins have a relative molecular mass of up to 10^6. In addition to proteins, smaller polymers of amino acids, containing up to about 50 amino acids, are important in the regulation of metabolism. Collectively these are known as polypeptides.

6.4.1 *The amino acids*

Twenty-one amino acids are involved in the synthesis of proteins, together with some that occur in proteins as a result of chemical modification after the protein has been synthesized. In addition, other amino acids occur as metabolic intermediates, but are not involved in proteins.

Chemically the amino acids all have the same basic structure – an amino group ($—NH_2$) and a carboxylic acid group (—COOH) attached to the same carbon atom (the α-carbon). As shown in Figure 6.13, what differs between the amino acids is the nature of the other group attached to the α-carbon. In the simplest amino acid, glycine, there are two hydrogen atoms; in all other amino acids there is one hydrogen atom and a side chain, varying in chemical complexity from the simple methyl group ($—CH_3$) of alanine to the aromatic ring structures of phenylalanine, tyrosine and tryptophan. Figure 6.13 also shows the three-letter abbreviations for the amino acids and single-letter codes used in protein sequences. The starred amino acids in Figure 6.13 are dietary essentials (see §10.1.3).

The amino acids can be classified according to the chemical nature of the side chain; whether it is hydrophobic (Figure 6.13, left) or hydrophilic (Figure 6.13, right) and the nature of the group:

- Small hydrophobic amino acids: glycine, alanine, proline.
- Branched-chain amino acids: leucine, isoleucine, valine.
- Aromatic amino acids: phenylalanine, tyrosine, tryptophan.

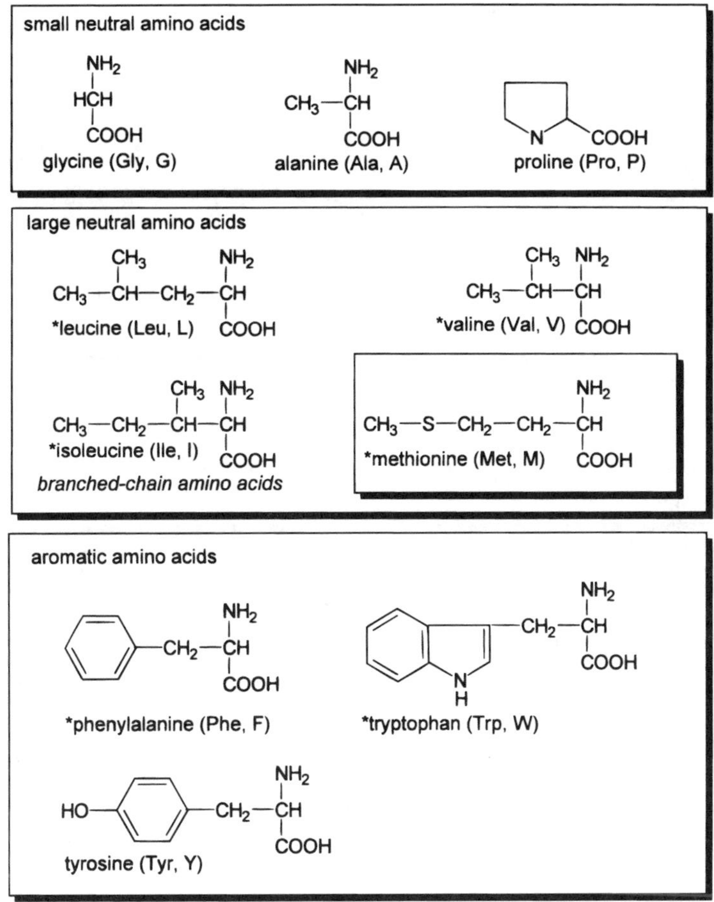

Figure 6.13 The amino acids arranged by the chemistry of their side chains; those with hydrophobic side chains are shown on the left, and those with hydrophilic side chains on the right. The three-letter abbreviations and single letter codes used in protein sequences are shown in parentheses. Starred amino acids are dietary essentials (see §10.1.3).

- Sulphur-containing amino acids: cysteine, methionine (and the selenium analogue of cysteine, selenocysteine, which is not shown in Figure 6.13).
- Neutral hydrophilic amino acids: serine and threonine.
- Acidic amino acids: glutamic and aspartic acids (the salts of these acids are glutamate and aspartate respectively).
- Amides of the acidic amino acids: glutamine and asparagine.
- Basic amino acids: lysine, arginine, histidine.

hydrophilic amino acids

neutral hydrophilic amino acids

$HO{-}CH_2{-}CH(NH_2)COOH$
serine (Ser, S)

$CH_3{-}CH(OH){-}CH(NH_2)COOH$
*threonine (Thr, T)

$HS{-}CH_2{-}CH(NH_2)COOH$
cysteine (Cys, C)

acidic amino acids

$HOOC{-}CH_2{-}CH(NH_2)COOH$
aspartate (Asp, D)

$HOOC{-}CH_2{-}CH_2{-}CH(NH_2)COOH$
glutamate (Glu, E)

amino acid amides

$H_2N{-}OC{-}CH_2{-}CH(NH_2)COOH$
asparagine (Asn, N)

$H_2N{-}OC{-}CH_2{-}CH_2{-}CH(NH_2)COOH$
glutamine (Gln, Q)

basic amino acids

$H_2N{-}CH_2{-}CH_2{-}CH_2{-}CH_2{-}CH(NH_2)COOH$
*lysine (Lys, K)

(imidazole ring)$-CH_2{-}CH(NH_2)COOH$
*histidine (His, H)

$HN{=}C(NH_2){-}NH{-}CH_2{-}CH_2{-}CH_2{-}CH(NH_2)COOH$
arginine (Arg, R)

Figure 6.13 *Continued*

6.4.2 *Protein structure and denaturation*

Proteins are composed of linear chains of amino acids, joined by condensation of the carboxyl group of one with the amino group of another to form a peptide bond (see Figure 3.12). Chains of amino acids linked in this way are known as polypeptides.

The sequence of amino acids in a protein is its primary structure. It is different for each protein, although proteins that are closely related to each other often have similar primary structures. The primary structure of a protein is determined by the gene containing the information for that protein (see §10.2).

Polypeptide chains fold up in a variety of ways. Two main types of chemical interaction are responsible for this folding: hydrogen bonds between the oxygen of one peptide bond and the nitrogen of another (see §3.5.1) and interactions between the side chains of the amino acids. Depending on the nature of the side chains, different regions of the chain may fold into one of the following patterns:

- α-Helix, in which the peptide backbone of the protein adopts a spiral (helix) form. The hydrogen bonds are formed between peptide bonds that are near each other in the primary sequence.
- β-Pleated sheet, in which regions of the polypeptide chain lie alongside one another, forming a 'corrugated' or pleated surface. The hydrogen bonds are between peptide bonds in different parts of the primary sequence.
- Hairpins and loops, in which small regions of the polypeptide chain form very tight bends.
- Random coil, in which there is no recognizable organized structure. Although this appears to be random, in that it is not an organized structure, for any one protein the shape of a random coil region will always be the same.

A protein may have several regions of α-helix, β-pleated sheet (with the peptide chains running parallel or antiparallel), hairpins and random coil, all in the same molecule.

Having formed regions of secondary structure, the whole protein molecule then folds up into a compact shape. This is the third (tertiary) level of structure, and is largely the result of interactions between the side chains of the amino acids, both with each other and with the environment. Proteins in an aqueous medium in the cell generally adopt a tertiary structure in which hydrophobic amino acid side chains are inside the molecule and can interact with each other, whereas hydrophilic side chains are exposed to interact with water. By contrast, proteins embedded in membranes (see Figure 3.9) have a hydrophobic region on the outside, to interact with the membrane lipids.

Two further interactions between amino acid side chains may be involved in the formation of tertiary structure, in this case forming covalent links between regions of the peptide chain (see Figure 6.14):

- The amino group on the side chain of lysine can form a peptide bond with the carboxyl group of aspartate or glutamate. This is nutritionally important, since the side chain peptide bond is not hydrolysed by digestive enzymes, and the lysine (and also the glutamate or aspartate) is not available for absorption and metabolism.
- The sulphydryl (–SH) groups of two cysteine molecules may be oxidized, to form a disulphide bridge between two parts of the protein chain.

Some proteins consist of more than one polypeptide chain; the way in which the chains interact with each other after they have separately coiled up

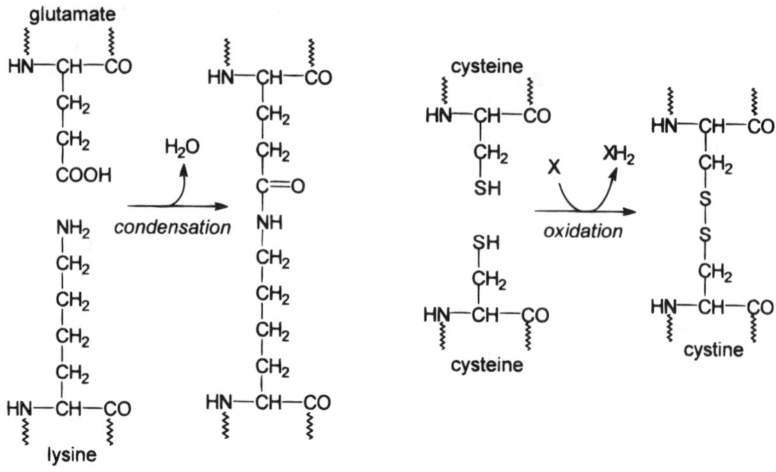

Figure 6.14 Formation of cross-links between protein chains: peptide bond formation between the side chains of glutamate and lysine (left) and oxidation of cysteine sulphydryl groups to form a disulphide bridge (right).

into their secondary and tertiary structures is the quaternary structure of the protein. Interactions between the subunits of multi-subunit proteins, involving changes in quaternary structure, are important in regulatory enzymes (see §4.2.1.3 and §11.1).

Because of their secondary and tertiary structures, most proteins are resistant to digestive enzymes – few bonds are accessible to the enzymes that catalyse hydrolysis of peptide bonds. However, apart from covalent links formed by reaction between the side chains of lysine and aspartate or glutamate, and disulphide bridges, the native structure of proteins is maintained by relatively weak non-covalent forces: ionic interactions, hydrogen bonding and van der Waals forces.

Like all molecules, proteins vibrate and, as the temperature increases, so the vibration increases. Eventually, this vibration disrupts the weak non-covalent forces that hold the protein in its organized structure. When this happens, proteins frequently become insoluble. This is the process of denaturation – a loss of the native structure of the protein. In denatured proteins most of the peptide bonds are accessible to digestive enzymes, and consequently denatured (i.e. cooked) proteins are more readily hydrolysed to their constituent amino acids. Gastric acid is also important, since relatively strong acid will also disrupt hydrogen bonds and denature proteins.

6.4.3 Protein digestion

Protein digestion occurs by hydrolysis of the peptide bonds between amino acids. There are two main classes of protein digestive enzymes (proteases), with different specificities for the amino acids forming the peptide bond to be hydrolysed, as shown in Table 6.2:

- Endopeptidases cleave proteins by hydrolysing peptide bonds between specific amino acids in the middle of the molecule.
- Exopeptidases remove amino acids one at a time from the end of the molecule, again by the hydrolysis of the peptide bond.

The first enzymes to act on dietary proteins are the endopeptidases: pepsin in the gastric juice and trypsin, chymotrypsin and elastase secreted by the pancreas into the small intestine. The result of the combined action of these enzymes is that the large protein molecules are broken down into medium-sized polypeptides, with many terminals for the exopeptidases to act on. There are two classes of exopeptidase:

- Carboxypeptidases, secreted in the pancreatic juice, release amino acids from the free carboxyl terminal of peptides.
- Aminopeptidases, secreted by the intestinal mucosal cells, release amino acids from the amino terminal of peptides.

The proteases are secreted as inactive precursors (zymogens); this is essential if they are not to digest themselves and each other, as well as tissue proteins, before they are secreted. In each case the active site of the enzyme is masked by a small region of the peptide chain, which has to be removed for the enzyme to have activity. This is achieved by hydrolysis of a specific peptide bond in the precursor molecule, releasing the blocking peptide and revealing the active site of the enzyme.

Pepsin is secreted in the gastric juice as pepsinogen, which is activated by the action of gastric acid, and also by the action of already activated pepsin. In the small intestine, trypsinogen, the precursor of trypsin, is activated by the

Table 6.2 Protein digestive enzymes

Enzyme	Secreted by	Specificity
Endopeptidases		
Pepsin	Gastric mucosa	Adjacent to aromatic amino acid, leucine or methionine
Trypsin	Pancreas	Lysine or arginine esters
Chymotrypsin	Pancreas	Aromatic esters
Elastase	Pancreas	Neutral aliphatic esters
Enteropeptidase	Intestinal mucosa	Trypsinogen → trypsin
Exopeptidases		
Carboxypeptidases	Pancreas	Carboxy-terminal amino acids
Aminopeptidases	Intestinal mucosa	Amino-terminal amino acids
Tripeptidases	Mucosal brush border	Tripeptides
Dipeptidases	Mucosal brush border	Dipeptides

action of a specific enzyme, enteropeptidase (sometimes known by its obsolete name of enterokinase), which is secreted by the duodenal epithelial cells; trypsin can then activate chymotrypsinogen to chymotrypsin, pro-elastase to elastase, procarboxypeptidase to carboxypeptidase, and pro-aminopeptidase to aminopeptidase.

The end-product of the action of these various proteases is a mixture of free amino acids, di- and tripeptides, and oligopeptides, all of which are absorbed:

- Free amino acids are absorbed across the intestinal mucosa by sodium-dependent active transport, as occurs in the absorption of glucose and galactose (see Figure 6.6). The different amino acid transport systems have specificity for the chemical nature of the side chain (acidic, basic, aromatic, large or small neutral; see Figure 6.13).
- Dipeptides and tripeptides enter the brush border of the intestinal mucosal cells, where they are hydrolysed to free amino acids, which are then transported into the bloodstream.
- Even relatively large oligopeptides may be absorbed intact, either by uptake into mucosal epithelial cells (the transcellular route) or by passing between epithelial cells (the paracellular route). Many such oligopeptides are large enough to stimulate antibody formation in the bloodstream; this is the basis of food allergy.

6.5 The absorption of vitamin B_{12}

Vitamin B_{12} (see §12.2.9) is released from the proteins to which it is bound in foods by the combined actions of gastric acid and pepsin in the stomach, and binds to the protein cobalophilin, which is secreted in the saliva. In the duodenum, cobalophilin is hydrolysed, and the vitamin B_{12} is liberated to bind to intrinsic factor, a protein secreted by the gastric mucosa. This binding to intrinsic factor is essential for absorption of the vitamin; the transport mechanism in the distal third of the ileum recognizes and binds the vitamin B_{12}–intrinsic factor complex, but not free vitamin B_{12}. It is not known whether the vitamin B_{12}–intrinsic factor complex enters the mucosal cells, or whether the vitamin is transferred by a membrane transport protein, leaving the intrinsic factor in the intestinal lumen. Vitamin B_{12} then leaves the mucosal cell and enters the bloodstream bound to transcobalamin, which is the major transport protein for the vitamin in plasma.

Intrinsic factor is so named because, in the early studies of pernicious anaemia (see §12.2.9.1), it was recognized that two factors were required: an extrinsic or dietary factor, now known to be vitamin B_{12}, and an intrinsic factor produced in the body. Dietary deficiency of vitamin B_{12} is rare, except among strict vegetarians (vegans), but pernicious anaemia as a result of failure to absorb the vitamin is relatively common. Three conditions may lead to failure of vitamin B_{12} absorption:

- Achlorhydria, a more or less complete failure of the secretion of gastric acid as a result of the production of antibodies against the gastric parietal cells which secrete both the gastric acid and intrinsic factor. This is the classic form of pernicious anaemia. The vitamin B_{12} deficiency may be treated either by injection of the vitamin or by oral administration of intrinsic factor.
- The production and secretion of antibodies against intrinsic factor itself. The resultant vitamin B_{12} deficiency cannot be treated by oral administration of intrinsic factor, since the secreted antibodies would bind to it, preventing it from binding vitamin B_{12} for absorption.
- Atrophic gastritis with advancing age: gradual atrophy of the gastric parietal cells, and hence reduced secretion of both gastric acid and intrinsic factor. Although there are normally relatively large reserves of vitamin B_{12} in the body, deficiency as a result of atrophic gastritis is a problem among elderly people.

6.6 The absorption of iron

Only about 10 per cent of dietary iron is absorbed, and only as little as 1–5 per cent of that in many plant foods. As discussed in §12.3.2.3, iron deficiency is a serious problem; some 10–15 per cent of women of childbearing age have iron losses in menstruation greater than can be met from a normal dietary intake. Haem iron in meat is absorbed better than is inorganic iron from plant foods, and by a separate transport system; little is known about the mechanism of haem absorption.

Inorganic iron is absorbed only in the Fe^{2+} (reduced) form. This means that a variety of reducing agents present in the intestinal lumen, together with dietary iron, will enhance its absorption. The most effective such compound is vitamin C (see §12.2.13), and although intakes of 40–60 mg of vitamin C per day are more than adequate to meet requirements, an intake of 25–50 mg per meal is sometimes recommended to enhance iron absorption.

Like other minerals, iron enters the mucosal cells by carrier-mediated passive diffusion and is accumulated in the cells by binding to a protein, ferritin. Once all the ferritin in the mucosal cell is saturated with iron, no more can be taken up from the gut lumen. Iron can leave the mucosal cell only if there is free transferrin in plasma for it to bind to, and once plasma ferritin is saturated with iron, any that has accumulated in the mucosal cells will be lost back into the intestinal lumen when the cells are shed at the tip of the villus (see §6.1).

Although compounds such as vitamin C, fructose and alcohol enhance the absorption of iron when they are in the intestinal lumen together with iron, other compounds present in foods inhibit the absorption of iron, sometimes quite severely. Such compounds include phytate (present in whole grain cereals, but inactivated by yeast in bread-making), some types of dietary fibre, tannic acid (present in tea) and calcium. Phytate, tannic acid and dietary fibre all affect iron absorption by binding it in the gut lumen, so that it is insoluble and not available for absorption. The mechanism by which calcium inhibits iron absorption is not clear, and the absorption of both inorganic and haem iron is similarly inhibited: a glass of milk drunk with a meal will reduce the absorption of iron from meat quite significantly.

The mucosal barrier to the absorption of iron has a protective function. Iron overload is a serious condition, leading to deposition of inappropriately large amounts of iron in tissues. Once the normal tissue iron-binding proteins are saturated, free iron ions will accumulate in tissues. As discussed in §2.5.1, iron ions in solution are able to generate tissue-damaging oxygen radicals, and this may be a factor in the development of cardiovascular disease and some forms of cancer. Indeed, one of the reasons why women are less at risk of atherosclerosis than are men may be that women generally have a lower iron status than men, because of menstrual blood losses.

7

Energy Nutrition: the Metabolism of Carbohydrates and Fats

If the intake of metabolic fuels is equivalent to energy expenditure, there is a state of energy balance. Overall there will be equal periods of fed state metabolism (during which nutrient reserves are accumulated as liver and muscle glycogen, adipose tissue triacylglycerols and labile protein stores), and fasting state metabolism, during which these reserves are utilized. Averaged out, certainly over several days, there will be no change in body weight or body composition.

By contrast, if the intake of metabolic fuels is greater than is required to meet energy expenditure, the body will spend more time in the fed state than the fasting state; there will be more accumulation of nutrient reserves than utilization. The result of this is an increase in body size; and especially an increase in adipose tissue stores. If continued for long enough, this will result in overweight or obesity, with potentially serious health consequences (see Chapter 8).

The opposite state of affairs is when the intake of metabolic fuels is lower than is required to meet energy expenditure. Now the body has to mobilize its nutrient reserves, and overall spends more time in the fasting state than in the fed state. The result of this is undernutrition, starvation and eventually death (see Chapter 9).

7.1 Estimation of energy expenditure

Energy expenditure can be determined directly, by measuring heat output from the body. This requires a thermally insulated chamber in which the temperature can be controlled so as to maintain the subject's comfort, and in which it is possible to measure the amount of heat produced, for example by the increase in temperature of water used to cool the chamber. Calorimeters of this sort are relatively small, so that it is possible for measurements of direct heat production to be made only for subjects performing a limited range of tasks and only for a relatively short time. Most estimates of energy expenditure are based on indirect measurements, either measurement of oxygen consumption and carbon dioxide production (indirect calorimetry, see §7.1.1) or indirect assessment of carbon dioxide production by use of dual isotopically labelled water (see §7.1.2). From the results of studies in which energy expenditure in different activities has been measured, it is possible to calculate people's energy expenditure from the time spent in each type of activity (see §7.1.3).

7.1.1 *Indirect calorimetry and the respiratory quotient*

Energy expenditure can be determined from the rate of consumption of oxygen. This is known as indirect calorimetry, since there is no direct measurement of the heat produced. As shown in Table 7.1, there is an output or expenditure of 20 kJ per L of oxygen consumed, regardless of whether the fuel being metabolized is carbohydrate, fat or protein. Measurement of oxygen consumption is quite simple using a respirometer. Such instruments are portable, so people can carry on more or less normal activities for several hours at a time, while their energy expenditure is being estimated.

Measurement of both oxygen consumption and carbon dioxide production at the same time, again a simple procedure using a respirometer, provides information on the mixture of metabolic fuels being metabolized. In the metabolism of starch, the same amount of carbon dioxide is produced as oxygen is consumed – i.e. the ratio of carbon dioxide produced to oxygen consumed (the respiratory quotient) = 1.0. This is because the overall reaction is:

$$C_6H_12O_6 + 6\ O_2 \rightarrow 6\ CO_2 + 6\ H_2O.$$

Proportionally more oxygen is required for the oxidation of fat. The major process involved is the oxidation of $—CH_2—$ units:

$$—CH_2 + 1\tfrac{1}{2}\ O_2 \rightarrow CO_2 + H_2O.$$

Allowing for the fact that in triacylglycerols there are also the glycerol and three carboxyl groups to be considered, overall for the oxidation of fat the respiratory quotient = 0.7.

Table 7.1 Oxygen consumption and carbon dioxide production in oxidation of metabolic fuels

	Energy yield ($kJ\ g^{-1}$)	Oxygen consumed ($L\ g^{-1}$)	Carbon dioxide produced ($L\ g^{-1}$)	Respiratory quotient (CO_2/O_2)	Energy/Oxygen consumption (kJ/L oxygen)
Carbohydrate	16	0.829	0.829	1.0	~20
Protein	17	0.966	0.782	0.809	~20
Fat	37	2.016	1.427	0.707	~20

The metabolism of proteins gives a ratio of carbon dioxide produced to oxygen consumed intermediate between that of carbohydrate and fat – this is because proteins contain more oxygen per carbon than do fats, although less than carbohydrates. For protein metabolism the respiratory quotient is 0.8. The amount of protein being oxidized can be determined quite separately by measurement of the excretion of urea, the end-product of amino acid metabolism (see §10.3.1.4).

Measurement of the respiratory quotient and urinary excretion of urea thus permits calculation of the relative amounts of fat, carbohydrate and protein being metabolized. In the fasting state (see §7.3.2), when a relatively large amount of fat is being used as a fuel, the respiratory quotient is around 0.8–0.85; after a meal, when there is more carbohydrate available to be metabolized (see §7.3.1), the respiratory quotient rises to about 0.9–1.0.

7.1.2 ***Long-term measurement of energy expenditure: the dual isotopically labelled water method***

Although indirect calorimetry has considerable advantages over direct calorimetry, it still only permits measurement of energy expenditure over a period of hours. A more recent technique permits estimation of total energy expenditure over a period of 1–2 weeks. This method depends on the administration of a sample of water labelled with stable isotopes (see §3.1.1). Both the hydrogen and oxygen of the water are labelled, the hydrogen as deuterium (^2H) and the oxygen as ^{18}O. The rate at which the labelled water is lost from the body is determined by measuring the amounts of these two isotopes in urine or saliva.

The deuterium (^2H) is lost from the body only as water. The labelled oxygen (^{18}O) is lost more rapidly. It can be lost as either water or carbon dioxide, because of the rapid equilibrium between carbon dioxide and bicarbonate:

$$H_2O + CO_2 \rightleftharpoons H^+ + HCO_3^-.$$

Since all three oxygen atoms in the bicarbonate ion are equivalent, label from $H_2{}^{18}O$ can be lost in both water and carbon dioxide.

The difference between the rate of loss of the two isotopes from body water (plasma, saliva or urine) thus reflects the total amount of carbon dioxide that has been produced. Estimating the respiratory quotient from the proportions of fat, carbohydrate and protein in the diet permits calculation of the total amount of oxygen that has been consumed, and hence the total energy expenditure over a period of 2–3 weeks.

7.1.3 ***Calculation of energy expenditure***

Energy expenditure depends on: the requirement for maintenance of normal body structure, function and metabolic integrity – the basal metabolic rate (see

§7.1.3.1); the energy required for work and physical activity (see §7.1.3.2); the energy cost of synthesizing reserves of fat and glycogen; and the increase in protein synthesis in the fed state (see §7.1.3.3).

7.1.3.1 Basal metabolic rate (BMR)

Basal metabolic rate is the energy expenditure by the body when at rest, but not asleep, under controlled conditions of thermal neutrality, and about 12 hours after the last meal. It is the energy requirement for the maintenance of metabolic integrity, nerve and muscle tone, circulation and respiration, and so on. It is important that the subject be awake since, when asleep, some people show an increased metabolic rate (and hence increased heat output) and others have a reduced metabolic rate and a slight fall in body temperature. Where the measurement of metabolic rate has been made under less strictly controlled conditions, the result is more correctly called the resting metabolic rate.

Table 7.2 shows average values of basal metabolic rate. Obviously, it depends on body weight, since there will be a greater amount of metabolically active tissue in a larger body. The decrease in BMR with increasing age is the result of changes in body composition. With increasing age, even when body weight remains constant, there is loss of muscle tissue and replacement by adipose tissue, which is metabolically very much less active, since 80 per cent of the weight of adipose tissue consists of reserves of triacylglycerol. Similarly, the gender difference (women have a significantly lower BMR than do men of the same body weight) is accounted for by differences in body composition. As shown in Table 7.3, the proportion of body weight that is adipose tissue reserves in lean women is considerably higher than in men. (See also §8.1.2 for

Table 7.2 The effects of age, gender and body weight on basal metabolic rate (MJ day^{-1})

	Men			Women		
Age (years)	60 kg	70 kg	80 kg	60 kg	70 kg	80 kg
10–17	7.19	7.93	8.67	6.26	6.82	7.38
18–29	6.68	7.31	7.94	5.76	6.38	6.99
30–59	6.53	7.01	7.49	5.58	5.92	6.26
60–74	5.92	6.42	6.92	5.19	5.58	5.96
>75	5.53	5.88	6.23	5.07	5.48	5.80

Table 7.3 Fat as a percentage of body weight

	Men	Women
Mean at age 25	16	30
Mean at age 65	24	36
Indicative of undernutrition	<10	<15

a discussion of methods of estimating the proportions of fat and lean tissue in the body.)

7.1.3.2 *Energy costs of physical activity*

The most useful way of expressing the energy cost of physical activities is as a multiple of BMR. The physical activity ratio (PAR) for an activity is the ratio of the energy expended while performing the activity to that expended at rest (=BMR). Very gentle, sedentary activities use only about 1.1–1.2 × BMR. By contrast, as shown in Table 7.4, vigorous exertion, such as climbing stairs, cross-country walking uphill, and so on, may use 6–8 × BMR.

Using data such as those in Table 7.4, and allowing for the time spent during each type of activity through the day permits calculation of an individual's physical activity level (PAL) – the sum of the PAR of each activity performed multiplied by the time spent in that activity. A desirable level of

Table 7.4 Physical activity ratios in different types of activity

PAR	Activity
1.0–1.4	Lying, standing or sitting at rest, e.g. watching television, reading, writing, eating, playing cards and board games
1.5–1.8	*Sitting*: sewing, knitting, playing piano, driving *Standing*: preparing vegetables, washing dishes, ironing, general office and laboratory work
1.9–2.4	*Standing*: mixed household chores, cooking, playing snooker or bowls
2.5–3.3	*Standing*: dressing, undressing, showering, making beds, vacuum cleaning *Walking*: 3–4 km h^{-1}, playing cricket *Occupational*: tailoring, shoemaking, electrical and machine tool industry, painting and decorating
3.4–4.4	*Standing*: mopping floors, gardening, cleaning windows, table tennis, sailing *Walking*: 4–6 km h^{-1}, playing golf *Occupational*: motor vehicle repairs, carpentry and joinery, chemical industry, bricklaying
4.5–5.9	*Standing*: polishing furniture, chopping wood, heavy gardening, volley ball *Walking*: 6–7 km h^{-1} *Exercise*: dancing, moderate swimming, gentle cycling, slow jogging *Occupational*: labouring, hoeing, road construction, digging and shovelling, felling trees
6.0–7.9	*Walking*: uphill with load or cross-country, climbing stairs *Exercise*: jogging, cycling, energetic swimming, skiing, tennis, football

physical activity, in terms of cardiovascular and respiratory health, is a PAL of 1.7.

Table 7.5 shows the classification of different types of occupational work by PAR. This is the average PAR during the 8-hour working day, and makes no allowance for leisure activities. From these figures it might seem that there would be no problem in achieving the desirable PAL of 1.7. However, in Britain the average PAL is only 1.4, and the desirable level of 1.7 is achieved by only 22 per cent of men and 13 per cent of women.

The energy cost of physical activity is obviously affected by body weight, because more energy is required to move a heavier body. Table 7.6 shows the effects of body weight on BMR and total energy expenditure at different levels of physical activity. Table 7.7 shows estimated average energy requirements at different ages, assuming average body weight and, for adults, the average PAL of 1.4 × BMR.

Table 7.5 Classification of types of occupational work by physical activity ratio; figures show the average PAR through an 8-hour working day, excluding leisure activities

Work intensity	PAR[a]	Occupation
Light	1.7	Professional, clerical and technical workers, administrative and managerial staff, sales representatives, housewives
Moderate	2.2–2.7	Sales staff, domestic service, students, transport workers, joiners, roofing workers
Moderately heavy	2.3–3.0	Machine operators, labourers, agricultural workers, bricklaying, masonry
Heavy	2.8–3.8	Labourers, agricultural workers, bricklaying, masonry where there is little or no mechanization

[a] Where a range of PAR is shown, the lower figure is for women and the higher for men.

Table 7.6 The effect of body weight and PAL on energy requirement

		Total energy expenditure (MJ day^{-1})		
Weight (kg)	BMR (MJ day^{-1})	PAL = 1.4	PAL = 1.7	PAL = 2.0
60	6.7	9.3	11.4	13.4
65	7.0	9.8	11.9	14.0
70	7.3	10.2	12.4	14.6
75	7.6	10.7	12.9	15.2
80	7.9	11.1	13.4	15.8

PAL = 1.7 is a desirable level of physical activity for health; the average in Britain is 1.4.

Table 7.7 Average requirements for energy, based on average weights, and for adults assuming PAL = 1.4

Age (Years)	Males (MJ day^{-1})	Females (MJ day^{-1})
1–3	5.2	4.9
4–6	7.2	6.5
7–10	8.2	7.3
11–14	9.3	7.9
15–18	11.5	8.8
Adults	10.6	8.0

7.1.3.3 *Diet-induced thermogenesis*

There is a considerable increase in metabolic rate in response to a meal. A small part of this is the energy cost of secreting digestive enzymes, and the energy cost of active transport of the products of digestion (see §5.2.2). The major part is the energy cost of synthesizing body reserves of glycogen (see §7.6.2) and triacylglycerol (see §7.6.1), as well as the increased protein synthesis that occurs in the fed state (see §10.2.3.3). The cost of synthesizing glycogen from glucose is about 5 per cent of the ingested energy, and that of synthesizing triacylglycerol from glucose is about 20 per cent of the ingested energy. Depending on the relative amounts of fat and carbohydrate in the diet, and the amounts of triacylglycerol and glycogen being synthesized, this diet-induced thermogenesis may account for 10 per cent or more of the total energy yield of a meal.

7.2 Energy balance and changes in body weight

When energy intake is greater than energy expenditure (positive energy balance), there is increased storage of excess metabolic fuel, largely as adipose tissue; similarly, if energy intake is inadequate to meet expenditure (negative energy balance), there is utilization of reserves of adipose tissue. Adipose tissue consists of 80 per cent triacylglycerol (with an energy yield of 37 kJ per g) and 5 per cent protein (energy yield 17 kJ per g); the remaining 15 per cent is water. Hence, adipose tissue reserves are equivalent to approximately 30 kJ per g, or 30 MJ per kg. This means that the theoretical change in body weight is 33 g per MJ energy imbalance per day, or 230 g per MJ energy imbalance per week. On this basis, it is possible to calculate that, even with total starvation, a person with an energy expenditure of 10 MJ per day would lose only 330 g body weight per day or 2.3 kg per week.

These calculations suggest that there should be a constant change of body weight with a constant excessive or deficient energy intake, but this is not observed in practice. With positive energy balance the rate of weight gain is never as great as would be predicted, and gradually slows down, so that after a time the subject regains energy balance, albeit with a higher body weight. Similarly, in negative energy balance, weight is not lost at a constant rate; the rate of loss slows down, and (assuming that the energy deficit is not too severe) levels off, and the subject regains energy balance, at a lower body weight. Several factors contribute to this adaptation in changing energy balance:

- As more food is eaten, so there is an increased energy cost of digestion and absorption.
- When food intake is in excess of requirements, a greater proportion is used for synthesis of adipose tissue triacylglycerol reserves, so there is a considerably greater diet-induced thermogenesis. Conversely, in negative energy balance there will be considerably less synthesis of adipose tissue reserves.
- The rate of protein turnover increases with greater food intake (see §10.2.3.3), and decreases with lower food intake.
- Although adipose tissue is less metabolically active than muscle, 5 per cent of its weight is metabolically active, and therefore the BMR changes as body weight changes, increasing as body weight rises and decreasing as it falls.
- As shown in Table 7.6, the energy cost of physical activity is markedly affected by body weight; so, even assuming a constant level of physical activity, total energy expenditure will increase with increasing body weight. Furthermore, there is some evidence that people with habitually low energy intakes are more efficient in their movements, and so have a lower cost of activity.

7.3 Metabolic fuels in the fed and fasting states

Energy expenditure is relatively constant throughout the day, but food intake normally occurs in two or three meals. There is therefore a need for metabolic regulation to ensure that there is a more or less constant supply of metabolic fuel to tissues, regardless of the variation in intake. (See §11.4 for a more detailed discussion of the hormonal control of metabolism in the fed and fasting states.)

7.3.1 *The fed state*

During the 3–4 hours after a meal, there is an ample supply of metabolic fuel entering the circulation from the gut (see Figure 7.1). Glucose from carbohydrate digestion and amino acids from protein digestion are absorbed into the portal circulation, and to a considerable extent the liver controls the amounts that enter the peripheral circulation. By contrast, the products of fat

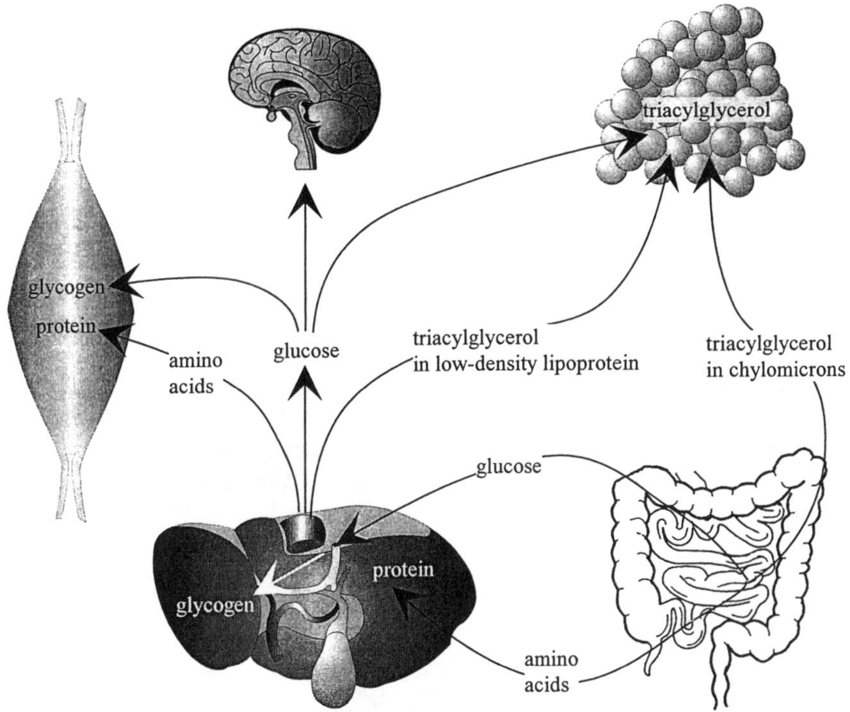

Figure 7.1 Metabolic fuels in the fed state.

digestion are absorbed into the lymphatic system as chylomicrons (see §6.3.2.2), and are available to peripheral tissues before the liver exerts control. Much of the triacylglycerol in chylomicrons goes directly to adipose tissue for storage; when there is a plentiful supply of glucose, it is the main metabolic fuel for all tissues.

The increased concentration of glucose and amino acids in the portal blood stimulates the β-cells of the pancreas to secrete insulin, and suppresses the secretion of glucagon by the α-cells of the pancreas. Insulin has four main actions:

- Stimulation of the uptake of glucose by muscle, so that it becomes the preferred fuel for muscle metabolism.
- Stimulation of the synthesis of glycogen (see §7.6.2) from glucose in both liver and muscle.
- Stimulation of glucose uptake into adipose tissue for synthesis of triacylglycerol (see §7.6.1).
- Stimulation of amino acid uptake into tissues, leading to an increased rate of protein synthesis.

The liver responds to increased glucose availability by increasing its rate of fatty acid and triacylglycerol synthesis; the triacylglycerols are exported from the liver in low-density lipoproteins for use as metabolic fuels in peripheral tissues, and for storage in adipose tissue.

7.3.2 The fasting state

In the fasting state (sometimes known as the postabsorptive state, since it begins about 4–5 hours after a meal, when the products of digestion have been absorbed) metabolic fuels enter the circulation from the reserves of glycogen, triacylglycerol and protein laid down in the fed state (see Figure 7.2).

As the concentration of glucose and amino acids in the portal blood falls, so the secretion of insulin by the β-cells of the pancreas decreases, and the secretion of glucagon by the α-cells increases. Glucagon has three main actions:

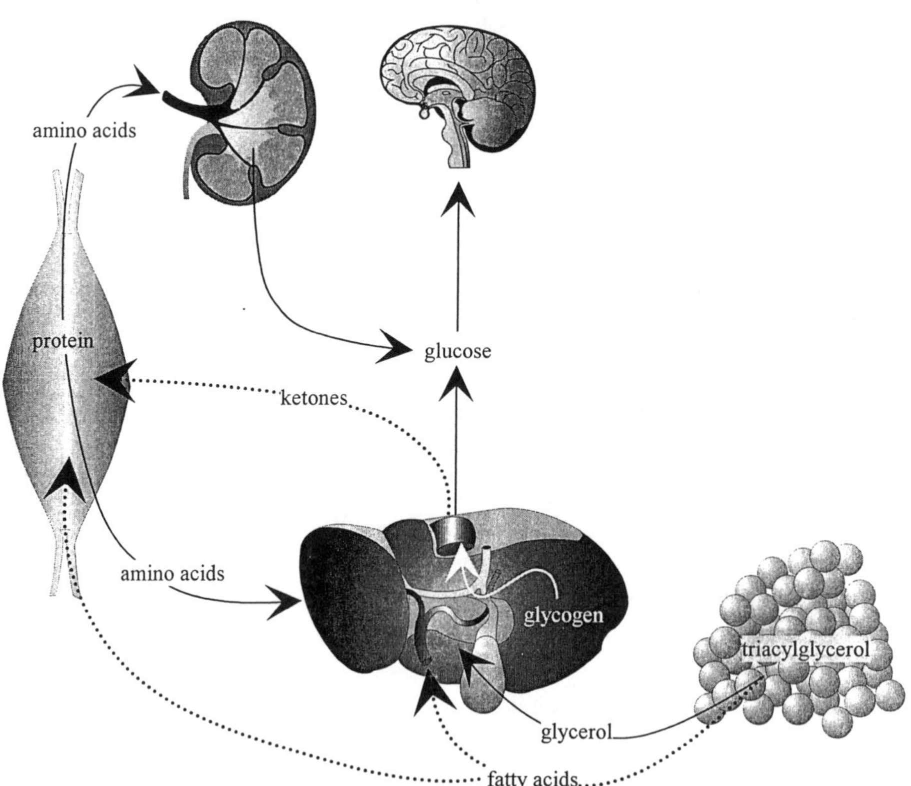

Figure 7.2 Metabolic fuels in the fasting state.

- Stimulation of the breakdown of glycogen in the liver, to release glucose into the circulation; as discussed in §7.7, muscle glycogen cannot be used directly as a source of free glucose.
- Stimulation of lipase in adipose tissue, resulting in the release of fatty acids into the circulation, bound to serum albumin.
- Stimulation of the synthesis of glucose from amino acids in liver and kidney (the process of gluconeogenesis, see §7.7).

At the same time, the reduced secretion of insulin results in a reduced rate of glucose uptake into muscle, and a reduced rate of protein synthesis, so that the amino acids arising from protein turnover are available for gluconeogenesis.

The metabolic problem in the fasting state is that the brain and red blood cells are entirely reliant on glucose as a metabolic fuel. Therefore, those tissues that can utilize other fuels do so, in order to spare glucose for the brain and red blood cells (see §11.4.2). Any metabolites that can be used for gluconeogenesis will be used to supplement the relatively small amount of glucose that is available from glycogen reserves – the total liver and muscle glycogen reserves would only meet requirements for 12–18 hours. The main substrates for gluconeogenesis are amino acids (see §10.3.2) and the glycerol of triacylglycerol.

Tissues other than the brain and red blood cells can utilize fatty acids as metabolic fuel, but only to a limited extent, and not enough to meet their energy requirements completely. By contrast, the liver has a greater capacity for the oxidation of fatty acids than is required to meet its own energy requirements. Therefore, in the fasting state the liver synthesizes ketones (acetoacetate and β-hydroxybutyrate, see §7.5.3), which it exports to other tissues for use as a metabolic fuel.

The result of these metabolic changes in the fasting state is shown in Table 7.8. The plasma concentration of glucose falls somewhat, but is maintained through fasting into starvation, as a result of gluconeogenesis; the concentration of free fatty acids in plasma increases in fasting, but does not increase any further in starvation; while the concentration of ketones increases continually through fasting into starvation. After about 2–3 weeks of starvation, the plasma concentration of ketones is high enough for them to enter the brain, and be used as a metabolic fuel – this means that in prolonged starvation there

Table 7.8 Changes of plasma concentrations of metabolic fuels in fasting and starvation

mmol L^{-1}	Fed	40-h fasting	7-day starvation
Glucose	5.5	3.6	3.5
Fatty acids	0.3	1.15	1.19
Ketones	Negligible	2.9	4.5

is reduction in the amount of tissue protein that needs to be catabolized for gluconeogenesis.

7.4 Energy-yielding metabolism

7.4.1 *Glycolysis: the metabolism of glucose*

Overall, the pathway of glycolysis is cleavage of the six-carbon glucose molecule into two three-carbon units. The key steps in the pathway are:

1 Two phosphorylation reactions to form fructose-bisphosphate.

2 Cleavage of fructose-bisphosphate to yield two molecules of triose (three-carbon sugar) phosphate.

3 Two steps in which phosphate is transferred from a substrate onto ADP, forming ATP (and hence a yield of 4 × ATP per mole of glucose metabolized).

4 One step in which NAD^+ is reduced to NADH (equivalent to 3 × ATP per mole of triose phosphate metabolized, or 6 × ATP per mol of glucose metabolized).

5 Formation of 2 mol of pyruvate per mole of glucose metabolized.

The immediate substrate for glycolysis is glucose 6–phosphate. This is formed from glucose, in a phosphorylation reaction catalysed by hexokinase, utilizing ATP. As discussed in §5.2.2.2, this represents metabolic trapping of the glucose in the cell, since glucose 6–phosphate does not cross cell membranes. In the liver, there are two isoenzymes of hexokinase; one, like that in all cells, has a low K_m, and is saturated at normal concentrations of glucose, so that it acts as a more or less constant rate. The other isoenzyme (sometimes called glucokinase) has a high K_m compared with the normal concentration of glucose, and only has significant activity in the fed state, when the concentration of glucose in the portal blood entering the liver may exceed 20 mmol per L. Glucokinase thus acts at times of high glucose availability, permitting the liver to regulate the concentration of glucose entering the peripheral circulation.

In liver and muscle, glucose 6–phosphate for gluconeogenesis is also formed from glycogen (Figure 7.3). Glycogen phosphorylase catalyses the removal of glucose units from glycogen, cleaving the terminal glycoside bond with inorganic phosphate to form glucose 1–phosphate, which is readily interconvertible with glucose 6–phosphate.

As shown in Figure 7.4, although the aim of glucose oxidation is to phosphorylate ADP to ATP, the pathway involves two steps in which ATP is used, one to form glucose 6–phosphate when glucose is the substrate, and the other to form fructose bisphosphate. In other words, there is a modest cost of ATP

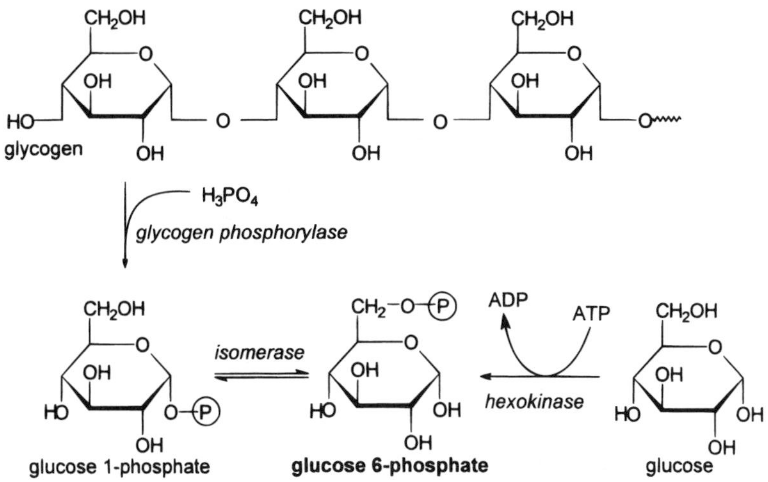

Figure 7.3 Formation of glucose 6–phosphate from glycogen or glucose.

to initiate the metabolism of glucose. The final yield of ATP is great enough for this investment to be worthwhile – overall, there is a net yield of 37 mol of ATP for each mole of glucose oxidized to carbon dioxide and water.

As discussed in §11.4.2, the formation of fructose bisphosphate, catalysed by phosphofructokinase, is an important step for the regulation of glucose metabolism. Once it has been formed, fructose bisphosphate is cleaved into two three-carbon compounds, which are interconvertible. The metabolism of these three-carbon sugars is linked to both the reduction of NAD^+ to NADH, and direct (substrate-level) phosphorylation of ADP to ATP (see §5.3). The result is the formation of 2 mol of pyruvate from each mole of glucose.

The oxidation of glucose to pyruvate thus requires the utilization of 2 mol of ATP (giving ADP) per mole of glucose metabolized, but yields 4 × ATP by direct phosphorylation of ADP, and 2 × NADH (formed from NAD^+), which is equivalent to a further 6 × ATP when oxidized in the electron transport chain (see §5.3.1.3). There is thus a net yield of 8 × ADP + phosphate → ATP from the oxidation of 1 mol of glucose to 2 mol of pyruvate.

The overall sequence of reactions from glucose to pyruvate is known as glycolysis – the process of splitting glucose. As discussed in §7.7, the reverse of this pathway is important as a means of glucose synthesis – the process of gluconeogenesis. Most of the reactions of glycolysis are readily reversible, but at three points (the reactions catalysed by hexokinase, phosphofructokinase and pyruvate kinase) there are separate enzymes involved in glycolysis and gluconeogenesis.

For both hexokinase and phosphofructokinase, the equilibrium of the reaction is in the direction of glycolysis, because of the utilization of ATP in the reaction and the high ratio of ATP to ADP in the cell (see §5.2.1). These two

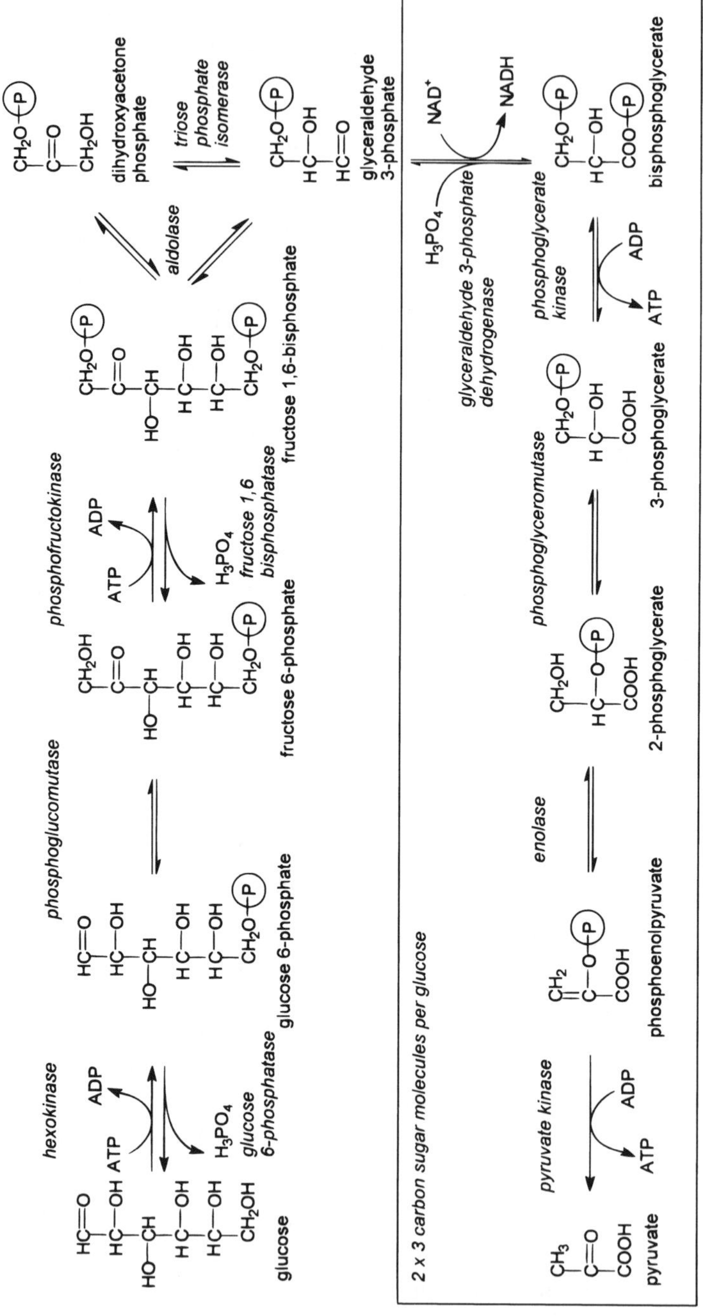

Figure 7.4 Glycolysis: the metabolism of glucose.

reactions are reversed in gluconeogenesis by simple hydrolysis of fructose bisphosphate → fructose 6–phosphate + phosphate (catalysed by fructose bisphosphatase) and of glucose 6–phosphate → glucose + phosphate (catalysed by glucose 6–phosphatase).

The equilibrium of pyruvate kinase is also strongly in the direction of glycolysis. In this case it is because the immediate product of the reaction is enolpyruvate, which is chemically unstable. As shown in Figure 7.19, enolpyruvate undergoes a rapid non-enzymic reaction to yield pyruvate. This means that the product of the enzymic reaction is not available to any significant extent to undergo the reverse reaction in the direction of gluconeogenesis. The conversion of pyruvate to phosphoenolpyruvate in gluconeogenesis is discussed in §7.7.

The glycolytic pathway also provides a route for the metabolism of fructose, galactose (which undergoes phosphorylation to galactose 1–phosphate and isomerization to glucose 1–phosphate) and glycerol. Some fructose is phosphorylated directly to fructose 6–phosphate by hexokinase, but most is phosphorylated to fructose 1–phosphate by a specific enzyme, fructokinase. Fructose 1–phosphate is then cleaved to yield dihydroxyacetone phosphate and glyceraldehyde; the glyceraldehyde can be phosphorylated to glyceraldehyde 3–phosphate by triose kinase.

Glycerol, arising from the hydrolysis of triacylglycerols can be phosphorylated and oxidized to dihydroxyacetone phosphate. In triacylglycerol synthesis (see §7.6.1.2), most glycerol phosphate is formed from dihydroxyacetone phosphate.

7.4.1.1 *The pentose phosphate pathway: an alternative to glycolysis*

There is an alternative pathway for the conversion of glucose 6–phosphate to fructose 6–phosphate, the pentose phosphate pathway (sometimes known as the hexose monophosphate shunt), shown in Figure 7.5.

Overall, the pentose phosphate pathway produces 2 mol of fructose 6–phosphate, 1 mol of glyceraldehyde 3–phosphate and 3 mol of carbon dioxide from 3 mol of glucose 6–phosphate, linked to the reduction of 6 mol of $NADP^+$ to NADPH. The sequence of reactions is as follows:

1 Three moles of glucose are oxidized to yield 3 mol of the five-carbon sugar ribulose 5–phosphate + 3 mol of carbon dioxide.

2 Two moles of ribulose 5–phosphate are isomerized to yield 2 mol of xylulose 5–phosphate.

3 One mole of ribulose 5–phosphate is isomerized to ribose 5–phosphate.

4 One mole of xylulose 5–phosphate reacts with the ribose 5–phosphate, yielding (ultimately) fructose 6–phosphate and erythrose 4–phosphate.

5 The other mole of xylulose 5–phosphate reacts with the erythrose 4–phosphate, yielding fructose 6–phosphate and glyceraldehyde 3–phosphate.

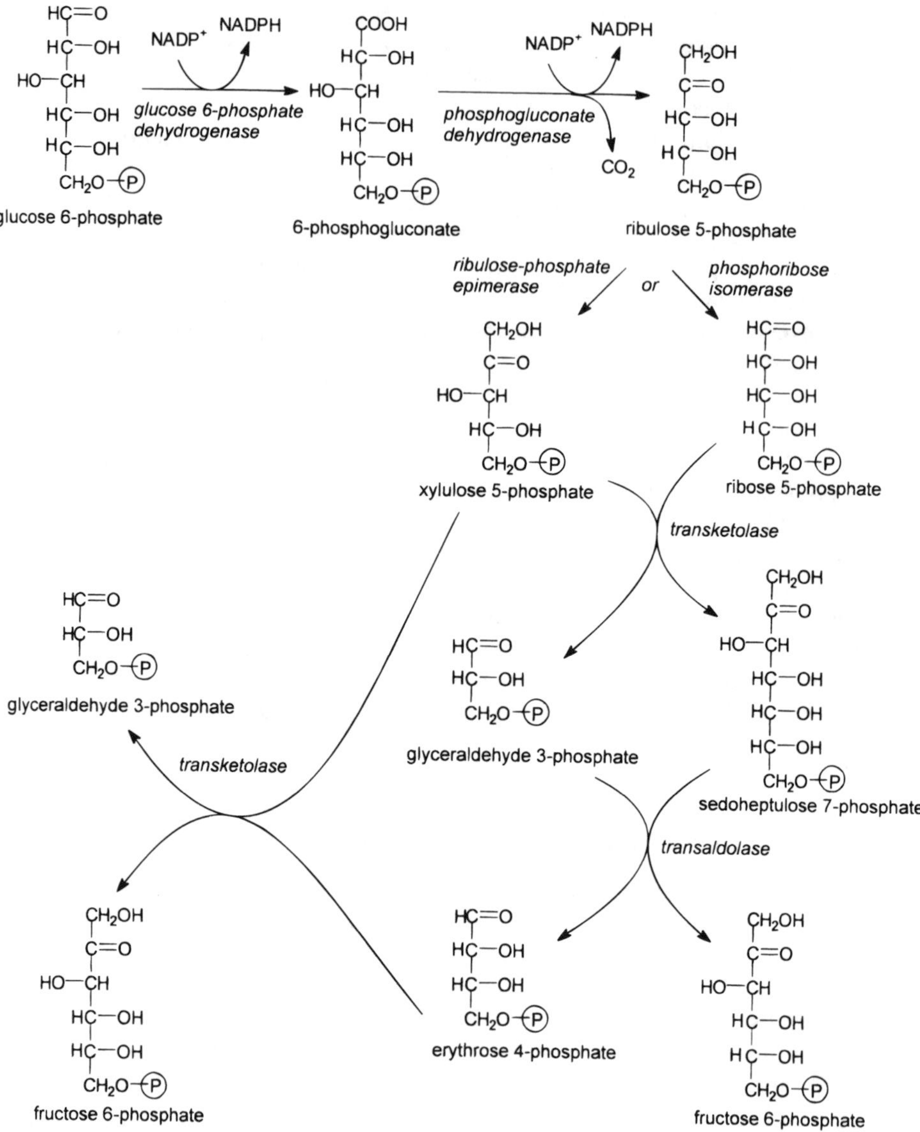

Figure 7.5 The pentose phosphate pathway of carbohydrate metabolism.

This is the pathway for the synthesis of ribose for nucleotide synthesis (see §5.1); more importantly, it is a major source of NADPH for fatty acid synthesis (see §7.6.1); tissues that synthesize large amounts of fatty acids have a high activity of the pentose phosphate pathway.

The pentose phosphate pathway is also important in the red blood cell, where the NADPH is required to maintain an adequate pool of reduced glutathione, which is used to remove hydrogen peroxide. Partial or total lack of glucose 6–phosphate dehydrogenase (and hence impaired activity of the pentose phosphate pathway) is the cause of favism, an acute haemolytic anaemia with fever and haemoglobinuria, precipitated in genetically susceptible people by the consumption of broad beans (fava beans) and a variety of drugs, all of which, like the toxins in fava beans, undergo redox cycling, producing hydrogen peroxide. Because of the low activity of the pentose phosphate pathway, there is a lack of NADPH in red blood cells, and hence an impaired ability to remove this hydrogen peroxide, which causes oxidative damage to the cell membrane lipids. Other tissues are unaffected because there are mitochondrial enzymes that can provide a supply of NADPH; red blood cells have no mitochondria.

The enzyme transketolase is thiamin diphosphate (vitamin B_1) dependent. One of the most sensitive tests of thiamin nutritional status is determination of the activity of transketolase in red blood cells. It is noteworthy that there is a strong correlation, both in time and in brain regions affected, between the neurological effects of thiamin deficiency (see §12.2.5.1) and loss of transketolase activity, suggesting that the pentose phosphate pathway is also important in brain metabolism.

7.4.2 *The metabolism of pyruvate*

Pyruvate arising from glycolysis (or from amino acids, see §10.3.2) can be metabolized in three different ways, depending on the metabolic state of the body:

- reduction to lactate
- complete oxidation to carbon dioxide and water
- as a substrate for gluconeogenesis (see §7.7)

7.4.2.1 *The reduction of pyruvate to lactate: anaerobic glycolysis*

As shown in Figure 7.6, the oxidation of glucose to pyruvate results in the reduction of 2 mol of NAD^+ to NADH. This is normally reoxidized to NAD^+ in the mitochondrial electron transport chain, linked to the phosphorylation of 3 × ADP → ATP for each NADH oxidized (see §5.3.1.3). However, under conditions of maximum exertion, for example in sprinting, the rate at which oxygen can be taken up into the muscle is not great enough to allow for the reoxidation of all the NADH being formed. In order to maintain the oxidation

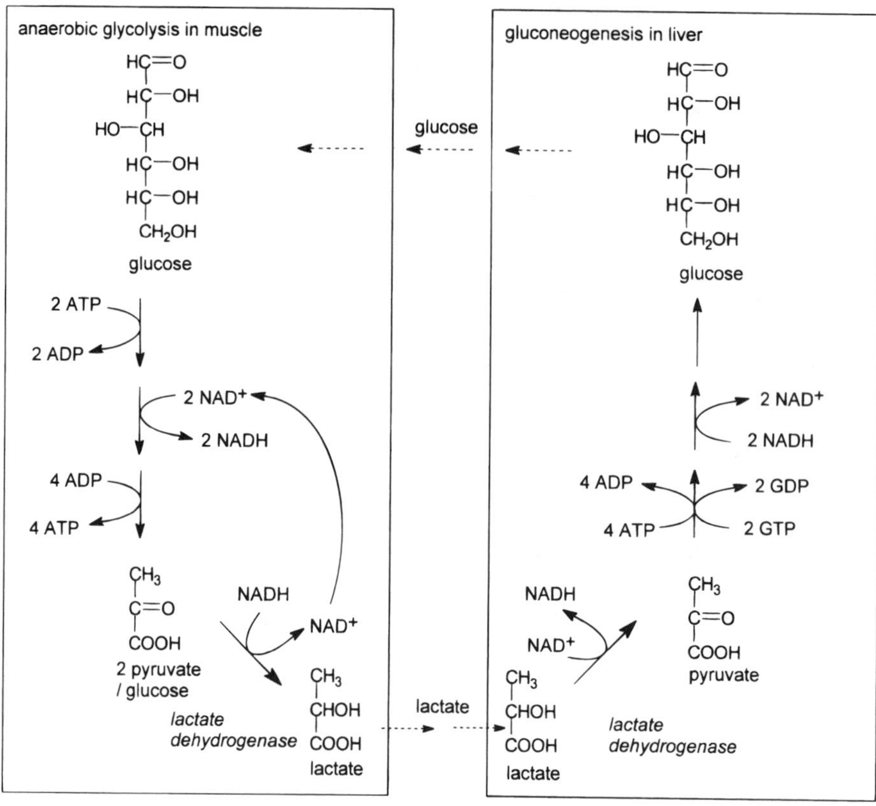

Figure 7.6 The Cori cycle: anaerobic glycolysis in muscle and gluconeogenesis in the liver.

of glucose, and the net yield of 2 × ATP per mole of glucose oxidized, NADH is oxidized back to NAD^+ by the reduction of pyruvate to lactate, catalysed by lactate dehydrogenase (see Figure 7.6).

The resultant lactate is exported from the muscle, and taken up by the liver, where it is used for the resynthesis of glucose. As shown on the right of Figure 7.6, synthesis of glucose from lactate is an ATP (and GTP) requiring process. The oxygen debt after strenuous physical activity is the result of an increased rate of energy-yielding metabolism to provide the ATP and GTP that are required to metabolize the lactate that has accumulated. Lactate can also be taken up by other tissues where oxygen availability is not a limiting factor under these conditions, such as the heart. Here it is oxidized to pyruvate, and the resultant NADH is oxidized in the mitochondrial electron transport chain, yielding 3 × ATP. The pyruvate is then a substrate for complete oxidation to carbon dioxide and water, as discussed below.

The conversion of glucose to lactate is known as anaerobic glycolysis, since it does not require oxygen. However, it is not true to say that human metabolism is ever wholly anaerobic. The formation of lactate is the fate of *some* of the pyruvate formed from glucose under conditions of maximum muscle exertion when oxygen is limiting, but as much as possible will continue to undergo complete oxidation.

Many tumours have a poor blood supply and hence a low capacity for oxidative metabolism, so that much of the energy-yielding metabolism in the tumour is indeed anaerobic. Lactate produced by anaerobic glycolysis in tumours is exported to the liver for gluconeogenesis; as discussed in §9.2.1.4, this increased cycling of glucose between anaerobic glycolysis in the tumour and gluconeogenesis in the liver may account for much of the weight loss (cachexia) that is seen in patients with advanced cancer. There is a net cost of $4 \times$ ATP per mole of glucose metabolized anaerobically and resynthesized in the liver.

Truly anaerobic glycolysis does occur in microorganisms that are capable of living in the absence of oxygen. Here there are two possible fates for the pyruvate formed from glucose, both of which involve the oxidation of NADH to NAD^+:

- *Reduction to lactate, as occurs in human muscle*: This is the pathway in lactic acid bacteria, which are responsible for the fermentation of lactose in milk to form yogurt and cheese, and also for the gastrointestinal discomfort after consumption of lactose in people who lack intestinal lactase (see §6.2.2.2).
- *Decarboxylation and reduction to ethanol*: This is the pathway of fermentation in yeast, which is exploited to produce alcoholic beverages. Human gastrointestinal bacteria normally produce lactate and other fatty acids rather than ethanol.

7.4.2.2 *The oxidation of pyruvate to acetyl CoA*

The first step in the complete oxidation of pyruvate is a complex reaction in which carbon dioxide is lost, and the resulting two-carbon compound is oxidized to acetate. The oxidation involves the reduction of NAD^+ to NADH. Since 2 mol of pyruvate are formed from each mole of glucose, this step represents the formation of 2 mol of NADH, equivalent to $6 \times$ ATP for each mole of glucose metabolized. The acetate is released from the enzyme esterified to coenzyme A, as acetyl CoA (see Figure 7.7). (Coenzyme A is derived from the vitamin pantothenic acid; see §12.2.12.)

The decarboxylation and oxidation of pyruvate to form acetyl CoA requires the coenzyme thiamin diphosphate, which is formed from vitamin B_1 (see §12.2.5). In thiamin deficiency this reaction is impaired, and deficient subjects are unable to metabolize glucose normally. Especially after a test dose of glucose or moderate exercise, they develop high blood concentrations of pyruvate and lactate. In some cases this may be severe enough to result in life-threatening acidosis.

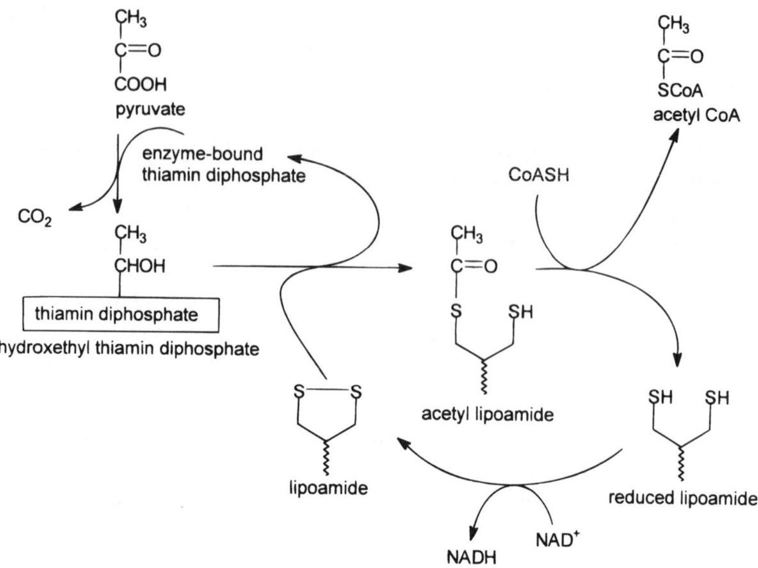

Figure 7.7 The reaction of pyruvate dehydrogenase.

7.4.2.3 *Complete oxidation of acetyl CoA: the citric acid cycle*

The acetate part of acetyl CoA undergoes a stepwise oxidation to carbon dioxide and water in a cyclic pathway, the citric acid cycle, shown in Figures 7.8 and 7.9. For each mole of acetyl CoA oxidized in this pathway, there is a yield of:

- 3 × NAD^+ reduced to NADH, equivalent to 9 × ATP
- 1 × flavoprotein reduced, equivalent to 2 × ADP
- 1 × GDP phosphorylated to GTP, equivalent to 1 × ATP

This is a total of 12 × ATP for each mole of acetyl CoA oxidized; since 2 mol of acetyl CoA are formed from each mole of glucose, this cycle yields 24 × ATP for each mole of glucose oxidized.

Although it appears complex at first sight, the citric acid cycle is a relatively simple pathway. A four-carbon compound, oxaloacetate, reacts with acetyl CoA to form a six-carbon compound, citric acid. The cycle is then a series of steps in which these two carbon atoms are oxidized and released as carbon dioxide, eventually reforming oxaloacetate. The CoA of acetyl CoA is released, and is available for further formation of acetyl CoA from pyruvate.

The citric acid cycle is also involved in the oxidation of acetyl CoA arising from other sources – mainly from the oxidation of fatty acids (see §7.5.2), but also the oxidation of ketones in fasting and starvation (see §7.5.3) and those amino acids that give rise to acetyl CoA (see §10.3.2).

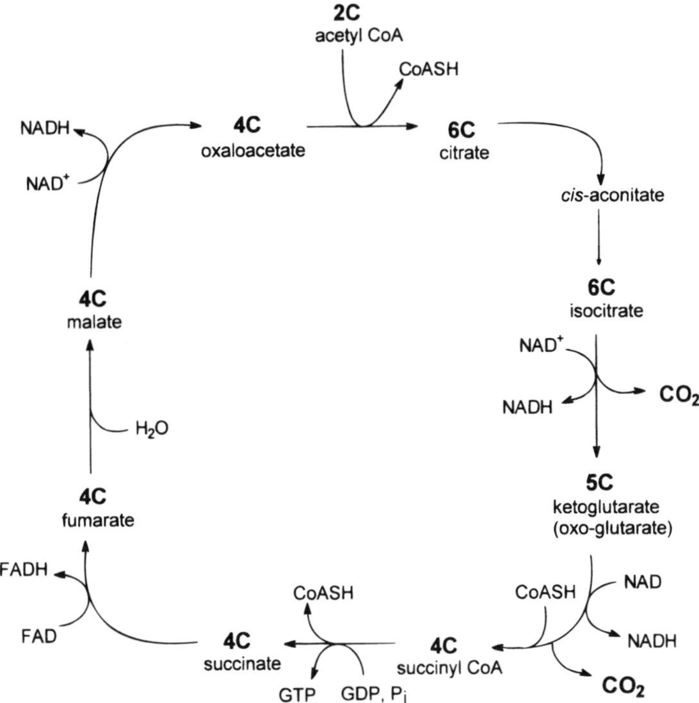

Figure 7.8 An overview of the citric acid cycle.

This cycle is an important central metabolic pathway, providing the link between carbohydrate, fat and amino acid metabolism. Many of the intermediates can be used for the synthesis of other compounds – for example, oxoglutarate and oxaloacetate can give rise to the amino acids glutamate and aspartate respectively; citrate is used as the source of acetyl CoA for fatty acid synthesis in the cytosol in the fed state (see §7.6.1) and oxaloacetate is an important precursor for glucose synthesis in the fasting state (see §7.7).

Obviously, if oxaloacetate is removed from the cycle for glucose synthesis, it must be replaced, since if there is not enough oxaloacetate available to form citrate, the rate of acetyl CoA metabolism will slow down. Although the cycle acts to interconvert the various intermediates, it cannot act as a net source of compounds unless there is some source of one of the intermediates (any one of them will do) to replace what is being lost. As discussed in §10.3.2, a variety of amino acids give rise to citric cycle intermediates such as oxoglutarate, fumarate and oxaloacetate.

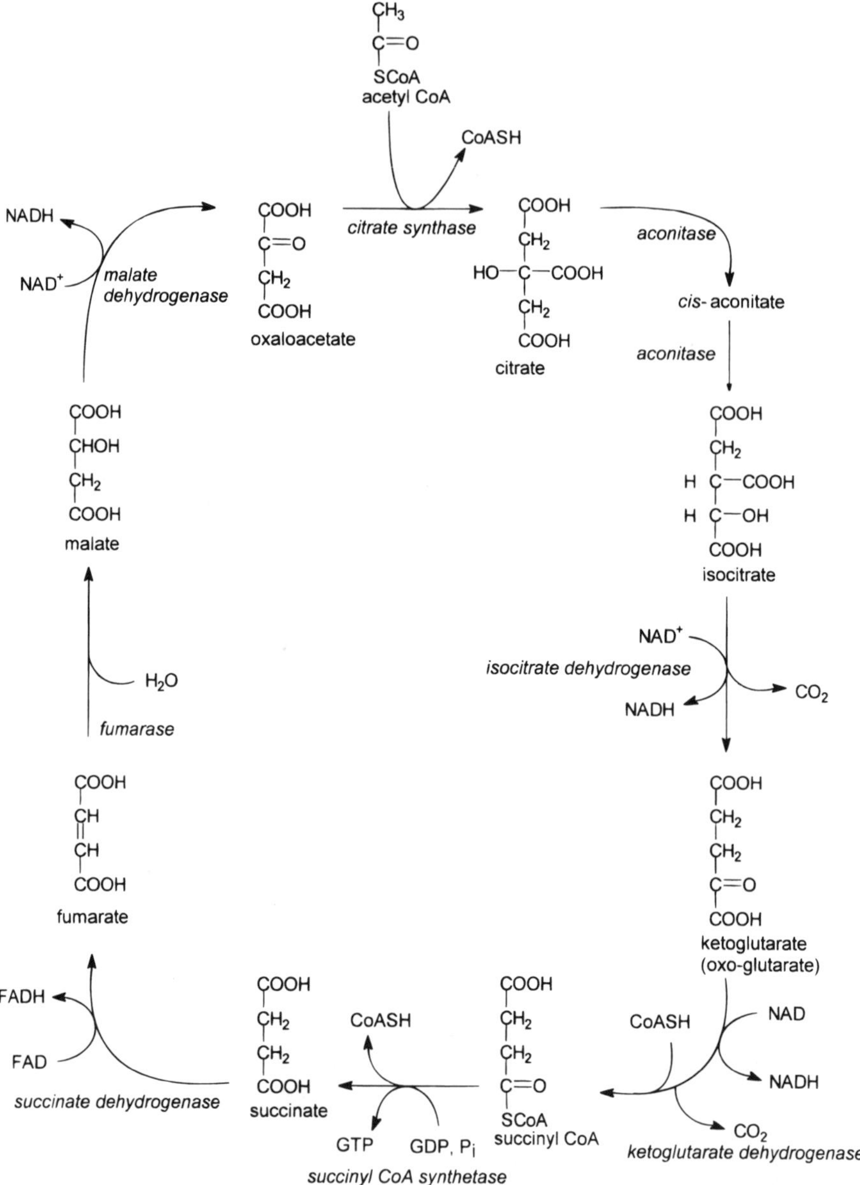

Figure 7.9 The citric acid cycle.

7.5 The metabolism of fats

As shown in Figure 7.10, fatty acids may be made available to cells in two ways:

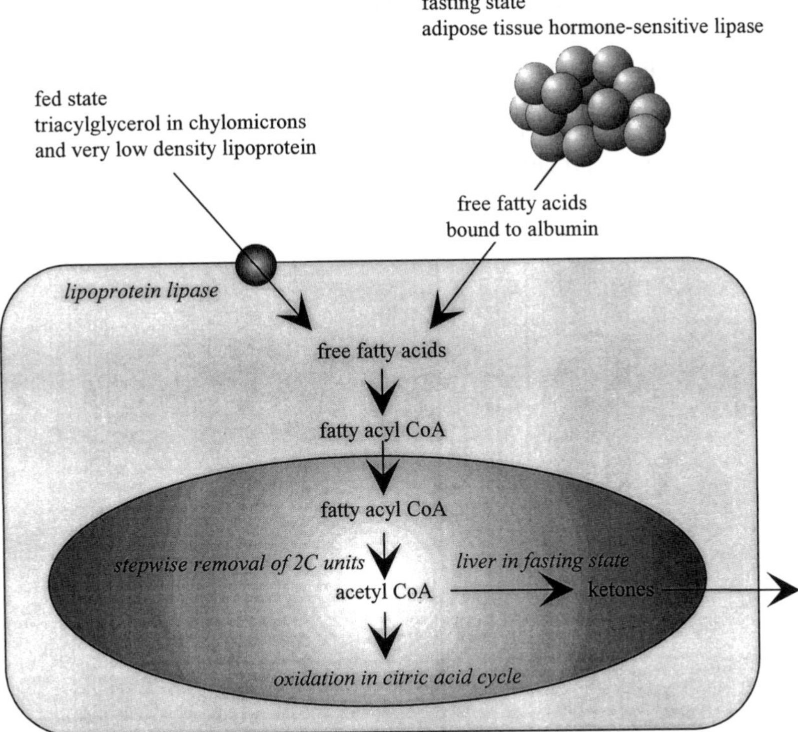

Figure 7.10 An overview of fatty acid metabolism.

- In the fed state, chylomicrons assembled in the small intestine (see §6.3.2.2) and low-density lipoproteins exported from the liver (see §7.6.1.2) bind to the cell surface, where lipoprotein lipase catalyses hydrolysis of triacylglycerols to glycerol and free fatty acids.
- In the fasting state, hormone-sensitive lipase in adipose tissue is activated in response to glucagon (see §7.3.2 and §11.4.1) and catalyses the hydrolysis of triacylglycerol, releasing free fatty acids into the bloodstream, where they bind to albumin, and are transported to tissues.

The glycerol is phosphorylated and converted to dihydroxyacetone phosphate (see Figure 7.4), which may be used either as a metabolic fuel (in the fed state) or for gluconeogenesis (in the fasting state).

The fatty acids are oxidized in the mitochondria by the β-oxidation pathway, in which two carbon atoms at a time are removed from the fatty acid chain as acetyl CoA. This acetyl CoA then enters the citric acid cycle, together with that arising from the metabolism of pyruvate.

7.5.1 Carnitine and the transport of fatty acids into the mitochondrion

As shown in Figure 7.11, fatty acids are esterified with coenzyme A, forming acyl CoA, as they enter the cell. This is necessary to protect the cell membranes against the lytic action of free fatty acids (see §3.5.3). Fatty acyl CoA will cross the outer mitochondrial membrane, but cannot cross the inner mem-

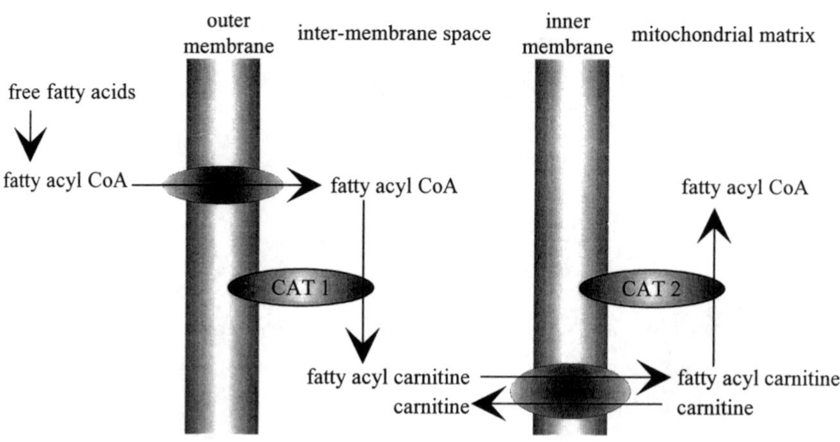

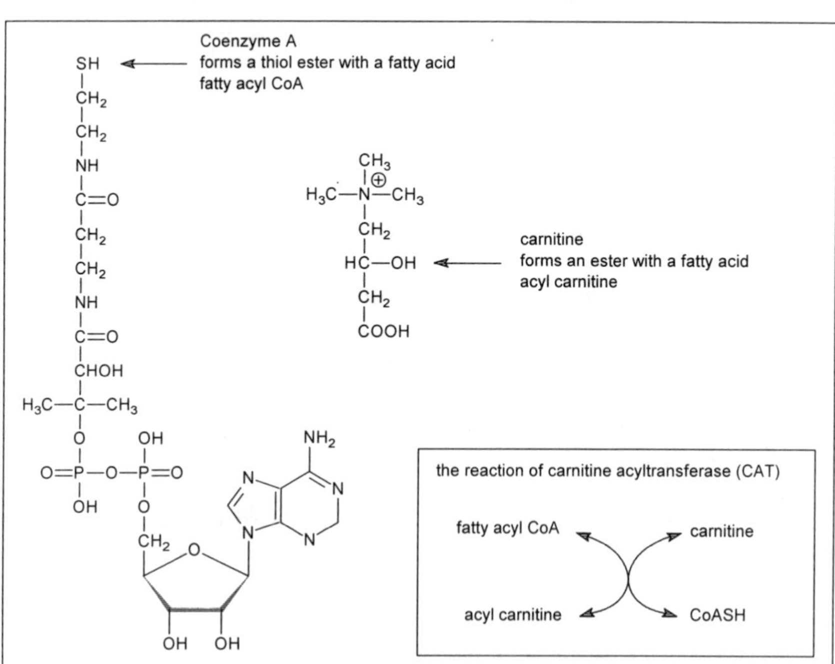

Figure 7.11 The role of carnitine in the uptake of fatty acids into the mitochondrion.

brane into the matrix, where the enzymes for β-oxidation are located.

On the inner face of the outer mitochondrial membrane, the fatty acid is transferred from CoA onto carnitine, forming acylcarnitine. This can cross the inner mitochondrial membrane, but only on a counter-transport system, which takes in acylcarnitine in exchange for free carnitine being returned to the intermembrane space. Once inside the mitochondrial inner membrane, acylcarnitine transfers the acyl group onto CoA. This provides a regulation of the uptake of fatty acids into the mitochondrion for oxidation. As long as there is free CoA available in the mitochondrial matrix, fatty acids can be taken up, and the carnitine returned to the outer membrane for uptake of more fatty acids. However, if most of the CoA in the mitochondrion is acylated, then there is no need for further fatty uptake immediately, and indeed, it is not possible.

This carnitine shuttle also serves to prevent uptake into the mitochondrion (and hence oxidation) of fatty acids synthesized in the cytosol in the fed state; malonyl CoA (an intermediate in fatty acid synthesis, see §7.6.1) is a potent inhibitor of carnitine acyltransferase in the outer mitochondrial membrane.

7.5.2 *The β-oxidation of fatty acids*

Once it has entered the mitochondria, fatty acyl CoA undergoes a series of four reactions, as shown in Figure 7.12, which result in the cleavage of the fatty acid molecule to give acetyl CoA and a new fatty acyl CoA which is two carbons shorter than the initial substrate. This new, shorter, fatty acyl CoA is then a substrate for the same sequence of reactions, which is repeated until the

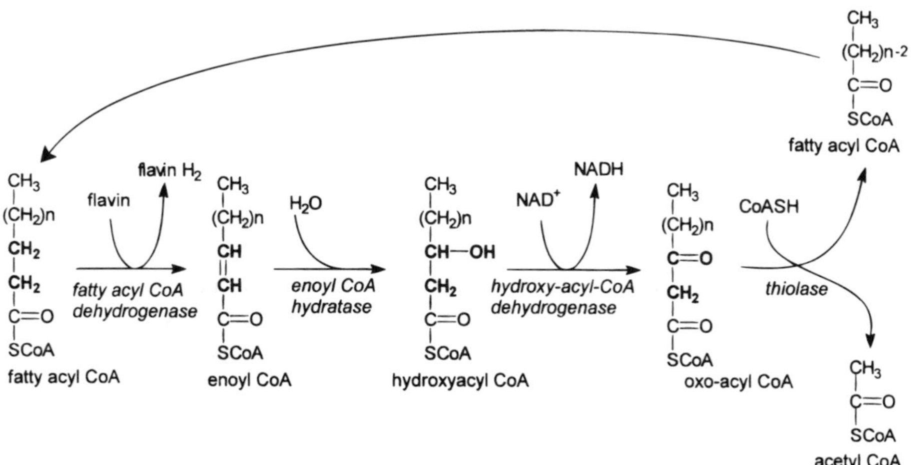

Figure 7.12 The β-oxidation of fatty acids.

final result is cleavage to yield two molecules of acetyl CoA. This is the pathway of β-oxidation, so called because it is the β-carbon of the fatty acid (carbon-3, see §3.7) that undergoes oxidation.

The reactions of β-oxidation are chemically the same as those in the conversion of succinate to oxaloacetate in the citric acid cycle (see Figure 7.9):

1 The first step is removal of two hydrogens from the fatty acid, to form a carbon–carbon double bond: an oxidation reaction that yields a reduced flavin, so for each double bond formed in this way there is a yield of 2 × ATP.
2 The newly formed double bond in the fatty acyl CoA then reacts with water, yielding a hydroxyl group: a hydration reaction.
3 The hydroxylated fatty acyl CoA undergoes a second oxidation in which the hydroxyl group is oxidized to an oxo group, yielding NADH (equivalent to 3 × ATP).
4 The oxo-acyl CoA is then cleaved by reaction with CoA, to form acetyl CoA and the shorter fatty acyl CoA, which undergoes the same sequence of reactions.

The acetyl CoA formed by β-oxidation then enters the citric acid cycle (see Figure 7.9). Almost all of the metabolically important fatty acids have an even number of carbon atoms, so that the final cycle of β-oxidation is the conversion of a four-carbon fatty acyl CoA (butyryl CoA) to two molecules of acetyl CoA.

7.5.3 *Ketone bodies*

Most tissues have a limited capacity for fatty acid oxidation, and in the fasting state cannot meet their energy requirements from fatty acid oxidation alone. By contrast, the liver is capable of forming considerably more acetyl CoA from fatty acids than is required for its own metabolism. It takes up fatty acids from the circulation and oxidizes them to acetyl CoA, then exports the four-carbon ketones formed from acetyl CoA to other tissues (especially muscle) for use as a metabolic fuel.

The reactions involved are shown in Figure 7.13. Acetoacetyl CoA is formed by reaction between two molecules of acetyl CoA. This is essentially the reverse of the final reaction of fatty acid β-oxidation (see Figure 7.12). Acetoacetyl CoA then reacts with a further molecule of acetyl CoA to form hydroxymethyl-glutaryl CoA, which then undergoes cleavage to release acetyl CoA and acetoacetate.

As well as being an intermediate in the synthesis of ketone bodies, hydroxymethyl-glutaryl CoA is the precursor for the synthesis of cholesterol (see §6.3.1.3). Inhibitors of the enzyme which commits hydroxymethyl-glutaryl CoA to cholesterol synthesis (hydroxymethyl-glutaryl CoA reductase) are

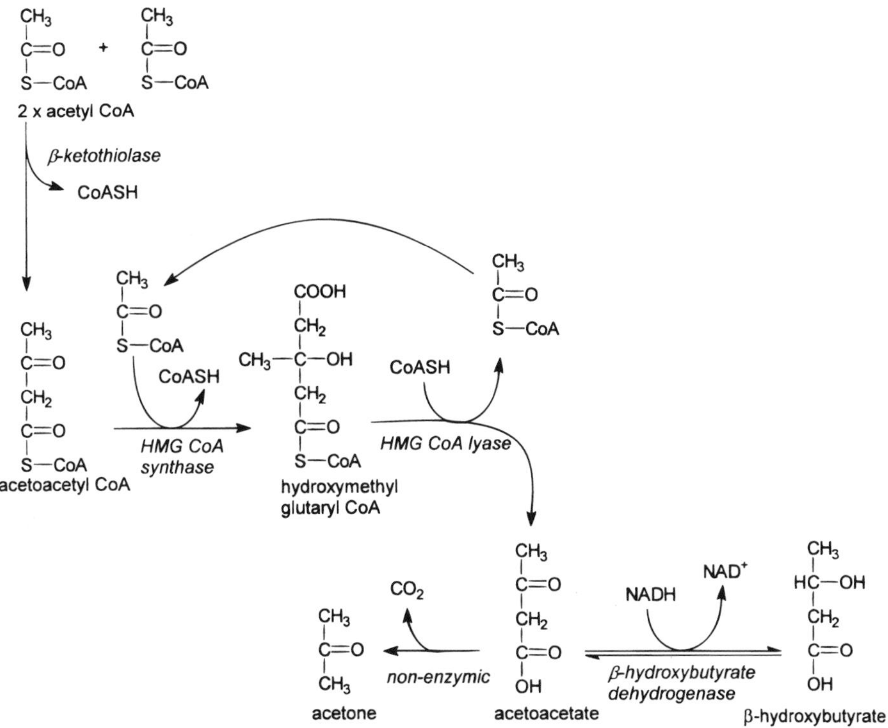

Figure 7.13 The formation of ketones in the liver.

commonly used in the treatment of patients with dangerously high plasma concentrations of cholesterol due to a genetic defect in the regulation of cholesterol synthesis.

Acetoacetate is chemically unstable and undergoes a non-enzymic reaction to yield acetone, which is metabolically useless. There is no pathway for its utilization; it is excreted in the urine and in exhaled air – a waste of valuable metabolic fuel reserves in the fasting state. To avoid this, much of the acetoacetate is reduced to *β*-hydroxybutyrate before being released from the liver.

The pathway for the utilization of *β*-hydroxybutyrate and acetoacetate in tissues other than the liver is shown in Figure 7.14. The utilization of acetoacetate is controlled by the activity of the citric acid cycle. The reaction of acetoacetate succinyl CoA transferase provides an alternative to the reaction of succinyl CoA synthase (see Figure 7.9), and there will only be an adequate supply of succinyl CoA to permit conversion of acetoacetate to acetoacetyl CoA as long as the rate of citric acid cycle activity is adequate.

Acetoacetate, *β*-hydroxybutyrate and acetone are collectively known as the ketone bodies, and the occurrence of increased concentrations of these three compounds in the bloodstream is known as ketosis. Although acetone and

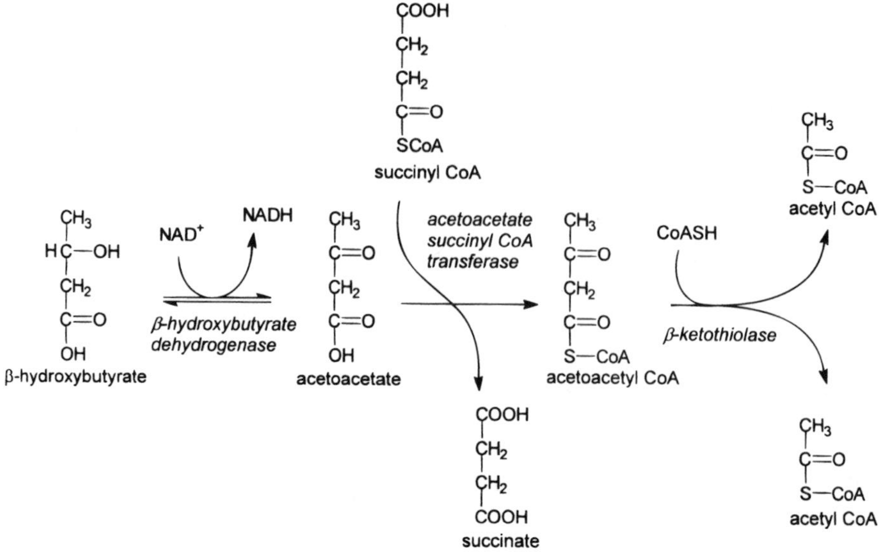

Figure 7.14 The metabolism of ketones in extrahepatic tissues.

acetoacetate are chemically ketones, having the —C=O grouping, hydroxy-butyrate is not chemically a ketone. It is classified with the other two because of its metabolic relationship. (See §11.5 for a discussion of the problems of ketoacidosis in uncontrolled diabetes mellitus.)

7.6 Tissue reserves of metabolic fuels

In the fed state, as well as providing for immediate energy needs, substrates are converted into storage compounds for use in the fasting state. There are two main stores of metabolic fuels:

- triacylglycerols in adipose tissue
- glycogen as a carbohydrate reserve in liver and muscle

In addition, there is an increase in the synthesis of tissue proteins in response to a meal, so that there is some increase in the total body content of protein. This can also be used as a metabolic fuel in the fasting state.

In the fasting state, which is the normal state between meals, these reserves are mobilized and used. Glycogen is a source of glucose, while adipose tissue provides both fatty acids and glycerol from triacylglycerol. Some of the relatively labile protein laid down in response to meals is also mobilized in fasting.

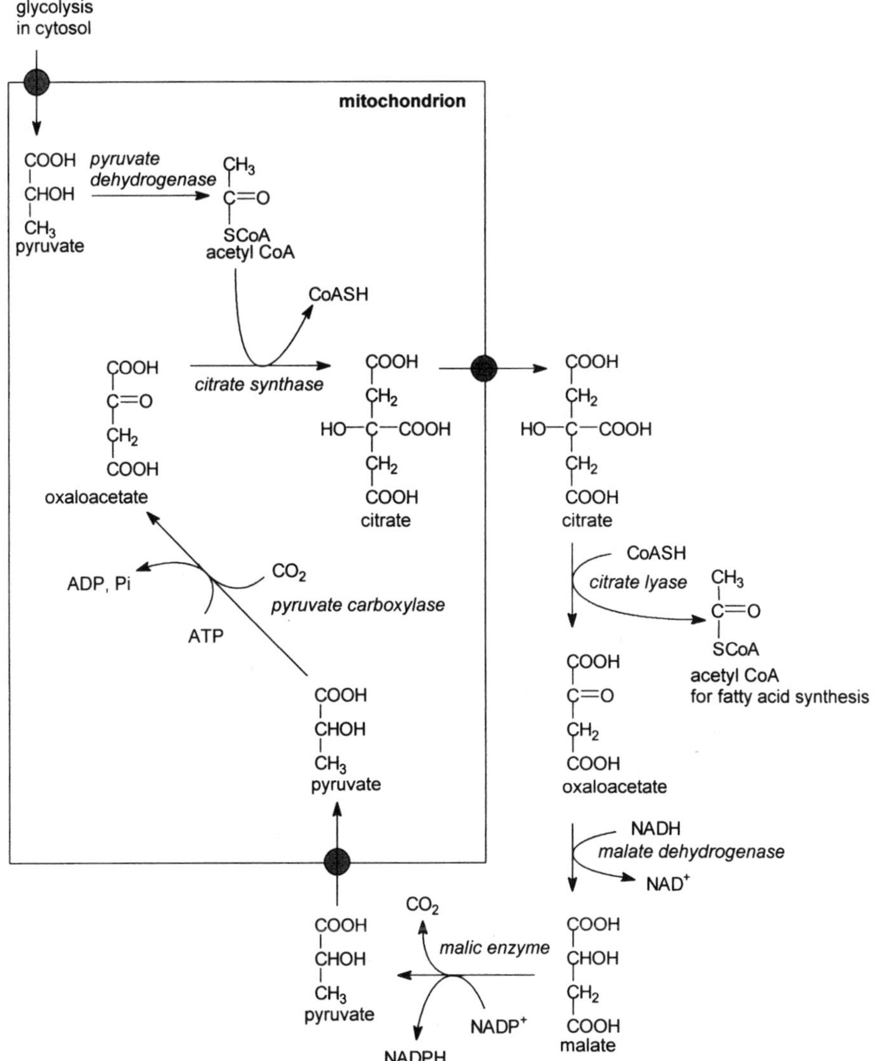

Figure 7.15 The source of acetyl CoA for fatty acid synthesis in the cytosol.

7.6.1 *Synthesis of fatty acids and triacylglycerols*

Fatty acids are synthesized by the successive addition of two-carbon units from acetyl CoA, followed by reduction. Unlike β-oxidation, which occurs in the mitochondrial matrix, fatty acid synthesis occurs in the cytosol. The enzymes required for fatty acid synthesis form a multi-enzyme complex, arranged in a ring around a central acyl carrier protein (ACP), which carries the growing fatty acid chain from one enzyme to the next. The functional group of the acyl carrier protein is the same as that of CoA, derived from the vitamin pantothenic acid and cysteamine (see §12.2.12).

The only source of acetyl CoA is in the mitochondrial matrix and, as discussed in §7.5.1, acetyl CoA cannot cross the mitochondrial inner membrane. For fatty acid synthesis, citrate is formed inside the mitochondria by reaction between acetyl CoA and oxaloacetate (see Figure 7.15), and is then transported out of the mitochondria, to undergo cleavage in the cytosol to yield acetyl CoA and oxaloacetate. The acetyl CoA is used for fatty acid synthesis, while the oxaloacetate (indirectly) returns to the mitochondria to maintain citric acid cycle activity. This means that fatty acid synthesis will occur only when there is a greater rate of formation of citrate than is required for energy-yielding metabolism – i.e. when there is a ready availability of substrates, in the fed state. Oxaloacetate cannot re-enter the mitochondrion directly. As shown in Figure 7.15, it is reduced to malate, which then undergoes oxidative decarboxylation to pyruvate, linked to the reduction of $NADP^+$ to NADPH. The resultant pyruvate enters the mitochondrion, and is carboxylated to oxaloacetate in a reaction catalysed by pyruvate carboxylase (see §7.7).

As shown in Figure 7.16, the first reaction in the synthesis of fatty acids is carboxylation of acetyl CoA to malonyl CoA. This is a biotin-dependent reaction (see §12.2.11). The malonyl group is transferred onto an acyl carrier protein, and then reacts with the growing fatty acid chain, bound to the central acyl carrier protein of the fatty acid synthase complex. The carbon dioxide that was added to form malonyl CoA is lost in this reaction. For the first cycle of fatty acid synthesis, the central acyl carrier protein carries an acetyl group, and the product of reaction with malonyl CoA is acetoacetyl-ACP; in subsequent reaction cycles, it is the growing fatty acid chain that occupies the central ACP, and the product of reaction with malonyl CoA is a keto-acyl-ACP.

The keto-acyl-ACP is then reduced to yield a hydroxyl group. In turn, this is dehydrated to yield a carbon–carbon double bond, which is reduced to yield a saturated fatty acid chain. Thus, the sequence of chemical reactions is the reverse of that in β-oxidation (see Figure 7.12). For both reduction reactions in fatty acid synthesis, NADPH is the hydrogen donor. One source of this NADPH is the pentose phosphate pathway (see §7.4.1.1) and the other is the indirect pathway, by which the oxaloacetate released by the citrate cleavage enzyme re-enters the mitochondrion as pyruvate (see Figure 7.15).

7.6.1.1 *Unsaturated fatty acids*

Although fatty acid synthesis involves the formation of an unsaturated intermediate, the next step, reduction to the saturated fatty acid derivative, is an obligatory part of the reaction sequence and cannot be omitted. The product of the fatty acid synthase multi-enzyme complex is always a saturated fatty acid, normally palmitate (C16). Some unsaturated fatty acids can be synthe-

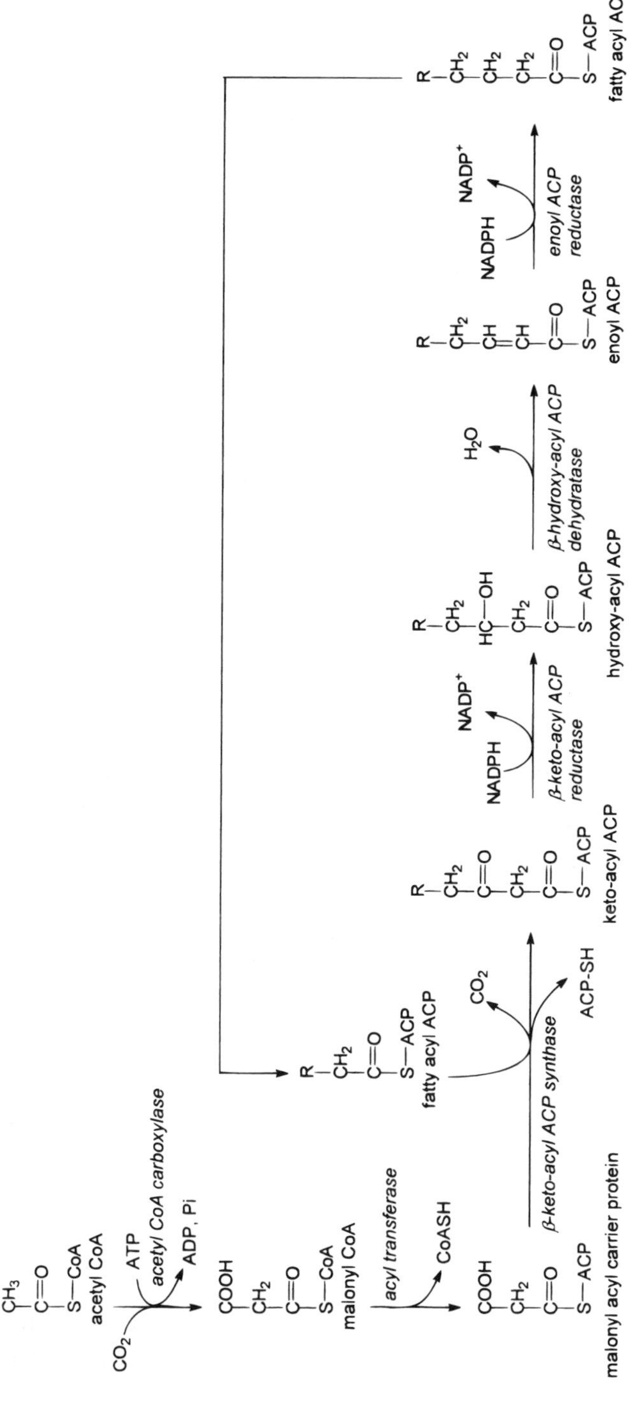

Figure 7.16 The synthesis of fatty acids.

sized from saturated fatty acids, by the removal of hydrogen to yield a carbon–carbon double bond. This fatty acid desaturation is a mitochondrial process, as is the elongation of fatty acids to longer than C16.

As discussed in §6.3.1.1, there is a dietary requirement for two unsaturated fatty acids which cannot be synthesized in the body: linoleic (C18:2 ω6) and α-linolenic (C18:3 ω3) acids. Each of these can undergo chain elongation and further desaturation in the mitochondrion, to yield the long-chain polyunsaturated fatty acids that are precursors of the prostaglandins.

7.6.1.2 *Synthesis of triacylglycerols*

The storage lipids in adipose tissue are triacylglycerols: glycerol esterified with three molecules of fatty acids; as discussed in §6.3.1, the three fatty acids in a triacylglycerol molecule are not always the same, and the fatty acid at carbon-2 is usually unsaturated.

Triacylglycerols are synthesized mainly in the liver, adipose tissue and small intestinal mucosa, as well as lactating mammary gland. As shown in Figure 7.17, the substrates for triacylglycerol synthesis are fatty acyl CoA esters (formed by reaction between fatty acids and CoA, linked to the conversion of ATP $\rightarrow$ AMP + pyrophosphate) and glycerol phosphate. The main source of glycerol phosphate is by reduction of dihydroxyacetone phosphate (an intermediate in glycolysis, see Figure 7.4), although the liver can also phosphorylate glycerol to glycerol phosphate.

Two molecules of fatty acid are esterified to the free hydroxyl groups of glycerol phosphate, by transfer from fatty acyl CoA, forming monoacylglycerol phosphate and then diacylglycerol phosphate (or phosphatidic acid). Diacylglycerol phosphate is then hydrolysed to diacylglycerol and phosphate before reaction with the third molecule of fatty acyl CoA to yield triacylglycerol. (The diacylglycerol phosphate can also be used for the synthesis of phospholipids; see §6.3.1.2).

It is obvious from Figure 7.17 that triacylglycerol synthesis incurs a considerable ATP cost; if the fatty acids are being synthesized from glucose, then overall some 20 per cent of the energy yield of the carbohydrate is expended in synthesizing triacylglycerol reserves. The energy cost is lower if dietary fatty acids are being esterified to form triacylglycerols.

Triacylglycerols synthesized in the liver are assembled into low-density lipoproteins, together with cholesterol, for export to extrahepatic tissues; as discussed in §6.3.2.2, triacylglycerols synthesized in the intestinal mucosa are assembled into chylomicrons and enter the lymphatic system.

7.6.2 ***Glycogen***

In the fed state, glycogen is synthesized from glucose in both liver and muscle. The reaction is a stepwise addition of glucose units onto the glycogen that is already present.

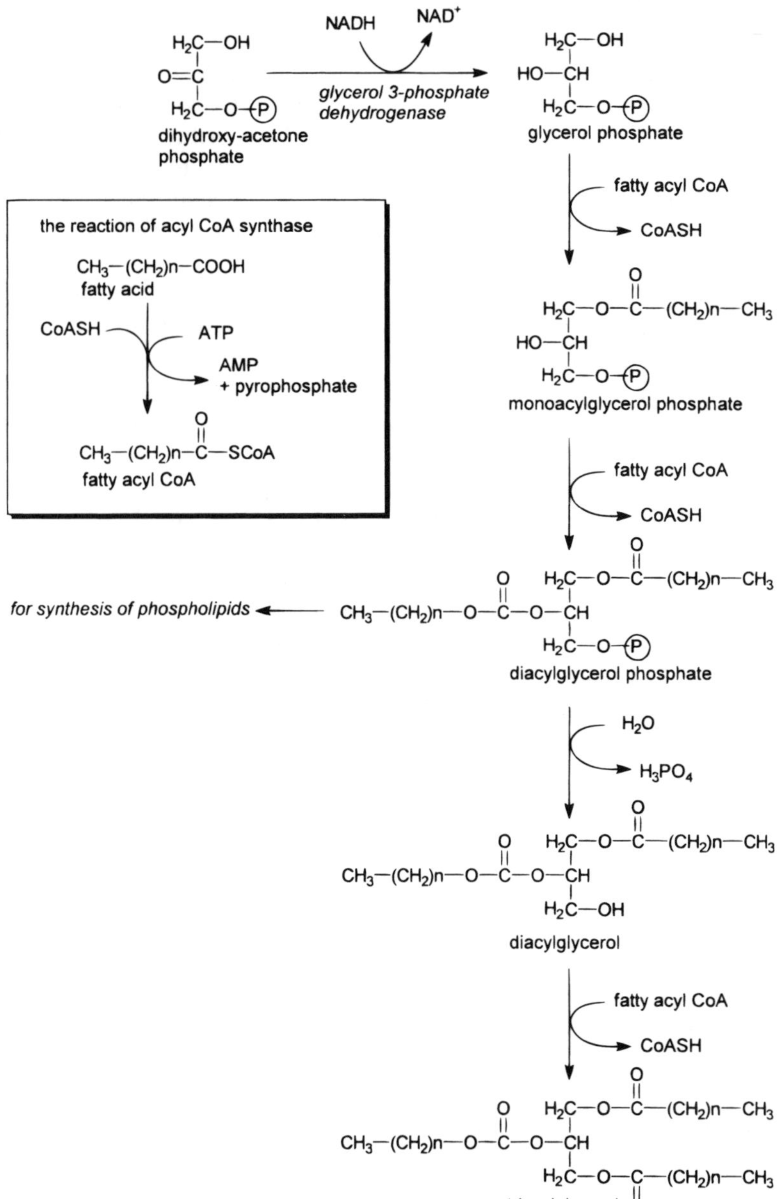

Figure 7.17 The synthesis of triacylglycerol.

As shown in Figure 7.18, glycogen synthesis involves the intermediate formation of UDP-glucose (uridine diphosphate glucose) by reaction between glucose 1–phosphate and UTP (uridine triphosphate). As each glucose unit is added to the growing glycogen chain, so UDP is released, and must be rephosphorylated to UTP by reaction with ATP. There is thus a significant cost of ATP in the synthesis of glycogen: 2 mol of ATP are converted to ADP + phosphate for each glucose unit added, and overall the energy cost of glycogen synthesis may account for 5 per cent of the energy yield of the carbohydrate stored.

Glycogen synthetase forms only the straight chains of glycogen. The branch points are introduced by the transfer of 6–10 glucose units in a chain from carbon-4 to carbon-6 of the glucose unit at the branch point.

In the fasting state, glycogen is broken down by the removal of glucose units, one at a time, from the many ends of the molecule. As shown in Figure 7.3, the reaction is a phosphorolysis – cleavage of the glycoside link between two glucose molecules by the introduction of phosphate. The product is glucose 1–phosphate, which is then converted to glucose 6–phosphate. In the

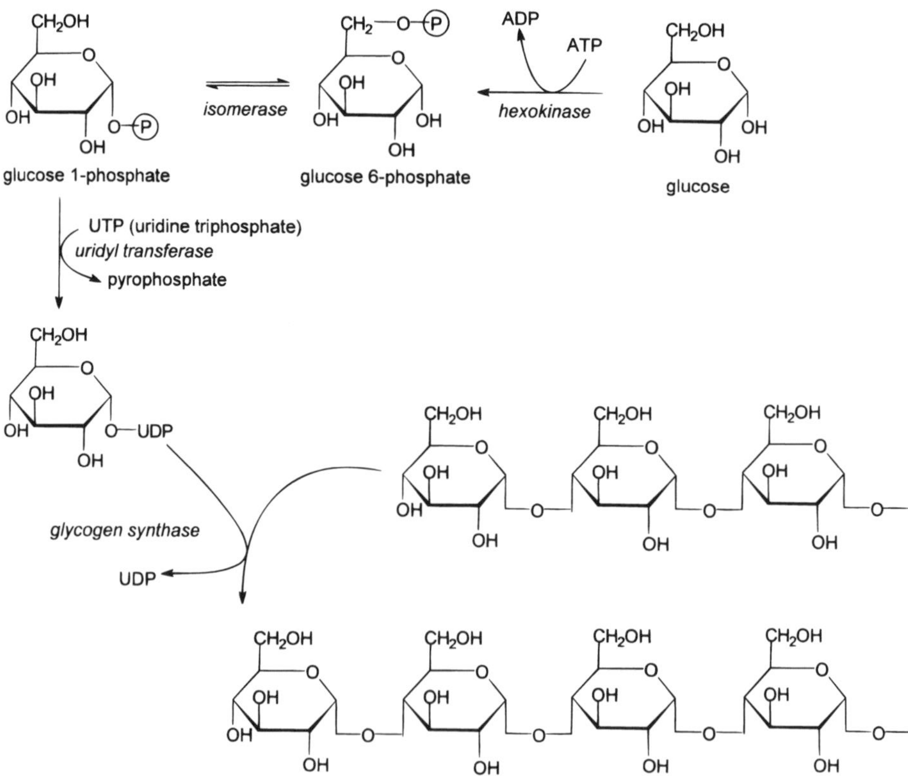

Figure 7.18 The synthesis of glycogen (for the structure of UTP, see Figure 5.2).

liver glucose 6–phosphatase catalyses the hydrolysis of glucose 6–phosphate to free glucose, which is exported for use by the brain and red blood cells. Muscle cannot release free glucose from the breakdown of glycogen, since it lacks glucose 6–phosphatase.

7.7 Gluconeogenesis: the synthesis of glucose from non-carbohydrate precursors

Because the brain and red blood cells are wholly reliant on glucose as their metabolic fuel, there is a need to maintain the blood concentration of glucose between about 3 and 5 mmol per L, even in the fasting state. If the plasma concentration of glucose falls below about 2 mmol per L there is a loss of consciousness: hypoglycaemic coma.

To a considerable extent the plasma concentration of glucose is maintained in short-term fasting by the use of liver glycogen as a source of free glucose, and by releasing free fatty acids from adipose tissues, and ketones from the liver, which are preferentially used by muscle, so sparing such glucose as is available, for use by the brain (see §11.4.2). In the fasting state, muscle uses its glycogen reserves to produce pyruvate (i.e. glycolysis), and then exports the three-carbon unit as the amino acid alanine (see §10.3.2) to the liver, where it is a substrate for gluconeogenesis.

However, there is only a relatively small amount of glycogen in the body, and the total body pool would be exhausted within 12–18 hours of fasting if there were no other source of glucose. The process of gluconeogenesis is the synthesis of glucose from non-carbohydrate precursors: amino acids from the breakdown of protein, and the glycerol of triacylglycerols. It is important to note that, although acetyl CoA, and hence fatty acids, can be synthesized from pyruvate (and therefore from carbohydrates), the decarboxylation of pyruvate to acetyl CoA cannot be reversed. Pyruvate cannot be formed from acetyl CoA. Since two molecules of carbon dioxide are formed for each two-carbon acetate unit metabolized in the citric acid cycle (see Figure 7.8), there can be no net formation of oxaloacetate from acetate. **It is not possible to synthesize glucose from acetyl CoA, and fatty acids cannot serve as a precursor for glucose synthesis under any circumstances.**

The pathway of gluconeogenesis is essentially the reverse of the pathway of glycolysis (Figure 7.4). However, at three steps there are separate enzymes involved in the breakdown of glucose (glycolysis) and gluconeogenesis. As discussed in §7.4.1, the reactions of pyruvate kinase, phosphofructokinase and hexokinase cannot readily be reversed (i.e. they have equilibria that are strongly in the direction of the formation of pyruvate, fructose bisphosphate and glucose 6–phosphate, respectively).

There are therefore separate enzymes, under distinct metabolic control, for the reverse of each of these reactions in gluconeogenesis:

- Pyruvate is converted to phosphoenolpyruvate for glucose synthesis by a two-step reaction, with the intermediate formation of oxaloacetate. As shown in Figure 7.19, pyruvate is carboxylated to oxaloacetate in an ATP-dependent reaction in which the vitamin biotin (see §12.2.11) is the coenzyme. This reaction can also be used to replenish oxaloacetate in the citric acid cycle when intermediates have been withdrawn for use in other pathways, and is involved in the return of oxaloacetate from the cytosol to the mitochondrion in fatty acid synthesis (see Figure 7.15). Oxaloacetate then undergoes a phosphorylation reaction, in which it also loses carbon dioxide, to form phosphoenolpyruvate. The phosphate donor for this reaction is GTP.
- Fructose bisphosphate is hydrolysed to fructose 6–phosphate by a simple hydrolysis reaction catalysed by the enzyme fructose bisphosphatase.
- Glucose 6–phosphate is hydrolysed to free glucose and phosphate by the action of glucose 6–phosphatase. The glucose is then exported from the liver for use by the nervous system and other tissues. Glucose 1–phosphate arising from the phosphorolysis of liver glycogen can readily be converted to glucose 6–phosphate, and then hydrolysed to glucose for release into the bloodstream.

The other reactions of glycolysis are readily reversible, and the overall direction of metabolism, either glycolysis or gluconeogenesis, depends mainly on the relative activities of phosphofructokinase and fructose bisphosphatase, as discussed in §11.4.2.

Many of the products of amino acid metabolism can also be used for gluconeogenesis as discussed in §10.3.2, since they are sources of pyruvate or one of

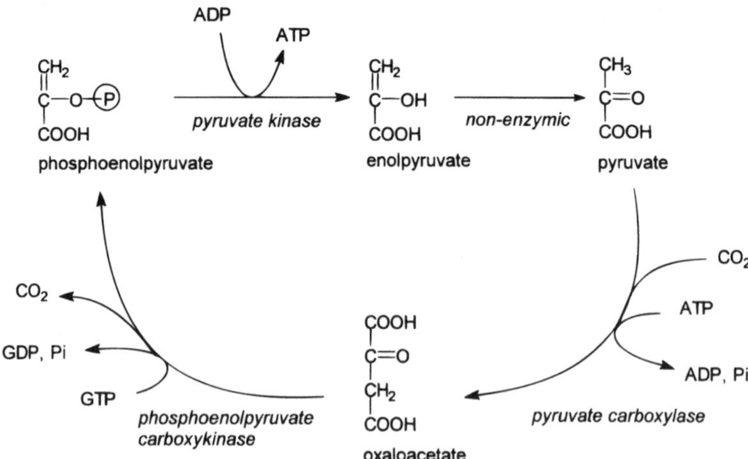

Figure 7.19 The utilization of pyruvate for gluconeogenesis, bypassing the irreversible reaction of pyruvate kinase.

the intermediates in the citric acid cycle, and hence give rise to oxaloacetate. The requirement for gluconeogenesis from amino acids, in order to maintain a supply of glucose for the brain and red blood cells, explains why there is often a considerable loss of muscle in prolonged fasting or starvation, even if there are apparently adequate reserves of adipose tissue to meet energy needs.

The controlling reaction in gluconeogenesis from amino acids is the conversion of oxaloacetate to phosphoenolpyruvate, catalysed by phosphoenolpyruvate carboxykinase (see Figure 7.19). Unusually, this reaction utilizes GTP, rather than ATP, as the phosphate donor. This regulates the withdrawal of oxaloacetate for gluconeogenesis, and ensures that there is always an adequate pool of oxaloacetate for maintenance of citric acid cycle activity. The only mitochondrial reaction for the phosphorylation of GDP to GTP is the reaction of succinyl CoA synthase, in the citric acid cycle. Therefore, if the rate of citric acid cycle activity falls, as a result of depletion of intermediates, there will be inadequate formation of GTP, and it will not be possible to withdraw oxaloacetate for gluconeogenesis.

8

Overweight and Obesity

As discussed in §7.2, if the intake of metabolic fuels (in other words the total intake of food) is greater than is required to meet energy expenditure, the result is storage of the excess, largely as triacylglycerols in adipose tissue.

It is normal and desirable to have some reserves of fat in the body. In lean men about 16 per cent of body weight is fat at age 25, increasing to 24 per cent by age 65. In lean women, about 30 per cent of body weight is fat at age 25, increasing to about 36 per cent by age 65. This chapter is concerned with the problems associated with excessive accumulation of body fat: overweight and obesity.

8.1 Desirable body weight

Figure 8.1 shows the relationship between body weight and premature death. It is based on a study of 750 000 people, who were classified according to their percentage of the average weight of the study group, then followed for 15 years. There is a steady increase in mortality with increasing body weight above average, so that people who are 50–60 per cent over average weight are twice as likely to die prematurely as those of average weight.

People who were significantly below average weight at the beginning of the study were also slightly more at risk of premature death. However, this may be because those people who were significantly underweight were already seriously ill (see §9.2.1.4), rather than implying that a moderate degree of underweight is undesirable or poses any health hazards.

Figure 8.1 also shows that people whose weight was about 90 per cent of the average, were less likely to die prematurely than those of average weight. Such data make it possible to define a range of body weight, somewhat below average weight, which is associated with optimum life expectancy. The ranges of desirable weight for height, based on insurance company data of life expectancy, are shown in Table 8.1.

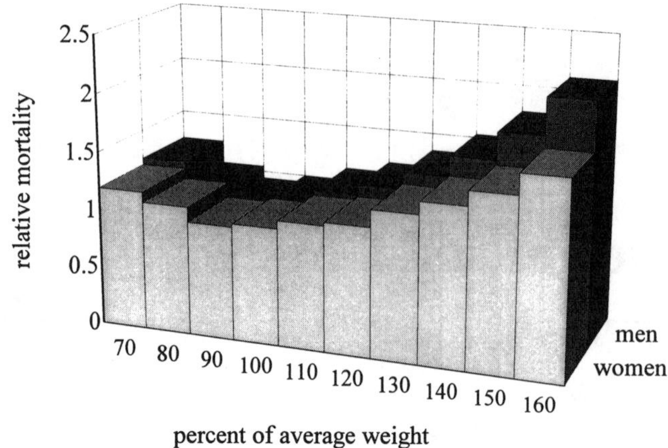

Figure 8.1 Body weight and premature death; mortality of 750 000 people over 15 years, relative to mortality at average weight = 1.0.

8.1.1 *Body mass index*

As an alternative to using tables of weight and height, it is possible to calculate a simple numerical index from height and weight, and use this to establish acceptable ranges. The most commonly used such index is the body mass index (BMI), sometimes also called Quetelet's index, after the man who first demonstrated its usefulness in nutritional studies.

Body mass index is calculated from the weight divided by the square of the height: BMI = weight (kg)/height^2 (m). The desirable range, associated with optimum life expectancy, is 20–25. As discussed in §9.1, values of BMI below 20 are associated with undernutrition. Table 8.2 shows the classification of overweight and obesity by BMI. For older people, there is some evidence that a higher body weight is associated with better health and survival; Table 8.3 shows the desirable ranges of BMI at different ages.

8.1.2 *Measurement of body fat*

Although weight for height, or BMI, is widely used to assess overweight and obesity, what is important for health and life expectancy is the body content of fat, and it is important to be able to determine the proportion of body weight that is fat. This is termed adiposity; several techniques are available for assessing adiposity, although most of them are research techniques and are inappropriate for routine screening of the general public.

Table 8.1 Ranges of weight for height

	Body weight (kg)		
	Desirable range	Obese	Severely obese
Height (cm)	BMI = 20 BMI = 25	BMI = 30	BMI = 40
150	45.0–56.3	67.5	90.0
152	46.2–57.8	69.3	92.4
154	47.4–59.3	71.1	94.9
156	48.7–60.8	73.0	97.3
158	49.9–62.4	74.9	99.9
160	51.2–64.0	76.8	102.4
162	52.5–65.6	78.7	105.0
164	53.8–67.2	80.7	107.6
166	55.1–68.9	82.7	110.2
168	56.4–70.6	84.7	112.9
170	57.8–72.3	86.7	115.6
172	59.2–74.0	88.8	118.3
174	60.6–75.7	90.8	121.1
176	62.0–77.4	92.9	123.9
178	63.4–79.2	95.1	126.7
180	64.8–81.0	97.2	129.6
182	66.2–82.8	99.4	132.5
184	67.7–84.6	101.6	135.4
186	69.2–86.5	103.8	138.4
188	70.7–88.4	106.0	141.4
190	72.2–90.3	108.3	144.4
192	73.7–92.2	110.6	147.5
194	75.3–94.1	112.9	150.5
196	76.8–96.0	115.2	153.7
198	78.4–98.0	117.6	156.8
200	80.0–100.0	120.0	160.0

BMI (body mass index) = weight (kg)/height^2 (m).

Table 8.2 Classification of overweight and obesity by body mass index

	BMI	Excess weight (kg)	% of desirable weight
Desirable	20–25	—	100
Acceptable but not desirable	25–27	< 5	100–110
Overweight	25–30	5–15	110–120
Obese	30–40	15–25	120–160
Severely obese	>40	>25	>160

Body mass index = weight (kg)/height^2 (m).

Table 8.3 Desirable ranges of body mass index with age

Age (years)	Desirable BMI
19–24	19–24
25–34	20–25
35–44	21–26
45–54	22–27
55–64	23–28
>65	24–29

Body mass index = weight (kg)/ height^2 (m).

8.1.2.1 *Determination of body density*

The density of body fat is 0.9 g per ml, and that of the fat-free body mass is 1.10 g per ml. This means that if the density of the body can be calculated, then the proportion of fat and lean tissue can be calculated.

Density is determined by weighing in air and then totally submerged in water (the density of water = 1.0 g per ml), or by determining the volume of the body by its displacement of water when submerged. Neither procedure is particularly pleasant for the experimental subject, and considerable precision is necessary in the measurements; at 10 per cent of body weight as fat, which is extremely low, density = 1.08 g per ml; at 50 per cent fat, which is very high, density = 1.00 g per ml. Direct determination of body density is the true standard, against which all the other techniques listed below must be calibrated.

8.1.2.2 *Determination of total body water or potassium*

The water content of fat (i.e. pure triacylglycerol, not adipose tissue) is zero and the fat-free mass of the body is 73 per cent water. The total amount of water in the body can be determined by giving a dose of water isotopically labelled with ^{2}H or ^{18}O (see §3.1.1) and then measuring the dilution of the label in urine or saliva.

An alternative approach is to measure the total body content of potassium; again fat contains no potassium, which occurs only in the fat-free mass of the body. There is a gender difference here: in males the fat-free mass contains 60 mmol potassium per kg, and in females 66 mmol per kg. The radioactive isotope of potassium, ^{40}K, occurs naturally as a small proportion of all potassium. It is a weak γ-emitter, and therefore total body potassium can be determined by measuring the γ-radiation of the appropriate wavelength emitted by the body. This requires total enclosure in a shielded, whole body counter for about 15 minutes to achieve adequate precision, and, because of this and the cost of the equipment required, this technique is confined to research work.

8.1.2.3 Imaging techniques

Fat, bone and lean tissues absorb X-rays and ultrasound to different extents, and therefore either an X-ray or an ultrasound image will permit determination of the amounts of different tissues in the body, by measuring the areas (or volumes if scanning imaging techniques are used) occupied by each type of tissue. Such imaging techniques permit not only determination of the total amount of fat in the body but also its distribution. As discussed in §8.2.3, the distribution of body fat is an important factor in the adverse effects of excess adiposity.

8.1.2.4 Measurement of whole body electrical conductivity

Fat is an electrical insulator, while lean tissue, being a solution of electrolytes (see §3.3.1.1) will conduct an electric current. If electrodes are attached to the hand and foot, and an extremely small alternating electric current (typically 80 μA at 50 MHz) is passed between them, measurement of the fall in voltage permits calculation of the conductivity of the body. The percentage of fat and lean tissue can be calculated from equations based on a series of studies in which this technique has been calibrated against direct determination of density (see §8.1.2.1).

At present, measurements of either total body electrical conductivity (TOBEC) or bioelectrical impedance (BIE) are used only in research, but as the equipment becomes more widely available, this will undoubtedly become the method of preference for routine estimation of body fat.

8.1.2.5 Measurement of skinfold thickness

The most widely used technique for estimating body fat reserves is measurement of the thickness of subcutaneous adipose tissue, using standardized calipers that exert a moderate pressure (10 g per mm^2 over an area of 20–40 mm^2) and hence cause some temporary discomfort. For greatest precision, the mean of the skinfold thickness at four sites should be calculated:

- Over the triceps, at the mid-point of the upper arm.
- Over the biceps, at the front of the upper arm, directly above the cubital fossa, at the same level as the triceps site.
- Subscapular, just below and laterally to the angle of the shoulder blade, with the shoulder and arm relaxed.
- Supra-iliac, on the mid-axillary line immediately superior to the iliac crest.

The approximate desirable ranges of mean skinfold thickness are: men 3–10 mm; women 10–22 mm. The precise relationship between skinfold thickness and percentage of body fat varies with age and gender, and in no case is it a simple linear relationship.

8.2 The problem of overweight and obesity

Historically, a moderate degree of overweight was considered desirable. In a society where food was scarce, fatness demonstrated greater than average wealth and prosperity. This attitude persists in many developing countries today; food is scarce, and few people have enough to eat, let alone too much.

There is a good biological (evolutionary) argument in favour of a modest degree of overweight. A person who has reserves of fat is more likely to be able to survive a period of food deprivation or famine than a person with smaller fat reserves. So, at least in times past, fatter people may have been at an advantage. This is no longer so in developed countries, where there are no longer seasonal shortages of food. Widespread hunger is not a problem in western Europe or North America, although, as discussed in Chapter 9, lack of food is still a major problem in many countries. Table 8.4 shows that in 1991 (the most recent year for which data are available) in Britain more than half of all men and nearly half of all women were classified as overweight (i.e. BMI > 25), and that 13 per cent of men and 16 per cent of women were classified as obese (i.e. BMI > 30). Perhaps more seriously, the proportion of people classified as obese doubled in the decade from 1980 to 1991, and there is no evidence of any reversal of this trend. There has been a similar increase in obesity in other developed countries since the mid-1970s.

8.2.1 Social problems of obesity

As food supplies have become more assured, so perceptions have changed. Fatness is no longer regarded as a sign of wealth and prosperity. No longer are the overweight in society envied. Rather, they are likely to be mocked, reviled and made deeply unhappy by the unthinking comments and prejudices of their lean companions.

Because society at large considers obesity undesirable, and fashion emphasizes slimness, many overweight and obese people have problems of a poor self-image, and low self-esteem. Obese people are certainly not helped by the all-too-common prejudice against them, the difficulty of buying clothes that

Table 8.4 The percentage of people classified as overweight or obese in Britain

	Overweight (BMI > 25)		Obese (BMI > 30)	
Year	Men	Women	Men	Women
1980	39	32	6	8
1987	45	36	8	12
1991	53	44	13	16

will fit, and the fact that they are often regarded as a legitimate butt of crude and cruel humour. This may lead to a sense of isolation and withdrawal from society, and may frequently result in increased food consumption, for comfort, thus resulting in yet more weight gain, a further loss of self-esteem, further withdrawal, and more eating for compensation.

The psychological and social problems of the obese spill over to people of normal weight as well. There is continual advertising pressure for 'slimness', and newspapers and magazines are full of propaganda for slimness, and 'diets' for weight reduction. This may be one of the factors in the development of major eating disorders such as anorexia nervosa and bulimia (see §9.2.1.1).

8.2.2 *The health risks of obesity*

As shown in Figure 8.1, people who are overweight are significantly more likely to die prematurely, and at 50 per cent over average weight there is a twofold risk of premature death. Table 8.5 shows the main causes of premature death that are associated with overweight and obesity, expressed as the ratio of that condition as a cause of death in obese people: the expected rate in lean people.

Table 8.5 Excess mortality with overweight and obesity. Figures show mortality relative to that for people between 90 and 110 per cent of average weight

	Body weight as percentage of mean					
	Men			Women		
Cause of death	120–129	130–149	>140	120–129	130–139	>140
All causes	1.27	1.46	1.87	1.29	1.46	1.89
Diabetes mellitus	2.56	3.51	5.19	3.34	3.78	7.90
Digestive diseases	1.88	2.89	3.99	1.61	2.19	2.29
Coronary heart disease	1.32	1.55	1.95	1.39	1.54	2.07
Cerebral vascular lesions	1.17	1.54	2.27	1.16	1.40	1.52
Cancer, all sites	1.09	1.14	1.33	1.19	1.23	1.55
Colorectal cancer	1.23	1.53	1.73	—	—	—
Prostate cancer	1.37	1.33	1.29	—	—	—
Endometrial cancer	—	—	—	1.85	2.30	5.42
All uterus cancer	—	—	—	1.81	1.40	4.65
Cervical cancer	—	—	—	1.51	1.42	2.39
Gall bladder cancer	—	—	—	1.74	1.80	3.58
Breast cancer	—	—	—	1.16	1.22	1.53

From data reported by Lew, E. A. and Garfinkel, L. (1979) Variation in mortality by weight among 750 000 men and women. *Journal of Chronic Diseases*, **12**, 563–76; and Garfinkel, L. (1986) Overweight and mortality. *Cancer*, **58**, 1826–9.

In addition to these diseases caused by, or associated with, obesity, obese people are considerably more at risk of death during surgery and post-operative complications. There are three main reasons for this:

- Surgery is longer and more difficult when the surgeon has to cut through large amounts of subcutaneous and intra-abdominal adipose tissue.
- Induction of anaesthesia is more difficult when veins are not readily visible through subcutaneous adipose tissue, and maintenance of anaesthesia is complicated by the solubility of anaesthetic agents in fat, so that there is a large buffer pool in the body, and adjustment of dose is difficult.
- Most importantly, anaesthesia depresses lung function (as does being in a supine position) in all subjects. Obese people suffer from impaired lung function under normal conditions, largely as a result of adipose tissue in the upper body segment; total lung capacity may be only 60 per cent of that in lean people, and the mechanical workload on the respiratory muscles may be twice that of lean people. Therefore, they are especially at risk during surgery.

Because of their impaired lung function, obese people are more at risk of respiratory distress, pneumonia and bronchitis than are lean people. In addition, excess body weight is associated with increased morbidity from such conditions as:

- Arthritis of the hips and knees, associated with the increased stress on weight-bearing joints.
- Varicose veins and haemorrhoids, associated with increased intra-abdominal pressure, and possibly attributable more to a low intake of dietary fibre (see §2.4.3.2 and §6.2.1.5), and hence straining on defecation, rather than directly a result of obesity.
- Maturity onset (non-insulin-dependent) diabetes mellitus and its complications (see §11.5). The underlying mechanisms involved are not well understood, but persistent high blood levels of lipids, as is common in obesity, are associated with resistance to the action of insulin, and in many cases weight reduction is all that is required to restore normal glycaemic control.

8.2.3 ***The distribution of excess adipose tissue***

The adverse effects of obesity are not attributable solely to the excessive amount of body fat but also to its distribution in the body. In most studies of coronary heart disease there is a threefold excess of men compared with women, a difference that persists even when the raw data are corrected for such known risk factors as blood pressure, cholesterol in low-density lipoproteins, body mass index, smoking and physical activity. However, if the data are corrected for the ratio of the diameter of waist to hip, there is now only a 1.4-fold excess of men over women.

The waist:hip ratio provides a convenient way of defining two patterns of adipose tissue distribution:

- Predominantly in the upper body segment (thorax and abdomen) – the classical male pattern of obesity, sometimes called apple-shaped obesity.
- Predominantly in the lower body segment (hips) – the classical female pattern of obesity, sometimes called pear-shaped obesity.

It is the male pattern of upper-body segment obesity that is associated with the major health risks, and in some studies assessment of the pattern of fat distribution by measurement of either the waist to hip ratio or the subscapular skinfold thickness (see §8.1.2.5) shows a greater correlation with the incidence of hypertension, diabetes and coronary heart disease than does BMI alone.

8.3 The causes and treatment of obesity

The cause of obesity is an intake of metabolic fuels greater than is required for energy expenditure, so that excess is stored, largely as fat in adipose tissue reserves. The simple answer to the problem of obesity is therefore to reverse the balance: reduce food intake and increase physical activity, and hence energy expenditure.

8.3.1 Energy expenditure

Part of the problem is the relatively low level of physical activity of many people in Western countries. As discussed in §7.1.3.2, the average physical activity level in Britain is only 1.4; physical activity accounts for only 40 per cent more energy expenditure than basal metabolic rate. At the same time, food is always readily available, with an ever-increasing array of attractive snack foods, which are easy to eat, and many of which are high in fat and sugar.

Sometimes, the problem can be attributed to a low rate of energy expenditure, despite a reasonable level of physical activity. There is a wide range of individual variation around the average BMR (see §7.1.3.1), perhaps as much as 30 per cent above and below the mean. This means that some people will have a very low BMR and hence a very low requirement for food. Despite eating very little compared with those around them, they may gain weight. Equally, there are people who have a relatively high BMR and are able to eat a relatively large amount of food without gaining weight.

Rarely, there are people who have a very low metabolic rate for a medical reason, for example, an underactive thyroid gland (the thyroid hormone controls the overall rate of metabolism). Here it is a matter of identifying and treating the underlying medical problem.

8.3.2 Control of energy balance

Most people manage to balance their food intake with energy expenditure remarkably precisely. Indeed, even people who are overweight or obese are in energy balance when their weight is more or less constant. The mechanisms involved in this natural control of energy balance are not known but involve control of appetite and energy expenditure.

8.3.2.1 Control of appetite

As discussed in §1.3, changes in the concentrations of glucose, free fatty acids, amino acids and ketones in the bloodstream have all been suggested to act as signals to the appetite control centres in the hypothalamus, as have changes in the hormones associated with the control of nutrient metabolism (insulin and glucagon, see §7.3). There is some evidence that the state of fullness or emptiness of the stomach and gastrointestinal tract may exert control over how much is eaten. Many of the peptide hormones that regulate gut function in response to food intake also act on the central nervous system. Certainly, as discussed in §8.3.3.6, weight-reducing diets that are high in dietary fibre are more successful than others, perhaps because they minimize feelings of hunger.

Very rarely, people are overweight or obese as a result of a physical defect of the appetite control centres in the brain; for example, some tumours can cause damage to the satiety centre, so that the patient feels hunger but not the sensation of satiety, and has no physiological cue to stop eating.

Part of the problem of obesity can be attributed to a psychological failure of appetite control. At its simplest, this can be blamed on the variety of attractive foods available. People can easily be tempted to eat more than they need, and it may take quite an effort of willpower to refuse a choice morsel. As discussed in §1.3, even when hunger has been satisfied, the appearance of a different dish can stimulate the appetite. Experimental animals, which normally do not become obese, can be persuaded to overeat and become obese by providing them with a 'cafeteria' array of attractive foods.

Studies comparing severely obese people with lean people have shown that some obese people do not sense the normal cues to hunger and satiety. Rather, in many cases, it is the sight of food that prompts them to eat, regardless of whether they are 'hungry' or not. If no food is visible, they will not feel hunger. Some obese people have a psychological dependence on eating and the actions of chewing and swallowing food, which is as severe a problem for them as is habituation or addiction to alcohol, tobacco or narcotics. There have been no such studies involving overweight or moderately obese people, so it is not known whether the apparent failure of appetite regulation is a general problem or whether it only affects the relatively few severely obese people with body mass index greater than 40 (see Table 8.2).

8.3.2.2 *Control of energy expenditure*

It is a common observation that many lean people are restless, fidgeting and making many small, often useless, movements, all of which increase their energy expenditure. By contrast, many obese people are much more restful companions, making fewer and more efficient movements, so conserving food energy.

Some people seem to be able to modify their energy expenditure to match their food intake. It is not known how important this is for maintenance of energy balance, but many people become quite hot after meals or when they are asleep. This is largely the result of uncoupling of electron transport from oxidative phosphorylation in the mitochondria of brown adipose tissue (see §5.3.1.4), so permitting oxidation of metabolic fuel that would otherwise be stored as fat in adipose tissue. Such people tend to be lean.

Other people seem to be much more energy efficient and their body temperature may drop slightly while they are asleep. This means that they are using less metabolic fuel to maintain body temperature and so are able to store more as adipose tissue. Such people tend to be overweight. (This response, lowering body temperature and metabolic rate to conserve food, is seen in a more extreme form in animals that hibernate. During their long winter sleep, these animals have a very low rate of metabolism, and hence a low rate of utilization of the fuel they have stored in adipose tissue reserves.)

8.3.3 *How obese people can be helped to lose weight*

In considering the treatment of obesity, two different aspects of the problem must be considered:

- The initial problem, which is to help the overweight or obese person to reduce his or her weight to within the desirable range, where life expectancy is maximum.
- The long-term problem of helping the now lean person to maintain desirable body weight.

This is largely a matter of education, increasing physical activity and changing eating habits. The same guidelines for a prudent diet (discussed in §2.4) apply to the slimmed-down, formerly obese, person as to anyone else.

8.3.3.1 *How fast can excess weight be lost?*

The aim of any weight reduction regime is to reduce the intake of food to below the level needed for energy expenditure, so that body reserves of fat will have to be used. As discussed in §7.2, the theoretical maximum possible rate of weight loss is 230 g per MJ energy imbalance per week; for a person with an energy expenditure of 10 MJ per day, total starvation would result in a loss of 2.3 kg per week. In practice, the rate of weight loss is lower than this theoretical figure, because of the changes in metabolic rate and energy expenditure that occur with changes in both body weight and food intake.

Very often, the first 1–2 weeks of a weight-reducing regime are associated with a very much greater loss of weight than this. Obviously, this cannot be attributable to loss of fat. In the early stages of severe restriction of energy intake there is a considerable utilization of glycogen reserves in liver and muscle. Glycogen is associated with very much more water than is fat, so a great deal of water is lost from the body. This does not continue for long and, after 1–2 weeks, when glycogen reserves are very much smaller, the rate of weight loss slows down to what would be expected from the energy deficit.

Although the initial rapid rate of weight loss is not sustained, it can be extremely encouraging for the obese person. The problem is to ensure that he or she realizes that it will not, and indeed cannot, be sustained. It also provides excellent advertising copy for less than totally scrupulous vendors of slimming diets, who make truthful claims about the weight loss in the first week or two, and omit any information about the later weeks and months needed to achieve goal weight.

8.3.3.2 *Starvation*

More or less total starvation has been used in a hospital setting to treat seriously obese patients, especially those who are to undergo elective surgery. Vitamins and minerals have to be supplied (see Chapter 12), as well as fluid, but apart from this an obese person can lose weight at about the predicted rate of 2.3 kg per week if starved completely. There are two major problems with total starvation as a means of rapid weight loss:

- *The problem of enforcement*: It is very difficult to deprive someone of food and to prevent them finding more or less devious means of acquiring it – by begging or stealing from other patients, visitors and hospital volunteers, or even by walking down to the hospital shop or out-patients' cafeteria.
- *A biochemical problem*: As discussed in §7.3.2, the brain and red blood cells are totally reliant on glucose, even in the fasting state. Once glycogen reserves are exhausted (and this will occur within a relatively short time) there will be increasing catabolism of tissue protein reserves to provide substrates for gluconeogenesis. As much as half the weight lost in total starvation may be muscle and other tissues, not adipose tissue. This is not

desirable; the stress of surgery causes a serious loss of protein (see §10.1.2.2) and it would be highly undesirable to start this loss before surgery.

8.3.3.3 Very low-energy diets

Many of the problems associated with total starvation can be avoided by feeding a very low energy intake, normally in a liquid formula preparation which provides adequate amounts of vitamins and minerals, together with some 1.0–1.5 MJ per day, largely as protein. Such regimes have shown excellent results in the treatment of severe obesity. There is very much less loss of tissue protein than in total starvation, and with this small intake people feel less hungry than those who are starved completely.

If very low-energy diets are used together with a programme of exercise, the rate of weight loss can be close to the theoretical maximum of 2–2.5 kg per week. Such diets should be regarded as a treatment of last resort, for people with a serious problem of obesity which does not respond to more conventional diet therapy. The manufacturers recommend that they should not be used for more than 3–4 weeks at a time without close medical supervision, because there is still some risk of loss of essential tissue proteins.

8.3.3.4 Conventional diets

For most people, the problem is not one of severe obesity, but of a more modest excess body weight. Even for people who have a serious problem of obesity, it is likely that less drastic measures than those discussed above will be beneficial. The aim is to reduce energy intake to below expenditure, and so ensure the utilization of adipose tissue reserves. To anyone who has not tried to lose weight, the answer would appear to be simply to eat less. Obviously, it is not so simple. As shown in Table 8.4, there is a considerable, and increasing, problem of obesity in Western countries, and a vast array of diets, slimming regimes, special foods, appetite suppressants, and so on.

The ideal approach to the problem of obesity and weight reduction would be to provide people with the information they need to choose an appropriate diet for themselves. This is not easy. It is not simply a matter of reducing energy intake, but of ensuring at the same time that intakes of protein, vitamins and minerals are adequate. The preparation of balanced diets, especially when the total energy intake is to be reduced, is a highly skilled job, and is one of the main functions of the professional dietitian. Furthermore, there is the problem of long-term compliance with dietary restrictions; the diet must not only be low in energy and high in nutrients, it must also be attractive and pleasant to eat in appropriate amounts.

Nevertheless, some degree of nutrition education can indeed help people to make informed choices of foods, and many people do manage to lose weight in just this way, both regaining a desirable body weight and altering their food and eating habits afterwards, to comply with the prudent diet discussed in §2.4.

People can be helped by describing specific types of diet changes. A simple way is to set up three lists of foods, based on food composition tables (see Appendix II):

- Energy-rich foods, which should be avoided. These are generally foods rich in fat and sugar, but providing little in the way of vitamins and minerals. Such foods include oils and fats, fried foods, fatty cuts of meat, cakes, biscuits, etc. and alcoholic beverages. They should be eaten extremely sparingly, if at all.
- Foods that are relatively high in energy yield, but also good sources of protein, vitamins and minerals. They should be eaten in moderate amounts.
- Foods that are generally rich sources of vitamins and minerals, high in starch and non-starch polysaccharide, and low in fat and sugars. These can be eaten (within reason) as much as is wanted.

8.3.3.5 Low carbohydrate diets

At one time, there was a vogue for low carbohydrate diets for weight reduction. These were soundly based on the fact that fat and protein are more slowly digested and absorbed than carbohydrates, and therefore have greater satiety value. At the same time, a severe restriction of carbohydrate intake would limit the intake of other foods as well; one argument was that, without bread, there was nothing on which to spread butter.

Nowadays a low carbohydrate diet would not be recommended for weight reduction, since the aim is to reduce the fat intake of the population as a whole, and this means that the proportion of metabolic fuel coming from carbohydrate must increase rather than decrease. Nevertheless, to those raised in the belief that carbohydrates are fattening (as is any food in excess), it is a strange concept that weight reduction is helped by increased starch consumption.

8.3.3.6 High fibre diets

One of the persistent problems raised by many people who are restricting their food intake to lose excess weight is that they continually feel hungry. Quite apart from true physiological hunger, the lack of bulk in the gastrointestinal tract may well be a factor here. This problem can be alleviated by increasing the intake of dietary fibre – increased amounts of whole grain cereal products, fruits and vegetables. Such regimes are certainly successful, and again represent essentially a more extreme version of the general advice for a prudent diet.

It is generally desirable that the dietary sources of non-starch polysaccharides should be ordinary foods, rather than 'supplements'. However, as an aid to weight reduction, preparations of dietary fibre are available. Some of these are more or less ordinary foods, but containing added fibre, which gives texture to the food, and increases the feeling of fullness and satiety. Some of the special slimmers' soups, biscuits and so on are of this type. They are formulated to provide about one-third of a day's requirement of protein, vitamins and minerals, but with a low energy yield. They are supposed to be taken in place of one meal each day, and to aid satiety they contain carboxymethylcellulose or another non-digested polysaccharide.

An alternative approach is to take tablets or a suspension of non-starch polysaccharide before a meal. This again creates a feeling of fullness, and so reduces the amount of food that is eaten.

8.3.3.7 'Diets' that probably won't work

Weight reduction depends on reducing the intake of metabolic fuels, but ensuring that the intake of nutrients is adequate to meet requirements. Equally important is the problem of ensuring that the weight that has been lost is not replaced; in other words, eating patterns must be changed after weight has been lost, to allow for maintenance of a body weight with a well balanced diet.

There is a bewildering array of different diet regimes on offer to help the overweight and obese to lose weight. Some of these are based on sound nutritional principles, as discussed above, and provide about half the person's energy requirement, together with adequate amounts of protein, vitamins and minerals. They permit a sustained weight loss of about 1–1.5 kg per week.

Other 'diets' are neither scientifically formulated nor based on sound nutritional principles and indeed often depend on pseudo-scientific mumbo-jumbo to attempt to give them some validity. They frequently make exaggerated claims for the amount of weight that can be lost, and rarely provide a balanced diet. Publication of testimonials from 'satisfied clients' cannot be considered to be evidence of efficacy, and publication in a best-selling book or in a magazine with wide circulation cannot correct the underlying flaws in many of these 'diets'.

Some of the more outlandish diet regimes depend on such nonsensical principles as eating protein and carbohydrates at different meals (so-called food combining), ignoring the fact that such 'carbohydrate' foods as bread and potatoes provide a significant amount of protein as well (see Table 10.3). Others depend on a very limited range of foods. The most extreme have allowed the client to eat bananas, grapefruit or peanuts (or some other food) in unlimited amounts, but little else. Other diet regimes ascribe almost magical properties to certain fruits (e.g. mangoes and pineapples), again with a very limited range of other foods allowed.

The idea is that if someone is permitted to eat as much as is wished of only a very limited range of foods, even desirable and much liked foods, they will end up eating very little, because even a favourite food soon palls if it is all that is permitted. In practice, these 'diets' do neither good nor harm. People get so bored that they give up before there can be any significant effect on body weight, or any adverse effects of a very unbalanced diet. This is all to the good; if people did stick to such diets for any length of time they might well encounter problems of protein, vitamin and mineral deficiency.

8.3.3.8 *Sugar substitutes*

As discussed in §2.4.3.1, the average consumption of sugar is considerably higher than is considered desirable. There is a school of thought that blames the ready availability of sugar for much of the problem of overweight and obesity in Western countries. Simply omitting the sugar in tea and coffee would make a significant contribution to reduction of energy intake – a teaspoon of sugar is 5 g of carbohydrate, and thus provides 80 kJ; in each of six cups of tea or coffee a day, two spoons of sugar would thus account for some 960 kJ – almost 10 per cent of the average person's energy expenditure. Quite apart from this obvious sugar, which people can see they are adding to their intake, there is a great deal of sugar in beverages; for example, a standard 330 ml can of lemonade provides 20 g of sugar (=320 kJ).

Because many people like their tea and coffee sweetened, and to replace the sugar in soft drinks, there is a range of sugar substitutes. These are synthetic chemicals that are very much sweeter than sugar, but are not metabolized as metabolic fuels. Even those that can be metabolized (e.g. aspartame, which is an amino acid derivative), are taken in such small amounts that they make no significant contribution to intake. Table 8.6 shows the commonly used synthetic sweeteners (also known as non-nutritive sweeteners or intense sweeteners), together with their sweetness compared with sugar. All of these compounds have been extensively tested for safety, but as a result of concerns about possible hazards, some are not permitted in some countries, although they are widely used elsewhere.

8.3.3.9 *Appetite suppressants*

Some compounds act either to suppress the activity of the hunger centre in the hypothalamus or to stimulate the satiety centre. Sometimes this is a highly undesirable side effect of drugs used to treat various diseases and it can contribute to the undernutrition seen in chronically ill people (see §9.2.1.4). As an aid to weight reduction, especially in people who find it difficult to control their food intake, drugs that suppress appetite can be useful. Three compounds are in relatively widespread use as appetite suppressants: fenfluramine (and more recently the D-isomer, dexfenfluramine), diethylpropion and mazindol. There is some evidence of psychiatric disturbance and possible problems of addiction with these drugs, and they should be used for only a limited time, and only under strict medical supervision. The action of appetite suppressants decreases after a few weeks, then tolerance or resistance to their action develops.

Table 8.6 Non-nutritive sweeteners and their sweetness compared with sucrose = 1.0

Sweetener	Relative sweetness
Cyclamate	30–40
Glycyrrhizin	50
Abrusides	50
Naringin dihydrochalcone	75
Aspartame	180–200
Acesulfame-K	150–200
Dulcin	200–300
Stevioside	300
Suosan	350
Rebaudioside A	450
Saccharin	300–550
Sucralose (trichlorosucrose)	600–650
Perillartine	750–2000
Trihalogenated benzamides	1000
Hernandulcin	1000
Neohesperidin dihydrochalcone	1500
Alitame	2000

Note that not all of these sweeteners are permitted as food additives in all countries.

8.3.3.10 *Surgical treatment of obesity*

Severe obesity may be treated by surgical removal of much of the excess adipose tissue – a procedure known as liposuction. Two further surgical treatments have also been used:

- Intestinal bypass surgery, in which the jejunum is connected to the distal end of the ileum, so bypassing much of the small intestine in which the digestion and absorption of food occurs (see §6.1). The resultant malabsorption means that the subject can, and indeed must, eat a relatively large amount of food, but will absorb only a small proportion. There are severe side effects of intestinal bypass surgery, including persistent foul-smelling diarrhoea and flatulence, and failure to absorb medication, as well as problems of mineral and vitamin deficiency. This procedure has been more or less completely abandoned in most centres.
- Gastroplasty, in which the physical capacity of the stomach is reduced to half or less. This limits the amount of food that can be consumed at any one meal. Although the results of such surgery appear promising, there have been no studies of the long-term outcome.

8.3.3.11 *Help and support*

Especially for the severely obese person, weight loss is a lengthy and difficult experience. Friends and family can be supportive, but specialist help and advice are often needed. To a great extent, this is the role of the dietitian and other healthcare professionals. In addition, there are organizations, normally of formerly obese people, who can offer a mixture of professional nutritional and dietetic advice together with practical help and counselling. The main advantage of such groups is that they provide a social setting, rather than the formal setting of the dietitian's office in a clinic, and all the members have experienced similar problems. Many people find the sharing of the problems and experiences of weight reduction extremely helpful.

9

Protein-energy Malnutrition: Problems of Undernutrition

If the intake of metabolic fuels is lower than is required for energy expenditure, the body's reserves of fat, carbohydrate (glycogen) and protein are used to meet energy needs. Especially in lean people, who have relatively small reserves of body fat, there is a relatively large loss of tissue protein when food intake is inadequate. As the deficiency continues, so there is an increasingly serious loss of tissue, until eventually essential tissue proteins are catabolized as metabolic fuels, a process that obviously cannot continue for long.

9.1 The classification of protein-energy malnutrition

The terms **protein-energy malnutrition** and **protein-energy deficiency** are widely used to mean a general lack of food, as opposed to specific deficiencies of vitamins or minerals (as discussed in Chapter 12). However, the problem is not one of protein deficiency, but rather a deficiency of metabolic fuels. Indeed, there may be a relative excess of protein, in that protein that might be used for tissue protein replacement, or for growth in children, is being used as a fuel because of the deficiency of total food intake. This was demonstrated in a series of studies in India in the early 1980s. Children whose intake of protein was just adequate were given additional carbohydrate (in sugary drinks). They showed an increase in growth and the deposition of new body protein. This was because their previous energy intake was inadequate, despite an adequate intake of protein. Increasing their intake of carbohydrate as a metabolic fuel both spared dietary protein for the synthesis of tissue proteins and also provided an adequate energy source to meet the high energy cost of protein synthesis (see §10.2.3.3). The body's first requirement, at all times, is for an adequate source of metabolic fuels. Only when energy requirements have been met can dietary protein be used for tissue protein synthesis.

The severity of protein-energy malnutrition in adults can be assessed from the body mass index (BMI; see §8.1.1), which gives an indication of the body's reserves of metabolic fuel, as shown in Table 9.1.

Table 9.1 Classification of protein-energy malnutrition by body mass index

BMI	
20–25	Acceptable/desirable range
17–18.4	Moderate protein-energy malnutrition
16–17	Moderately severe protein-energy malnutrition
<16	Severe protein-energy malnutrition

BMI = weight (kg)/height^2(m).

There are two extreme forms of protein-energy malnutrition:

- Marasmus can occur in both adults and children, and occurs in vulnerable groups of the population in developed countries as well as in developing countries. It is the predictable end-result of prolonged negative energy balance.
- Kwashiorkor only affects children, and has been reported only in developing countries. The distinguishing feature of kwashiorkor is that there is fluid retention, leading to oedema.

Protein-energy malnutrition in children can therefore be classified by both the deficit in weight compared with what would be expected for age, and also the presence or absence of oedema (Table 9.2). The most severely affected group, and therefore the priority group for intervention, are those suffering from marasmic kwashiorkor, who are both severely undernourished and also oedematous.

9.2 Marasmus

Marasmus is a state of extreme emaciation; the name is derived from the Greek for wasting away. Not only have the body's fat reserves been exhausted, but there is wastage of muscles as well. As the condition progresses, so there is loss of protein from the heart, liver and kidneys, although as far as possible essential tissue proteins are protected.

There is a general reduction in protein synthesis. As a result of this there is a considerable impairment of the immune response, so that undernourished

Table 9.2 Classification of protein-energy malnutrition in children

	No oedema	Oedema
60–80% of expected weight for age	Underweight	Kwashiorkor
<60% of expected weight for age	Marasmus	Marasmic kwashiorkor

people are more at risk from infections that those who are adequately nourished. Diseases that are minor childhood illnesses in developed countries can often prove fatal to undernourished children in developing countries. Measles is commonly cited as the cause of death, although it would be more correct to give the true cause of death as malnutrition, infection being simply the final straw.

Among the proteins secreted by the liver, one that is most severely affected by protein-energy malnutrition is the plasma retinol-binding protein, which transports vitamin A from liver stores to tissues where it is required (see §12.2.1.1). As the synthesis of retinol-binding protein is reduced, so there are increasing signs of vitamin A deficiency, although there may be adequate reserves of the vitamin in the liver. The problem is that, without adequate synthesis of the binding protein, these liver reserves cannot be transported to the tissues where they are required. It is quite common for signs of vitamin A deficiency to be associated with protein-energy malnutrition, but supplements of vitamin A have no effect, since the problem is in the transport and utilization of the vitamin. Nevertheless, as discussed in §12.2.1.3, dietary deficiency of vitamin A is also a serious problem in many developing countries and it contributes to the impaired immune response seen in protein-energy malnutrition.

A more serious effect of protein-energy malnutrition is impairment of the regeneration of the intestinal mucosa. As discussed in §6.1, intestinal mucosal cells turn over rapidly. In protein-energy malnutrition the villi are very much shorter than usual and in severe cases the intestinal mucosa is almost flat. This results in a very considerable reduction in the surface area of the intestinal mucosa, and hence a considerable reduction in the absorption of such nutrients as are available from the diet. As a result, diarrhoea is a common feature of protein-energy malnutrition. Thus, not only does the undernourished person have an inadequate intake of food, but the absorption of what is available is impaired, so making the problem worse.

9.2.1 Causes of marasmus, and vulnerable groups of the population

In developing countries, the causes of marasmus are either a chronic shortage of food or the more acute problem of famine, where there will be very little food available at all. All too frequently, famine comes on top of a long-term shortage of food, so its effects are all the more rapid and serious. Table 9.3 shows the total food energy available per head of population in various regions of the world; these figures take no account of food losses and wastage. A simple lack of food is unlikely to be a problem in developed countries, although the most socially and economically disadvantaged in the community are at risk of hunger and perhaps even protein-energy undernutrition in extreme cases.

Table 9.3 Food energy theoretically available per person per day

	MJ per head per day
Global average	11.1
North America	14.4
Europe	14.2
Middle East	12.2
Oceania	11.9
Latin America/Caribbean	10.7
Asia	10.4
Africa	9.5

Three different factors may cause marasmus in developed countries: disorders of appetite and eating behaviour, impairment of the absorption of nutrients, and increased metabolic rate.

9.2.1.1 *Disorders of appetite: anorexia nervosa and bulimia*

As discussed in §8.2.1, there is considerable pressure on people in Western countries to be slim. People are bombarded with well-informed or ill-informed articles about the evils of obesity, in magazines, newspapers, and on radio and television, and many of the fashion models and media stars who provide role models to young people are extremely thin. Although obesity is indeed a serious health problem, one side effect of the propaganda is to put considerable pressure on some people to reduce their body weight, even though they are within the acceptable and healthy weight range. In some cases this pressure may be a factor in the development of anorexia nervosa, a major psychological disturbance of appetite and eating behaviour. The group most at risk are adolescent girls, although similar disturbances of eating behaviour can occur in older women and (more rarely) in adolescent boys and men.

The main feature of anorexia nervosa is a refusal to eat, with the obvious result of very considerable weight loss. Despite all evidence and arguments to the contrary, the anorectic subject is convinced that she is overweight, and restricts her eating very severely. Dieting becomes the primary focus of her life. She has a preoccupation with, and often a considerable knowledge of, food, and often has a variety of stylized compulsive behaviour patterns associated with food. As a part of her pathological obsession with thinness, the anorectic subject may take a great deal of strenuous exercise, often exercising to exhaustion in solitude. She will go to extreme lengths to avoid eating, and when forced to eat may induce vomiting soon afterwards. Many anorectics also make excessive use of laxatives.

Surprisingly, many anorectic people are adept at hiding their condition, and it is not unknown for the problem to remain unnoticed, even in a family setting. Food is played with, but little or none is actually eaten; excuses are made to leave the table in the middle of the meal, perhaps on the pretext of going into the kitchen to prepare the next course.

Some anorectic subjects also exhibit a further disturbance of eating behaviour: bulimia or binge eating. After a period of eating little or nothing, they suddenly eat an extremely large amount of food (40 MJ or more in a single meal, compared with an average daily requirement of 8–12 MJ), sometimes followed by deliberate induction of vomiting and heavy doses of laxatives. This is followed by a further prolonged period of anorexia.

Bulimia also occurs in the absence of anorexia nervosa – a person of normal weight will consume a very large amount of food (commonly 40–80 MJ over a period of a few hours), again followed by induction of vomiting and excessive use of laxatives. In severe cases such binges may occur five or six times a week.

Anorexia nervosa is a psychological problem, rather than a simple nutritional one, and it requires sensitive specialist treatment. It is not simply a matter of persuading the patient to eat. One theory is that the root cause of the problem, at least in adolescent girls, is a reaction to the physical changes of puberty. By refusing food, the girl believes that she can delay or prevent these changes. To a considerable extent this is so. Breast development slows down or ceases as the energy balance becomes more negative, and as body weight falls below about 45 kg, menstruation also ceases. The considerable pressure for slimness from both the media and her peers, and the continual discussion of 'diets', place an additional stress on the anorectic subject.

On some estimates, almost 2 per cent of adolescent girls go through at least a short phase of anorexia. In most cases it is self-limiting, and normal eating patterns are re-established as the emotional crises of adolescence resolve themselves. Others may require specialist counselling and treatment, and in an unfortunate few, problems of eating behaviour persist into adult life.

9.2.1.2 *Malabsorption*

Any clinical condition that impairs the absorption of nutrients from the intestinal tract will lead to undernutrition, although in this case the intake is apparently adequate. The problem is one of digestion and/or absorption of the food.

Obviously, major intestinal surgery will result in a reduction in the amount of intestine available for the digestion and absorption of nutrients. Here the problem is known in advance, and precautionary measures can be taken: a period of intravenous feeding, to supplement normal food intake, and careful counselling by a dietitian, so as to ensure adequate nutrient intake despite the problems.

A variety of infectious diseases can cause malabsorption and diarrhoea. In many cases this lasts only a few days, and so has no long-term consequences. However, some intestinal parasites can cause long-lasting diarrhoea and damage to the intestinal mucosa, leading to malnutrition if the infection remains untreated for too long.

9.2.1.3 Food intolerance and allergy

Allergic reactions to foods may cause a wide variety of signs and symptoms, including dermatitis, eczema and urticaria, asthma, allergic rhinitis, muscle pain, rheumatoid arthritis and migraine, as well as having effects on the gastrointestinal tract. All of these will be likely to impair the sufferer's appetite, and hence may contribute to undernutrition. There can be serious damage to the intestinal mucosa, leading to severe malabsorption, and hence malnutrition despite an apparently adequate intake of food. One of the best understood such conditions is coeliac disease.

Coeliac disease is an allergy to one specific protein in wheat, the gliadin fraction of wheat gluten. The result is a considerable loss of intestinal mucosa, and flattening of the intestinal villi, so that the appearance of the intestine is similar to that seen in marasmus. This reduction in the absorptive surface of the intestine leads to persistent diarrhoea and a failure to absorb nutrients. The result is undernutrition; although the intake of food is apparently adequate, there is inadequate digestion and absorption of nutrients. Severe emaciation can occur in patients with untreated coeliac disease.

Once the diagnosis is established, and the immediate problems of undernutrition have been dealt with, treatment is relatively simple – avoidance of all wheat- and rye-based products. In practice, this is less easy than it sounds; apart from the obvious foods, such as bread and pasta, wheat flour is used in a great many food products. There is therefore a need for counselling from a dietitian, and careful reading of labels for lists of ingredients. Certain products have the symbol of the Coeliac Society on the label, to show that they are known to be free from gluten, and therefore safe for patients to eat.

Other intolerances or allergic reactions to foods can also lead to similar persistent diarrhoea, loss of intestinal mucosa and hence malnutrition. The problem of disaccharide intolerance was discussed in §6.2.2.2. In general, once the offending food has been identified, the patient's condition has stabilized and body weight has been restored, continuing treatment is relatively easy, although avoidance of some common foods may provide significant problems.

It is the identification of the offending food that provides the greatest problem, and frequently calls for lengthy investigations, maintaining the patient on a very limited range of foods, then gradually introducing additional foods, until the offending item is identified.

Patients with food intolerances or allergies are generally extremely ill after they have eaten the offending food, and this may persist for several days. Even after the offending foods have been identified, and the patient's condition has been stabilized, there may be continuing problems of appetite and eating behaviour.

9.2.1.4 Cachexia

Patients with advanced cancer, HIV infection and AIDS, and other chronic diseases are frequently undernourished. Physically they show all the signs of marasmus, but there is considerably more loss of body protein than occurs in starvation. The condition is called cachexia, from the Greek for 'in a poor condition'. Several factors contribute to the problem:

- The patients are extremely sick, and because of this their wish to eat may be impaired.
- Many of the drugs used in chemotherapy can cause nausea, loss of appetite and alteration of the senses of taste and smell, so that foods that were appetizing are now either unappetizing or even repulsive.
- There is a considerable increase in basal metabolic rate, to the extent that patients are described as being hypermetabolic. Even a mild fever causes an increase in basal metabolic rate of about 13 per cent per degree Celsius increase in body temperature. In advanced cancer there is also the problem of the relatively anaerobic metabolism of many tumours, so that there is increased activity of the Cori cycle – anaerobic glycolysis in the tumour producing lactate, and gluconeogenesis in the liver (see Figure 7.6). There is a net cost of 4 × ATP for each mole of glucose cycled in this way.
- One of the reactions of the body to infection and cancer is the secretion of cytokines, including cachectin (also known as tumour necrosis factor). Although these have beneficial effects in fighting infection and slowing the development of tumours, they both increase metabolic rate and increase the rate of breakdown of tissue protein. In starvation the rate of protein breakdown remains more or less constant; it is the rate of replacement synthesis that is impaired by the lack of metabolic fuel. By contrast, in response to trauma, infection and cancer, there is an increase in the rate at which tissue proteins are broken down (see §10.1.2.2).

There has been considerable success with nutritional support of patients. In addition to such food as they are able to eat, their nutritional status is enhanced by providing nutrients by either intravenous or intragastric tubes.

9.3 Kwashiorkor

Kwashiorkor was first described in Ghana (West Africa) in 1932, and the name is the Ga name for the condition. In addition to the wasting of muscle tissue, loss of intestinal mucosa and impaired immune responses seen in marasmus, children with kwashiorkor show characteristic features that distinguish this disease:

- Fluid retention and hence severe oedema, associated with a decreased concentration of plasma proteins. The puffiness of the limbs, caused by the oedema, masks the severe wasting of arm and leg muscles.
- Enlargement of the liver. This is because of the accumulation of abnormally large amounts of fat in the liver, to the extent that, instead of its normal

reddish-brown colour, the liver is pale yellow when examined at autopsy or during surgery. The metabolic basis for this fatty infiltration of the liver is not known. It is the enlargement of the liver that causes the paradoxical 'pot-bellied' appearance of children with kwashiorkor; together with the oedema, they appear from a distance to be plump, yet they are starving.

- Characteristic changes in the texture and colour of the hair. This is most noticeable in African children; instead of tightly curled black hair, children with kwashiorkor have sparse, wispy hair, which is less curled than normal, and poorly pigmented – it is often reddish or even grey.
- A sooty, sunburn-like skin rash.
- A characteristic expression of deep misery.

9.3.1 Factors in the aetiology of kwashiorkor

The underlying cause of kwashiorkor is an inadequate intake of food, as is the case for marasmus. Kwashiorkor traditionally affects children aged 3–5 years. In many societies a child continues to suckle until about this age, when the next child is born. As a result, the toddler is abruptly weaned, frequently onto very unsuitable food. In some societies, children are weaned onto a dilute gruel made from whatever is the local cereal; in others the child may be fed on the water in which rice has been boiled; it may look like milk, but has little nutritional value. Sometimes the child is given little or no special treatment, but has to compete with the rest of the family for a share from the stew-pot. A small child has little chance of an adequate meal under such conditions, especially if there is little food for the whole family.

There is no satisfactory explanation for the development of kwashiorkor rather than marasmus. At one time it was believed that it was caused by a lack of protein, with a more or less adequate intake of energy. However, analysis of the diets of children suffering from kwashiorkor shows clearly that this is not so. Furthermore, children who are protein deficient have a slower rate of growth and are therefore stunted (see §10.1.2.1); children who have kwashiorkor are generally less stunted that those with marasmus. Finally, many of the signs of kwashiorkor, and especially the oedema, begin to improve early in treatment, when the child is still receiving a low protein diet (see §9.3.2).

Very commonly, an infection precipitates kwashiorkor in children whose nutritional status is inadequate, even if they are not yet showing signs of malnutrition. Indeed, paediatricians in developing countries expect an outbreak of kwashiorkor a few months after an outbreak of measles.

The most likely cause of kwashiorkor is that, superimposed on general food deficiency, there is a deficiency of the antioxidant nutrients such as zinc, copper, carotene and vitamins C and E. These nutrients are involved in preventing or overcoming the toxic effects of oxygen radicals (see §2.5), both those generated during normal metabolism and those produced by cells of the immune system as a part of the process of killing bacteria. Thus, in deficient children, the added oxidant stress of an infection may well trigger the sequence of events that leads to the development of kwashiorkor.

9.3.2 *Rehabilitation of malnourished children*

The intestinal tract of the malnourished patient is in a very poor state. This means that the child is not able to deal at all adequately with a rich diet or a large amount of food. Rather, treatment begins with frequent feeding of small amounts of liquid – a dilute sugar solution for the first few days, followed by diluted milk, and then full strength milk. This may be achieved by use of a nasogastric tube, so that the dilute solution can be provided at a slow and constant rate throughout the day and night. Where such luxuries are not available, the malnourished infant is fed from a teaspoon, a few drops at a time, more or less continually.

Once the patient has begun to develop a more normal intestinal mucosa (when the diarrhoea ceases), ordinary foods can gradually be introduced. Recovery is normally rapid in children and they soon begin to grow at a normal rate.

10

Protein Nutrition and Metabolism

The need for protein in the diet was demonstrated early in the nineteenth century, when it was shown that animals that were fed only on fats, carbohydrates and mineral salts were unable to maintain their body weight, and showed severe wasting of muscle and other tissues. It was known that proteins contain nitrogen (mainly in the amino groups of their constituent amino acids, see §6.4.1), and methods of measuring total amounts of nitrogenous compounds in foods and excreta were soon developed. Figure 10.1 shows an overview of protein metabolism.

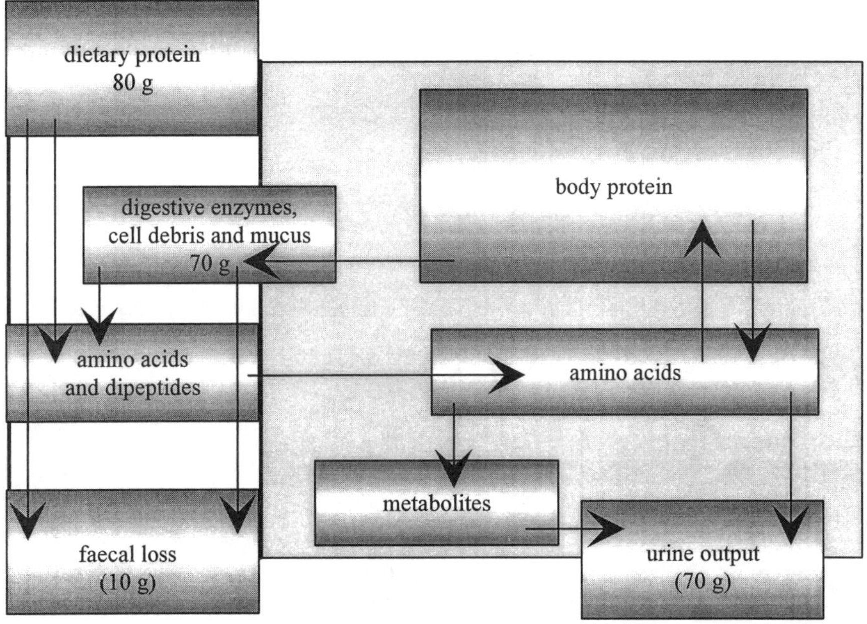

Figure 10.1 An overview of protein metabolism.

10.1 Nitrogen balance and protein requirements

The state of protein nutrition, and the overall state of body protein metabolism, can be determined by measuring the dietary intake of nitrogenous compounds and their output from the body. Although nucleic acids also contain nitrogen (see §10.2.1 and §10.2.3), protein is the major dietary source of nitrogenous compounds, and measurement of total nitrogen intake gives a good estimate of protein intake.

The output is largely in the urine and faeces, but significant amounts may also be lost in sweat and shed skin cells; and in longer experiments the growth of hair and nails must also be taken into account. Obviously, any loss of blood or tissue will also involve a loss of protein. Although the intake of nitrogenous compounds is mainly protein, the output is not. Most of the nitrogenous output from the body is urea (see §10.3.1.4), although small amounts of other products of amino acid metabolism are also excreted, as shown in Table 10.1.

The difference between intake and output of nitrogenous compounds is known as nitrogen balance. Three states can be defined:

- Under normal conditions, an adult in good health loses the same amount of nitrogen from the body each day as is taken in from the diet. This is nitrogen balance or nitrogen equilibrium: intake = output, and there is no change in the total body content of protein.
- In a growing child, a pregnant woman or someone recovering from protein loss, the output of nitrogenous compounds is less than the dietary intake; there is a net retention of nitrogen in the body, and an increase in the body content of protein. This is positive nitrogen balance: intake exceeds output, and there is a net gain in total body protein.
- In response to trauma or infection (see §10.1.2.2) or if the intake of protein is inadequate to meet requirements, there is a net loss of nitrogen from the

Table 10.1 Average daily excretion of nitrogenous compounds in the urine

Urea	10–35 g	150–600 mol	Depends on the intake of protein
Ammonium	340–1200 mg	20–70 mmol	Depends on the state of acid–base balance
Amino acids, peptides and conjugates	1.3–3.2 g	—	
Protein	<60 mg	—	Significant proteinuria indicates kidney damage
Uric acid	250–750 mg	1.5–4.5 mmol	Major product of purine metabolism
Creatinine	Male 1.8 g Female 1.2 g	Male 16 mmol Female 10 mmol	Depends on muscle mass
Creatine	<50 mg	<400 mmol	Higher levels indicate muscle catabolism

body: the output is greater than the intake. This is negative nitrogen balance: intake less than output, and there is a net loss of body protein.

10.1.1 Dynamic equilibrium

The proteins of the body are continually being broken down and replaced. As shown in Table 10.2, some proteins (especially the enzymes that have a role in controlling the activity of metabolic pathways) may turn over within a matter of minutes or hours; others last for longer before they are broken down, perhaps days or weeks. Some proteins only turn over very slowly; for example, the connective tissue protein collagen is broken down and replaced so slowly that it is almost impossible to measure the rate – perhaps half of the body's collagen is replaced in a year.

This continual breakdown and replacement is dynamic equilibrium. Superficially, there is no change in the body protein. In an adult there is no detectable change in the amount of protein in the body or the relative amounts of different proteins from one month to the next. Nevertheless, if an isotopically labelled amino acid is given, the process of turnover can be followed. The label rapidly becomes incorporated into newly synthesized proteins, and is gradually lost as the proteins are broken down. The rate at which the label is lost from any one protein depends on the rate at which that protein is broken down and replaced; the time for the labelling to fall to half its peak is the half-life of that protein (Table 10.2).

The process of protein breakdown is enzymic hydrolysis to release free amino acids, as occurs in the gastrointestinal tract in digestion (see §6.4.3). The mechanism by which individual proteins are targeted for breakdown, and why

Table 10.2 Half-lives of tissue proteins

Ornithine decarboxylase	11 min
Lipoprotein lipase	1 h
Tyrosine transaminase	1.5 h
Phosphoenolpyruvate carboxykinase	2 h
Tryptophan oxygenase	2 h
HMG CoA reductase	3 h
Glucokinase	12 h
Alanine transaminase	0.7–1 day
Glucokinase	1.25 day
Serum albumin	3.5 day
Arginase	4–5 day
Lactate dehydrogenase	16 day
Adult collagen	300 day
Infant collagen	1–2 and 150 day

some last so much longer than others, is poorly understood compared with the mechanisms involved in the control of new protein synthesis (see §10.2 and §11.3).

Studies with isotopically labelled amino acids have shown that tissue protein breakdown occurs at a more or less constant rate throughout the day, and an adult catabolizes and replaces some 3–6 g of protein per kg body weight per day. This turnover is also important in growing children, who synthesize considerably more protein per day than the net increase in body protein. Even children recovering from severe protein-energy malnutrition, and increasing their body protein rapidly, still synthesize two to three times more protein per day than the net increase.

The rate of replacement synthesis is lower than that of breakdown in the fasting state, so that what is observed is a net loss of tissue protein, liberating amino acids for gluconeogenesis (see §7.7 and §10.3.2). In the fed state, when there is an abundant supply of metabolic fuel, the rate of protein synthesis increases, and exceeds that of breakdown, so that what is observed is a net increase in tissue protein, replacing that which was lost in the fasting state. Even in severe undernutrition, the rate of protein breakdown remains more or less constant, while the rate of replacement synthesis falls, as a result of the low availability of metabolic fuels. It is only in cachexia (see §9.2.1.4) that there is increased protein catabolism as well as reduced replacement synthesis.

10.1.2 ***Protein requirements***

It is the continual catabolism of tissue proteins that creates the requirement for dietary protein. Although some of the amino acids released by breakdown of tissue proteins can be reused, most are metabolized to yield a variety of intermediates that can be used as metabolic fuels and for gluconeogenesis (see §7.7 and §10.3.2), and urea, which is excreted. This means that there is a need for dietary protein to replace the lost tissue proteins, even in an adult who is not growing. In addition, relatively large amounts of protein are lost from the body in mucus, enzymes and other proteins which are secreted into the gastro-intestinal tract and are not completely digested and reabsorbed.

Current estimates of protein requirements are based on studies of the amount required just to maintain nitrogen balance. If the intake is not adequate to replace the protein that has been broken down, then there is negative nitrogen balance: a greater output of nitrogen from the body than the dietary intake. Once the intake is adequate to meet requirements, nitrogen balance is restored. The proteins that have been broken down can be replaced, and any surplus intake of protein can be used as a metabolic fuel.

Such studies show that for adults the average daily requirement is 0.6 g of protein per kg body weight. Allowing for individual variation, the reference nutrient intake (RNI, see §12.1.1) is 0.75 g per kg body weight, or 50 g per day for a 65 kg adult. Average intakes of protein by adults in developed countries are considerably greater than requirements, of the order of 80–100 g per day. The reference intake of protein is sometimes called the safe level of intake, meaning that it is safe and (more than) adequate to meet requirements, not implying that there is any hazard from higher levels of intake.

Protein requirements can also be expressed as the percentage of total energy intake that must be met from protein. The energy yield of protein is 17 kJ per g, and the reference intake of protein represents some 7–8 per cent of energy intake. In Western countries protein provides on average 15 per cent of the energy intake. It is unlikely that adults in any country will suffer from protein deficiency if they are eating enough food to meet their energy requirements. Table 10.3 shows the protein content of cereals and other starchy foods, as a percentage of the energy they provide. It is obvious that almost all of these provide enough protein to meet requirements, if enough is eaten to meet energy needs. Only cassava, yam and possibly rice provide insufficient protein (as a percentage of energy) to meet adult requirements. The shortfall in protein provided by a diet based on yam or rice would be made up by small amounts of other foods that are good sources of protein, such as those shown in Table 10.4. With diets based largely on cassava there is a more serious problem in meeting protein requirements.

Table 10.4 shows the proportion of the protein that comes from different sources on average in Western countries. Meat, fish, eggs, and dairy produce are generally regarded as 'protein foods', whereas bread and potatoes are regarded as 'starchy foods'. However, cereal products (mainly bread and pasta) account for a significant proportion of average protein intake. Fish accounts for only a relatively small proportion of the protein on average because not many people eat much fish. On average, potatoes provide as much of our

Table 10.3 The protein content of dietary staples, as a percentage of energy yield

		Protein	
	Energy (kJ/100 g)	(g/100 g)	(% energy)
Wheat, wholemeal	1350	13.2	16.6
Wheat, white flour	1430	11.3	13.4
Spaghetti	1610	13.6	14.3
Maize	520	4.1	13.5
Oatmeal	1700	12.4	12.4
Semolina	1490	10.7	12.2
Rye	1430	8.2	9.8
Potato	370	2.1	9.6
Barley	1540	7.9	8.7
Rice	1540	6.5	7.2
Yam	560	2.0	6.1
Cassava	460	0.9	3.3

Table 10.4 Sources of protein in the average British diet

	(%)
Meat and meat products	36
Cereal products, including bread	23
Bread	14
Milk and milk products	17
Fruit and vegetables	10
Fish	6
Eggs	4

The figures show the percentage of the total intake of protein obtained from various foods in the average diet. They thus combine both the protein content of different foods and the amounts of various foods that people eat.

protein intake as fish. Although potatoes are relatively low in protein, they are widely eaten in relatively large amounts.

As is apparent from Tables 10.3 and 10.4, it is unlikely that vegetarians will be short of protein. Even people who eat meat or fish daily get half of their protein from vegetable sources, and anyway the average diet provides twice as much protein as is required. If the meat or fish is replaced with increased amounts of vegetables and nuts, then it is obvious that vegetarians are able to maintain a more than adequate intake of protein.

10.1.2.1 *Protein deficiency in children*

Since children are growing and increasing the total amount of protein in the body, they have a proportionally greater requirement for protein than do adults. A child should be in positive nitrogen balance while growing. Even so, the need for protein for growth is relatively small compared with the requirement to replace proteins that are turning over. Table 10.5 shows the protein requirements of children at different ages. As for adults, children in Western countries consume more protein than is needed to meet their requirements.

If a child has a protein-deficient diet, as may well occur in developing countries, the result is a slowing of the rate of growth. A protein-deficient child will grow more slowly than one receiving an adequate intake of protein; this is stunting of growth. As discussed in §9.1 and §9.3.1, the protein-energy deficiency diseases, marasmus and kwashiorkor, result from a general lack of food (and hence metabolic fuels), not a specific deficiency of protein.

10.1.2.2 *Protein requirements in convalescence*

One of the metabolic reactions to a major trauma, such as a burn, a broken limb or surgery, is an increase in the net catabolism of tissue proteins. As

Table 10.5 Reference nutrient intakes for protein (g per day)

Age (years)	Males	Females
1–3	15	15
4–6	20	20
7–10	28	28
11–14	42	41
15–18	55	45
19–50	56	45
Over 50	53	47

shown in Table 10.6, together with the loss of blood associated with injury, total losses of body protein may be as much as 750 g, equivalent to about 6–7 per cent of the total body protein content. Even prolonged bedrest results in a considerable loss of protein, because there is atrophy of muscles that are not used. Muscle protein is catabolized as normal, but without the stimulus of exercise it is not completely replaced.

This protein loss is mediated by the cytokines released in response to trauma; three mechanisms are involved:

- There is an increase in metabolic rate, leading to an increased rate of oxidation of amino acids as metabolic fuel, so reducing the amount available for protein synthesis.
- There may be an increase in the rate of protein catabolism, as occurs in cachexia (see §9.2.1.4).
- The cytokines are richer in two essential amino acids (see §10.1.3), cysteine and threonine, than most tissue proteins, and cytokine synthesis leads to a disproportionate depletion of these two amino acids, and hence an excess of others that cannot be used for protein synthesis, but are oxidized.

This loss of protein has to be made good as a part of the process of convalescence, and therefore patients who are convalescing will be in positive nitrogen balance. However, this does not mean that a convalescent patient requires a diet richer in protein than usual. As discussed in §10.1.2, average protein

Table 10.6 Protein losses (g) over 10 days after trauma or infection

	Tissue loss	Blood loss	Catabolism	Total
Fracture of femur	—	200	700	900
Muscle wound	500–750	150–400	750	1350–1900
Burns (35%)	500	150–400	750	1400–1650
Gastrectomy	20–180	20–10	625–750	645–850
Typhoid fever	—	—	675	685

intakes are twice requirements; a normal diet will provide adequate protein to permit replacement of the losses caused by illness and hospitalization.

10.1.3 ***Essential amino acids***

Early studies of nitrogen balance showed that not all proteins are the same. With some proteins more is needed for the maintenance of nitrogen balance than with others. This is because different proteins contain different amounts of the various amino acids (see §6.4.1). The body's requirement is not just for protein, but for the amino acids that make up proteins, in the correct proportions to replace the body proteins.

As shown in Table 10.7, the amino acids can be divided into two groups:

- The dispensable, or non-essential amino acids that can readily be synthesized from common metabolic intermediates, as long as there is enough total protein in the diet. If one of these amino acids is omitted from the diet, nitrogen balance can still be maintained.
- The nine essential or indispensable amino acids, which cannot be synthesized in the body. If one of these is lacking or provided in inadequate amount, then regardless of the total intake of protein or amino acids, it will not be possible to maintain nitrogen balance, since there will not be an adequate amount of the amino acid for protein synthesis.

For premature infants, and possibly also for full-term infants, a tenth amino acid is essential: arginine. Although adults can synthesize adequate amounts of arginine to meet their requirements, the capacity for arginine synthesis is low in infants, and may not be adequate to meet the requirements for growth.

Two amino acids occupy an intermediate position, in that they can be synthesized in the body, but only from an essential amino acid. They are cysteine, which is formed from methionine, and tyrosine, which is formed from phenylalanine. Adequate amounts of cysteine and tyrosine can be formed only if there is an adequate intake of the precursor essential amino acids, methionine and phenylalanine. The amount of cysteine and tyrosine provided in the diet

Table 10.7 Essential and non-essential amino acids

Essential	Essential precursor	Non-essential	Semi-essential
Histidine		Alanine	Arginine
Isoleucine		Aspartate	Asparagine
Leucine		Glutamate	Glutamine
Lysine			Glycine
Methionine	Cysteine		Proline
Phenylalanine	Tyrosine		Serine
Threonine			
Tryptophan			
Valine			

will affect the requirement for the precursor amino acids. If the intake of cysteine is relatively high, then less methionine will be used for the formation of cysteine, and more can be used as methionine. Similarly, an adequate dietary intake of tyrosine reduces the requirement for phenylalanine, since less will have to be used for the synthesis of tyrosine.

There is controversy over requirements for the essential amino acids. Most experimental studies of requirements have been performed on young adults, whose requirement is for maintenance, using studies of nitrogen balance. The figures usually used for assessing protein quality are the requirements of children, who have higher requirements, because of the needs for growth and net new protein synthesis. However, more recent studies, investigating the rate of irreversible oxidation of isotopically labelled amino acids, suggest that requirements of adults may be considerably higher. It is difficult to interpret the results of these studies because the amounts of labelled amino acids that were used were relatively large, and distorted the normal pools of amino acids available for metabolism.

10.1.3.1 *Protein quality and complementation*

A protein that contains at least as much of each of the essential amino acids as is required will be completely usable for tissue protein synthesis, whereas one that is relatively deficient in one or more of the essential amino acids will not. More of such a protein will be required to maintain nitrogen balance or growth.

The limiting amino acid of a protein is the essential amino acid that is present in lowest amount relative to the requirement. In cereal proteins the limiting amino acid is lysine; in animal and most other vegetable proteins it is methionine. (Correctly, the sum of methionine plus cysteine, since cysteine is synthesized from methionine, and the presence of cysteine, reduces the requirement for methionine.)

The nutritional value or quality of individual proteins depends on whether or not they contain the essential amino acids in the amounts that are required. Different ways of determining and expressing protein quality have been developed: methods 1–4 below are biological assays; methods 5 and 6 are based on chemical analysis:

1 Biological value (BV) is the proportion of absorbed protein retained in the body. A protein that is completely usable (e.g. egg and human milk) has BV = 0.9–1; meat and fish have BV = 0.75–0.8; wheat protein 0.5; gelatine (which totally lacks tryptophan) = 0.

2 Net protein utilization (NPU) is the proportion of dietary protein retained in the body under specified experimental conditions (i.e. it takes account of the digestibility of the protein). By convention NPU is measured at 10 per cent dietary protein (NPU_{10}), at which level the protein synthetic mechanism of the animal can utilize all of the protein so long as the balance of essential amino acids is correct.

3 Protein efficiency ratio (PER) is the gain in weight of growing animals per gram of protein eaten. Until 1991 this was the legally required way of expressing protein quality for nutritional labelling in the USA.
4 Relative protein value (RPV) is the ability of a test protein, fed at various levels of intake, to support nitrogen balance, compared with a standard protein.
5 Chemical score is based on chemical analysis of the protein; it is the amount of the limiting amino acid compared with the amount of the same amino acid in egg protein (which is completely usable for tissue protein synthesis).
6 Protein score (also known as amino acid score) is similar to chemical score, but uses the reference pattern of amino acid requirements of children as the standard. With a correction for the digestibility of the protein, the amino acid score is now the legally required method for nutritional labelling in USA.

Although protein quality is important when considering individual dietary proteins, it is not particularly relevant when considering total diets, because different proteins are limited by different amino acids and have a relative excess of other essential amino acids.

The result of mixing different proteins in a diet is to give an unexpected increase in the nutritional value of the mixture. For example, wheat protein provides only 62 per cent of the requirement for lysine, and thus has a protein score of 0.62. However, it provides more than enough methionine plus cysteine to meet requirements. Pea protein provides only 49 per cent of the requirement for methionine plus cysteine, and thus has a protein score of 0.49. However, it provides more than the requirement of lysine. A mixture of equal parts of wheat and pea proteins is limited by methionine plus cysteine, but provides 77 per cent of the requirement. In other words, the mixture has a protein score of 0.77; this is as high as the protein score of meat.

The result of this complementarity between proteins, which might individually be of low quality, to give mixtures of high nutritional value, means that the average Western diet, made up of the mixture of protein sources shown in Table 10.4, has a protein score of 0.73. The poorest diets in developing countries, with a restricted range of foods, and very little milk, meat or fish, have a protein score of 0.6. Since people eat mixtures of different types of protein, it is not useful to divide individual proteins into 'first class' and 'second class' categories. Most diets have very nearly the same protein quality, regardless of the individual protein sources.

10.2 Protein synthesis

The information for the amino acid sequence of each of the 50 000 different proteins in the body is contained in the DNA in the nucleus of each cell. As required, a working copy of the information for an individual protein is transcribed, as RNA, and this is then translated into protein on the ribosomes.

Both DNA and RNA are linear polymers of nucleotides (Figure 10.2). In RNA the sugar is ribose; in DNA it is deoxyribose (see Figure 6.3). The molecule consists of a backbone of alternating sugar and phosphate units, with the phosphate groups forming links from carbon-3 of one sugar to carbon-5 of the next. The bases of the nucleotides project from this sugar phosphate backbone.

10.2.1 ***The structure and information content of DNA***

As shown in Figure 10.3, DNA consists of two strands of deoxyribonucleotides, held together by hydrogen bonds (see §3.5.1) formed between a purine (adenine or guanine) and a pyrimidine (thymidine or cytosine): adenine forms two hydrogen bonds to thymidine, and guanine forms three hydrogen bonds to cytosine. The double strand coils into a helix, the so-called 'double

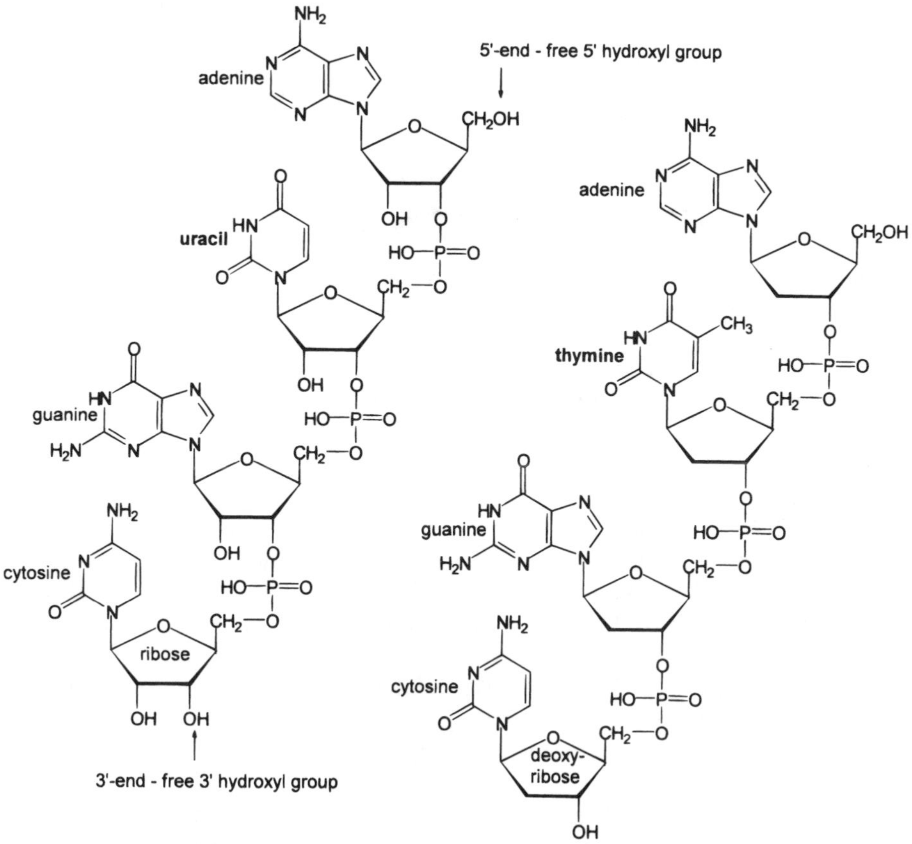

Figure 10.2 The structures of RNA (ribonucleic acid, left) and DNA (deoxyribonucleic acid, right). Both contain the purines adenine and guanine; in RNA the pyrimidines are uracil and cytosine; in DNA thymine replaces uracil.

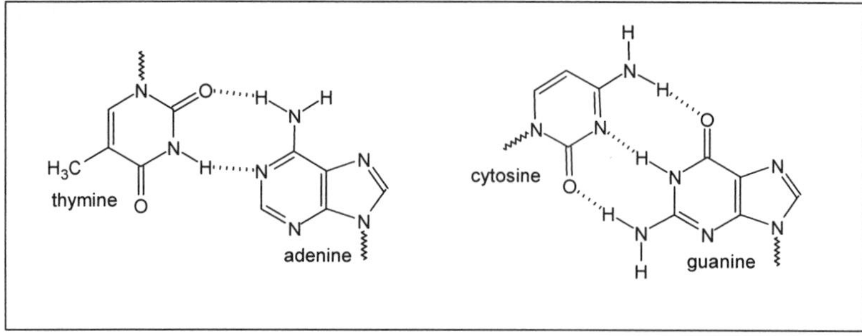

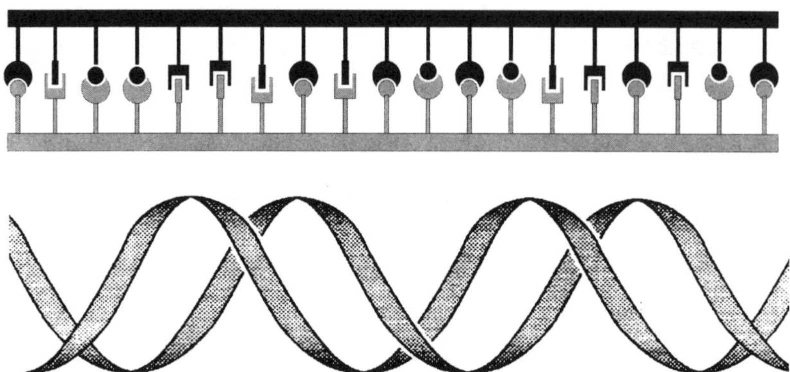

Figure 10.3 The structure of DNA. The two strands are held together by hydrogen bonds between thymine and adenine and between cytosine and guanine, then coil into the double helix shown below.

helix'. The two strands of a DNA molecule run in opposite directions. In other words, where one strand has a 3′-hydroxyl group at the end, on the complementary chain there is a free 5′-hydroxyl group. The information of DNA is always read from the 3′ end towards the 5′ end.

The DNA in a human cell contains some 1.2×10^{10} base pairs. The total length in each cell would about 2 m if it were stretched out. Obviously, since it is to be contained within a nucleus which is only 5 μm in diameter, the DNA must be folded tightly. The double helix can be bent into smooth curves, or supercoiled upon itself, with little or no disruption of the underlying conformation of the helix itself. This is like coiling, twisting and knotting a rope made up of twisted strands. The arrangement of the strands relative to each other is unaffected, but a considerable length of rope (or DNA) can be fitted into a small space.

The DNA in the nucleus is not only coiled upon itself, but is wrapped around a variety of proteins. At the beginning of cell division, when DNA is about to undergo replication (see §10.2.1.2) the DNA–protein complexes are clearly visible under the microscope as densely staining bodies inside the nucleus, the chromosomes. Altogether there are 46 chromosomes in human cells: two copies of each of 22 chromosomes, and one pair known as the sex chromosomes – two X chromosomes in females or an X plus a Y in males. Ova and sperm cells contain only one copy of each chromosome, and only one sex chromosome: always X in the ovum, and either X or Y in the sperm.

Not all of the DNA carries information for genes. Indeed, only 10 per cent of the DNA in a human cell actually carries information for the 50 000 genes that make up the human genome. The remainder is made up of:

- Control regions, which promote or enhance the expression of individual genes, and include regions that respond to hormones and other factors that control gene expression (see §11.3), as well as sites for the initiation and termination of DNA replication (see §10.2.1.2).
- Spacer regions, both between and within genes, which carry no translatable message but serve to link those regions that do carry a translatable message. When such regions occur within a gene sequence, they are called introns.
- Pseudo-genes, which seem to be genes that have undergone mutation in our evolutionary past, and are now untranslatable. Presumably these are a reminder of evolutionary history.

10.2.1.1 *The genetic code*

It is difficult at first sight to understand how a code made up of only four letters (A, G, C and T) can carry the information that must be contained in the nucleus of the cell for the 21 different amino acids that make up the 50 000 different proteins to be synthesized. The answer is that the bases are read in groups of three, not singly. Since each group of three can contain any one of the four bases in each position, there are 64 possible combinations. This means that four bases give a code consisting of 64 words. Each group of three nucleotides is a codon – a single unit of the genetic code.

Although 64 codons might not seem many to carry complex information, there is a need for only 23 codons. The information that has to be coded for in DNA is the sequence of the 21 amino acids in proteins, together with codes for the beginning and end of messages. The genetic code, as transcribed from DNA into RNA, is shown in Tables 10.8 and 10.9.

10.2.1.2 *The replication of DNA*

Cells replicate by division. The single cell which is the fertilized ovum grows and undergoes repeated divisions to yield the approximately 2×10^{12} cells in the body of the newborn infant. Cell division then continues throughout life, both for growth and because there is turnover and replacement of cells after growth has ceased.

When cells divide, each of the two new cells has a complete copy of the DNA of the parent cell. This means that, before cell division, the whole of the DNA of the cell has to be copied.

The replication of DNA requires an extremely high degree of precision and fidelity. Any changes in the information carried by DNA will be transmitted to future generations of cells. Considering the number of cell divisions that must occur throughout life, it is obvious that mistakes in replicating DNA could result in garbling of the information.

The key to the very high fidelity in replicating DNA is the base-pairing responsible for the double helical structure of the molecule. Replication involves the unwinding of a section of DNA, separation of the hydrogen-bonded base pairs, then binding of complementary bases onto each strand of the parent DNA. The result of this process is that each of the two copies of the DNA that are formed (one of which will end up in the nucleus of each new cell) has one newly synthesized strand and one from the parent molecule.

As the strands of DNA are unwound for replication, so the nucleotide triphosphates with bases complementary to those present on the strand to be copied form hydrogen bonds. If the hydrogen bonding to form base pairs is correct (A pairs with C, and G pairs with T) then the phosphates undergo a condensation reaction, forming the sugar–phosphate backbone of the new strand of DNA. If the base-pairing is not correct, this will distort the shape of the molecule, and the sugar–phosphate bonds cannot be formed. The mistaken base is removed and replaced by the correct one before the formation of the phosphate bond can occur.

Despite the checking before the formation of the sugar–phosphate bonds, and proofreading of the newly synthesized DNA, the rate of replication is of the order of 30 000 nucleotides incorporated per minute. However, the total human DNA to be replicated consists of some 1.2×10^{10} base pairs. If DNA replication simply started at one end of the molecule, it would take some 6700 hours to make a complete copy. Even allowing for the fact that the 46 chromosomes could be copied simultaneously, it would take about 6 days to make a complete set of copies. What happens is that replication starts at several hundred sites in each molecule of DNA, so that at any time during replication there are several hundred areas of unwinding and replication. In this way, replication of the whole of the DNA of a cell can occur in only about 7 hours.

10.2.2 ***Ribonucleic acid (RNA)***

In RNA the sugar is ribose, rather than deoxyribose as in DNA, and RNA contains the pyrimidine uracil where DNA contains thymidine. There are three main types of RNA in the cell:

- Messenger RNA (mRNA) is made in the nucleus, as a copy of one strand of DNA (the process of transcription, see §10.2.2.1). After some editing of the message, it is transferred into the cytosol, where it binds to ribosomes. The information carried by the mRNA is then translated into the amino acid sequence of proteins: the process of protein synthesis.

- Ribosomal RNA (rRNA) is part of the structure of the ribosomes on which protein is synthesized (see §10.2.3.2).
- Transfer RNA (tRNA) provides the link between mRNA and the amino acids required for protein synthesis on the ribosome (see §10.2.3.1).

10.2.2.1 *Transcription to form messenger RNA (mRNA)*

In the transcription of DNA to form mRNA, a part of the desired region of DNA is uncoiled, and the two strands of the double helix are separated. A complementary copy of one DNA strand is then made, in the same way as happens in DNA replication (see §10.2.1.2), except that in this case it is ribonucleotides that form the growing strand, rather than deoxyribonucleotides. There are three main differences between the replication of DNA and transcription:

- Only one of the two strands of DNA is transcribed to form messenger RNA, whereas in DNA replication both strands are copied at the same time.
- In replication, the whole of the DNA is copied. In transcription only specific regions (individual genes, corresponding to the individual proteins) are copied.
- Only one copy of the DNA is made in the process of replication, whereas in transcription multiple copies of the gene are made.

Transcription control sites in DNA include start and stop messages, and promoter and enhancer sequences. The main promoter region for any gene is about 25 bases before (upstream of) the beginning of the gene to be transcribed. It is the signal that what follows is a gene to be transcribed.

Enhancer and promoter regions may be found further upstream of the message, downstream or sometimes even in the middle of the message. The function of these regions, and of hormone response elements (see §11.3), is to increase the rate at which the gene is transcribed.

The first step in the transcription of a gene is to uncoil that region of DNA from its associated proteins, so as to allow the various enzymes involved in transcription to gain access to the DNA. The enzyme RNA polymerase moves along the DNA strand that is to be transcribed, and matches complementary ribonucleotide triphosphates one at a time to the bases in the DNA. Adenine in DNA is matched by guanosine triphosphate, guanine by adenosine triphosphate and thymine by cytosine triphosphate. However, cytidine in DNA is matched by uridine triphosphate; RNA contains uridine rather than thymidine as in DNA.

Although it is obviously important that the mRNA should be a good copy of the DNA, occasional mistakes would be less important than in DNA replication, so there is no need for the meticulous proofreading that occurs in DNA replication (see §10.2.1.2). DNA must be copied as correctly as possible, since it is the master copy of information in the cell, whereas messenger RNA

Table 10.8 The genetic code, showing the codons in mRNA

Amino acid		Codon(s)
Alanine	Ala	GCU GCC GCA GCG
Arginine	Arg	CGU CGC CGA CGG AGA AGG
Asparagine	Asn	AAU AAC
Aspartic acid	Asp	GAU GAC
Cysteine	Cys	UGU UGC
Glutamic acid	Glu	GAA GAG
Glutamine	Gln	CAA CAG
Glycine	Gly	GGU GGC GGA GGG
Histidine	His	CAU CAG
Isoleucine	Ile	AUU AUC AUA
Leucine	Leu	UUA UUG CUU CUC CUA CUG
Lysine	Lys	AAA AUG
Methionine	Met	AUG
Phenylalanine	Phe	UUU UUC
Proline	Pro	CCU CCC CCA CCG
Serine	Ser	UCU UCC UCA UCG AGU AGC
Threonine	Thr	ACU ACC ACA ACG
Tryptophan	Trp	UGG
Tyrosine	Tyr	UAU UAC
Valine	Val	GUU GUC GUA GUG
STOP		UAA UAG UGA[a]

[a] UGA also codes for selenocysteine in a specific context.

has a short life, turning over within a few hours, and an occasional faulty copy would have no serious consequences.

There are three steps in the processing of the RNA that is formed by RNA polymerase before it can be exported from the nucleus as messenger RNA:

- The 5′ end of the RNA is blocked by the formation of the unusual base 7-methyl-guanosine. This is called the 'cap' and it has an important role in the initiation of protein synthesis (see §10.2.3.2). The 5′ end of the RNA is the first to be synthesized, and the cap is added before transcription has been completed.
- A tail is added to the 3′ end of the RNA, after the termination codon. This tail is a sequence of 20–250 adenosine residues, and therefore is called the poly(A) tail. The poly(A) tail of messenger RNA has been extremely useful to molecular biologists, providing a simple way of separating mRNA from the other forms of RNA in the cell. Its function *in vivo* is not known. Experimental systems can be manipulated to produce tailless mRNA, which is transported from the nucleus to the cytosol like normal mRNA, and is translated equally well.
- Before the newly transcribed RNA can be translated, it undergoes editing and splicing to remove the introns that have been copied from DNA, which

do not carry information for protein synthesis. The final product is messenger RNA, which is then transported out of the nucleus into the cytosol to be used for protein synthesis.

10.2.3 ***Translation of mRNA: the process of protein synthesis***

The process of protein synthesis consists of translating the message carried by the sequence of bases on mRNA into amino acids, and then forming peptide bonds between the amino acids to form a protein. This occurs on the ribosome and requires a variety of enzymes, as well as specific transfer RNA molecules for each amino acid.

The genetic code, the base triplets (codons) for each amino acid, is shown in Tables 10.8 and 10.9. Most amino acids (apart from methionine and tryptophan) are coded for by more than one codon. In many cases only the first two bases of the codon have to be read to identify the amino acid; the third base can be either purine (A or G) or either pyrimidine (C or U). In some cases, it makes no difference which base is in the third position (A, G, C or U).

Three codons (UAA, UAG and UGA) do not code for amino acids, but act as stop signals to show the end of the message to be translated and so terminate protein synthesis. However, UGA also codes for the selenium analogue of

Table 10.9 The genetic code, showing the codons in mRNA

	Second base				
First base	U	C	A	G	Third base
U	Phe	Ser	Tyr	Cys	U
U	Phe	Ser	Tyr	Cys	C
U	Leu	Ser	STOP	STOP[a]	A
U	Leu	Ser	STOP	Trp	G
C	Leu	Pro	His	Arg	U
C	Leu	Pro	His	Arg	C
C	Leu	Pro	Gln	Arg	A
C	Leu	Pro	Gln	Arg	C
A	Ile	Thr	Asn	Ser	U
A	Ile	Thr	Asn	Ser	C
A	Ile	Thr	Lys	Arg	A
A	Met	Thr	Lys	Arg	G
G	Val	Ala	Asp	Gly	U
G	Val	Ala	Asp	Gly	C
G	Val	Ala	Glu	Gly	A
G	Val	Ala	Glu	Gly	G

[a] UGA also codes for selenocysteine in a specific context.

cysteine, selenocysteine, in some genes; whether UGA is read as stop or selenocysteine depends on the other information contained in the mRNA.

10.2.3.1 *Transfer RNA (tRNA)*

The key to translating the message carried by the codons on mRNA into amino acids is transfer RNA. There are 56 different types (species) of tRNA in the cell. They all have the same general structure, RNA twisted into a cloverleaf shape, and consisting of some 70–90 nucleotides. About half the bases in tRNA are paired by hydrogen bonding, which maintains the shape of the molecule. The 3′ and 5′ ends of the molecule are adjacent to each other as a result of this folding.

The different species of tRNA have many regions in common with each other, and all have a –CCA tail at the 3′ end, which reacts with the amino acid. Two regions are important in providing the specificity of the tRNA species:

- The anticodon, a sequence of three bases at the base of the clover leaf. The bases in the anticodon are complementary to the bases of the codons of mRNA, and each species of tRNA binds specifically to one codon, or in some cases, two closely related codons for the same amino acid.
- The region at the 5′ end of the molecule, which again contains a base sequence specific for the amino acid, and hence repeats the information contained in the anticodon.

Amino acids bind to activating enzymes (amino acyl-tRNA synthetases), which recognize both the amino acid and the appropriate tRNA molecule. The first step is reaction between the amino acid and ATP, to form amino acyl AMP, releasing pyrophosphate. The amino acyl AMP then reacts with the –CCA tail of tRNA to form amino acyl-tRNA, releasing AMP.

The specificity of these enzymes is critically important to the process of translation. Each enzyme recognizes only one amino acid, but will bind and react with all the various tRNA species that carry an anticodon for that amino acid. Mistakes are extremely rare. The easiest possible mistake would be the attachment of valine to the tRNA for isoleucine, or vice versa, because of the close similarity between the structures of these two amino acids (see Figure 6.13). However, it is only about once in every 3000 times that this mistake occurs. Amino acyl-tRNA synthetases have a second active site which checks that the correct amino acid has been attached to the tRNA, and if not, hydrolyses the newly formed bond, releasing tRNA and the amino acid.

10.2.3.2 *Protein synthesis on the ribosome*

The subcellular organelle concerned with protein synthesis is the ribosome. This consists of two subunits composed of RNA with a variety of associated proteins. The ribosome permits the binding of the anticodon region of amino acyl tRNA to the codon on mRNA, and aligns the amino acids for formation of peptide bonds. As shown in Figure 10.4, the ribosome binds to mRNA, and has two tRNA binding sites. One, the P site, contains the growing peptide chain, attached to tRNA; the other, the A site, binds the next amino acyl tRNA to be incorporated into the peptide chain.

The first codon of mRNA (the initiation codon) is always AUG, the codon for methionine. This means that the amino terminal of all newly synthesized proteins is methionine, although this may well be removed in post-translational modification of the protein (see §10.2.3.4).

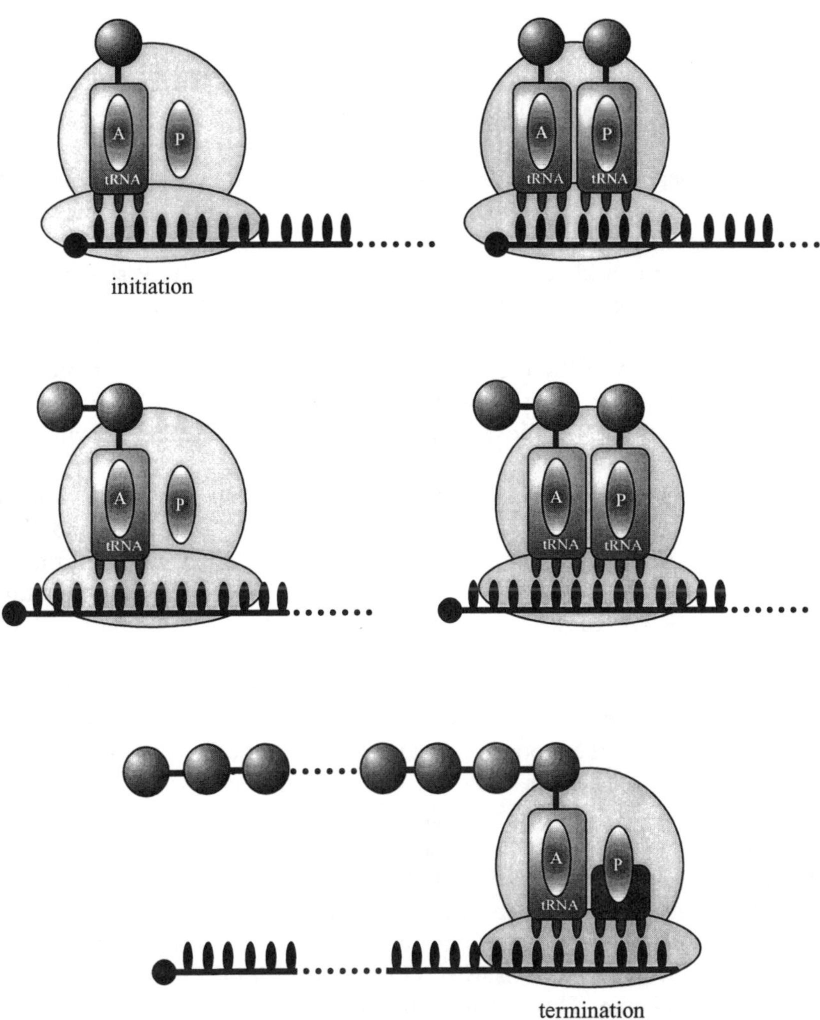

Figure 10.4 Protein synthesis on the ribosome.

An initiator methionine-tRNA forms a complex with the small ribosomal subunit, then together with a variety of initiation factors (enzymes and other proteins) binds to the initiator codon of mRNA, and finally to a large ribosomal subunit, to form the complete ribosome. The 5′ cap of mRNA is important for this process, since it marks the position of the initiator codon. AUG is the only codon for methionine, and anywhere else in mRNA, it binds the normal methionine-tRNA. It is only immediately adjacent to the cap that AUG binds the initiator methionine-tRNA.

After the ribosome has been assembled, with the initiator tRNA bound at the P site and occupying the AUG initiator codon, the next amino acyl tRNA binds to the A site of the ribosome, with its anticodon bound to the next codon in the sequence.

The methionine is released from the initiator tRNA at the P site, and forms a peptide bond to the amino group of the amino acyl tRNA at the A site of the ribosome. The initiator tRNA is then released from the P site, and the growing peptide chain, attached to its tRNA, moves from the A site to the P site. Since the peptide chain is attached to tRNA, which occupies a codon on the mRNA, this means that as the peptide chain moves from the A site to the P site, so the whole assembly moves one codon along the mRNA.

As the growing peptide chain moves from the A site to the P site, and the ribosome moves along the mRNA chain, so the next amino acyl tRNA occupies the A site, covering its codon. The growing peptide chain is transferred from the tRNA at the P site, forming a peptide bond to the amino acid at the A site. Again the free tRNA at the P site is released, and the growing peptide, attached to tRNA, moves from the A site to the P site, moving one codon along the mRNA as it does so.

The stop codons (UAA, UAG and UGA) are not read by tRNA, but by protein release factors. These occupy the A site of the ribosome, and they hydrolyse the peptide–tRNA bond. This releases the finished protein from the ribosome. As the protein leaves, so the two subunits of the ribosome separate and leave the mRNA; they are now available to bind another initiator tRNA and begin the process of translation over again.

Just as several molecules of RNA polymerase can transcribe the same gene at the same time, so several ribosomes translate the same molecule of mRNA at the same time. As the ribosomes travel along the mRNA, so each has a longer growing peptide chain than the one before. Such assemblies of ribosomes on a molecule of mRNA are called polysomes.

Termination and release of the protein from the ribosome require the presence of a stop codon and the protein release factors. However, protein synthesis can also come to a halt if there is not enough of one of the amino acids bound to tRNA. In this case, the growing peptide chain is not released from the ribosome, but remains, in arrested development, until the required amino acyl tRNA is available. This means that if the intake of one of the essential amino acids is inadequate, then once supplies are exhausted, protein synthesis will come to a halt.

10.2.3.3 *The energy cost of protein synthesis*

The minimum estimate of the energy cost of protein synthesis is four ATP equivalents per peptide bond formed, or 2.8 kJ per gram of protein synthesized:

- Formation of the amino acyl tRNA requires the formation of amino acyl AMP, with the release of pyrophosphate, which again breaks down to yield phosphate. Hence, for each amino acid attached to tRNA there is a cost equivalent to 2 mol of ATP → ADP + phosphate.
- The binding of each amino acyl tRNA to the A site of the ribosome involves the hydrolysis of GTP → GDP + phosphate, which is equivalent to ATP → ADP + phosphate.
- Movement of the growing peptide chain from the A site of the ribosome to the P site again involves the hydrolysis of ATP → ADP + phosphate.

If allowance is made for the energy cost of active transport of amino acids into cells, the cost of protein synthesis is increased to 3.6 kJ per g. Allowing for the nucleoside triphosphates required for mRNA synthesis gives a total cost of 4.2 kJ per gram of protein synthesized.

In the fasting state, when the rate of protein synthesis is relatively low, about 8 per cent of total energy expenditure (i.e. about 12 per cent of the basal metabolic rate) is accounted for by protein synthesis. After a meal, when the rate of protein synthesis increases, it may account for 12–20 per cent of total energy expenditure.

10.2.3.4 *Post-translational modification of proteins*

Proteins which are to be exported from the cell, or are to be targeted into subcellular organelles such as the mitochondrion, are synthesized with a hydrophobic signal sequence of amino acids at the amino terminal to direct them through the membrane. This is removed in the process of post-translational modification. Many other proteins have regions removed from the amino or carboxyl terminal during post-translational modification, and the initial (amino terminal) methionine is removed from most newly synthesized proteins.

Many proteins contain carbohydrates and lipids, covalently bound to amino acid side chains. Others contain covalently bound cofactors and prosthetic groups, such as vitamins and their derivatives, metal ions or haem. Again the attachment of these non-amino acid parts of the protein is part of the process of post-translational modification to form the active protein.

Some proteins contain unusual amino acids, for which there is no codon, and no tRNA. These are formed by modification of the protein after translation is complete. Such amino acids include:

- Methyl-histidine in the contractile proteins of muscle.

- Hydroxyproline and hydroxylysine in the connective tissue proteins. The formation of hydroxyproline and hydroxylysine requires vitamin C as a cofactor. This explains why wound healing, which requires new synthesis of connective tissue, is impaired in vitamin C deficiency (see §12.2.13.1).
- Interchain links in collagen and elastin, formed by the oxidation of three or four lysine residues. This reaction is catalysed by a copper-dependent enzyme, and copper deficiency leads to fragility of bones and loss of the elasticity of connective tissues (see §12.3.2.2).
- γ-Carboxyglutamate is present in several of the blood-clotting proteins, and in osteocalcin in bone. The formation of γ-carboxyglutamate requires vitamin K, and this explains the role of vitamin K in blood clotting (see §12.2.4.1).

10.3 The metabolism of amino acids

An adult has a requirement for a dietary intake of protein because there is continual oxidation of amino acids as a source of metabolic fuel and for gluconeogenesis (in the fasting state). Even in the fed state, amino acids that are not immediately required for protein synthesis are oxidized. Overall, for an adult in nitrogen balance, the total amount of amino acids being metabolized will be equal to the total intake of amino acids in dietary proteins. Amino acids are also required for the synthesis of a variety of important metabolic products, including:

- purines and pyrimidines for nucleic acid synthesis; here it is the nitrogen of amino acids that is required (see §10.3.1.5)
- haem, synthesized from glycine
- the catecholamine neurotransmitters, dopamine, noradrenaline and adrenaline, synthesized from tyrosine
- the thyroid hormones thyroxine and tri-iodothyronine, synthesized from tyrosine
- melanin, the pigment of skin and hair, synthesized from tyrosine
- the nicotinamide ring of the coenzymes NAD and NADP, synthesized from tryptophan (see §12.2.7)
- the neurotransmitter serotonin (5-hydroxytryptamine), synthesized from tryptophan
- the neurotransmitter histamine, synthesized from histidine
- the neurotransmitter GABA (γ-aminobutyrate), synthesized from glutamate
- carnitine (see §7.5.1), synthesized from lysine and methionine
- creatine, synthesized from arginine, glycine and methionine
- the phospholipid bases ethanolamine and choline (see §6.3.1.2), synthesized from serine and methionine; choline, as acetyl choline, also functions as a neurotransmitter

- taurine, synthesized from cysteine.

In general, the amounts required are small in comparison with the requirement for maintenance of nitrogen balance and protein turnover.

10.3.1 *Metabolism of the amino nitrogen*

The initial step in the metabolism of amino acids is the removal of the amino group ($-NH_2$), leaving the carbon skeleton of the amino acid. Chemically, these carbon skeletons are keto-acids (more correctly, they are oxo-acids). A keto-acid has a $-C{=}O$ group in place of the $HC{-}NH_2$ group of an amino acid; the metabolism of keto-acids is discussed in §10.3.2.

10.3.1.1 *Deamination*

Some amino acids can be directly oxidized to their corresponding keto-acids, releasing ammonia: the process of deamination (see Figure 10.5). There is a general amino acid oxidase which catalyses this reaction, but it has a low activity. There is also an active D-amino acid oxidase, which functions to deaminate, and hence inactivate, small amounts of D-amino acids that arise from bacterial proteins.

Four amino acids are deaminated by specific enzymes:

- glycine is deaminated to its keto-acid, glyoxylic acid, and ammonium ions by glycine oxidase

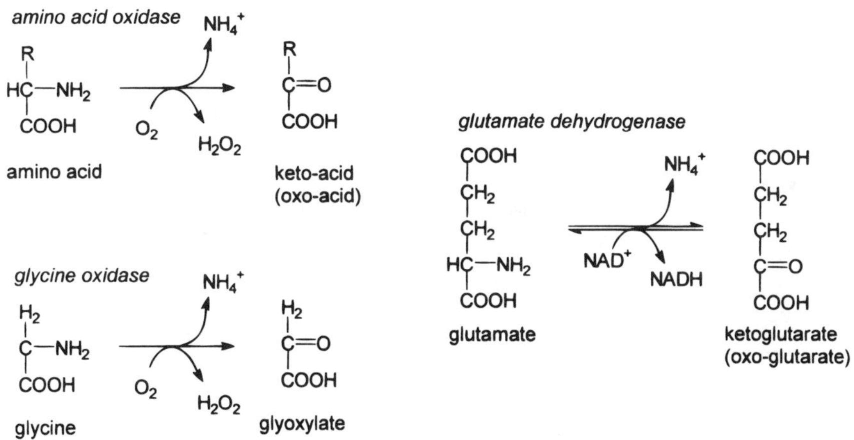

Figure 10.5 The oxidative deamination of amino acids.

- glutamic acid is deaminated to ketoglutarate and ammonium ions by glutamate dehydrogenase
- serine is deaminated and dehydrated to pyruvate by serine deaminase (sometimes called serine dehydratase)
- threonine is deaminated and dehydrated to oxo-butyrate by threonine deaminase.

10.3.1.2 *Transamination*

Most amino acids are not deaminated, but undergo the process of transamination. The amino group of the amino acid is transferred onto the enzyme, leaving the keto-acid. In the second half of the reaction, the enzyme transfers the amino group onto an acceptor, which is a different keto-acid, so forming the amino acid corresponding to that keto-acid. The acceptor for the amino group at the active site of the enzyme is pyridoxal phosphate, the metabolically active coenzyme derived from vitamin B_6 (see §12.2.8). The reaction of transamination is shown in Figure 10.6, and the keto-acids corresponding to the amino acids in Table 10.10.

Many of the keto-acids listed in Table 10.10 are common metabolic intermediates, such as pyruvate (see Figure 7.4), ketoglutarate and oxaloacetate (see Figure 7.9). Therefore, these amino acids can readily be synthesized by transamination of their keto-acids, provided that there is a source of amino groups available. This means that the non-essential amino acids (see §10.1.3) can be defined as those whose keto-acids can be synthesized from common metabolic pathways, whereas the essential amino acids are those whose keto-acids can only be derived form the amino acid itself.

Probably only three of the non-essential amino acids shown in Table 10.7 are totally dispensable, in that they can be synthesized in unlimited quantities, provided that there is an adequate source of amino groups for transamination:

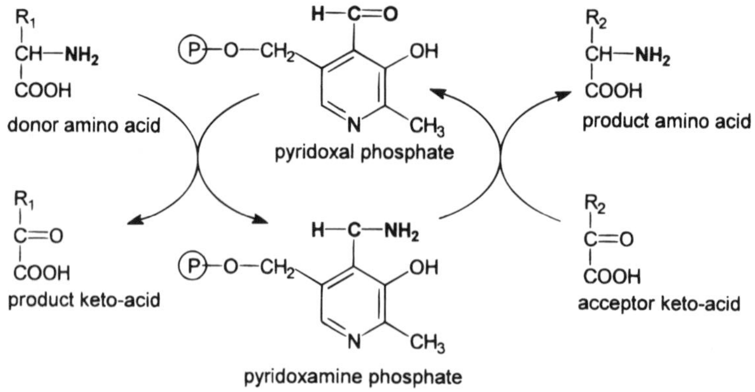

Figure 10.6 Transamination of amino acids.

Table 10.10 Transamination products of the amino acids

Amino acid	Keto-acid
Alanine	Pyruvate
Arginine	α-Keto-γ-guanidoacetate
Aspartic acid	Oxaloacetate
Cysteine	β-Mercaptopyruvate
Glutamic acid	α-Ketoglutarate
Glutamine	α-Ketoglutaramic acid
Glycine	Glyoxylate
Histidine	Imidazolepyruvate
Isoleucine	α-Keto-β-methylvalerate
Leucine	α-Keto-isocaproate
[Lysine[a]	α-Keto-ε-aminocaproate → pipecolic acid]
Methionine	*S*-Methyl-β-thiol 1α-oxopropionate
Ornithine	Glutamic-γ-semialdehyde
Phenylalanine	Phenylpyruvate
Proline	γ-Hydroxypyruvate
Serine	Hydroxypyruvate
Threonine	α-Keto-β-hydroxybutyrate
Tryptophan	Indolepyruvate
Tyrosine	*p*-Hydroxyphenylpyruvate
Valine	α-Keto-isovalerate

[a] Lysine does not normally undergo transamination; the keto-acid cyclizes non-enzymically to pipecolic acid.

alanine (formed from pyruvate), glutamate (formed from ketoglutarate) and aspartate (formed from oxaloacetate). For the other non-essential amino acids, synthesis of the keto-acid may be inadequate to meet requirements under conditions of metabolic stress, if none of the amino acid is supplied in the diet.

If the acceptor keto-acid in a transamination reaction is ketoglutarate, then glutamate is formed, and glutamate can readily be oxidized back to ketoglutarate, catalysed by glutamate dehydrogenase, with the release of ammonia. Similarly, if the acceptor keto-acid is glyoxylate, then the product is glycine. Again glycine can be oxidized back to glyoxylate and ammonia, catalysed by glycine oxidase. Thus, by means of a variety of transaminases, and using the reactions of glutamate dehydrogenase and glycine oxidase, all of the amino acids can, indirectly, be converted to their keto-acids and ammonia (see Figure 10.7). Aspartate can also act as an intermediate in the indirect deamination of a variety of amino acids, as shown in Figure 10.10.

10.3.1.3 *The metabolism of ammonia*

The deamination of amino acids (and some other reactions in the body) results in the formation of ammonium ions. Ammonia is highly toxic. The normal plasma concentration is less than 50 μmol per L. An increase to only 80–100 μmol per L (far too little to have any detectable effect on plasma pH) results in

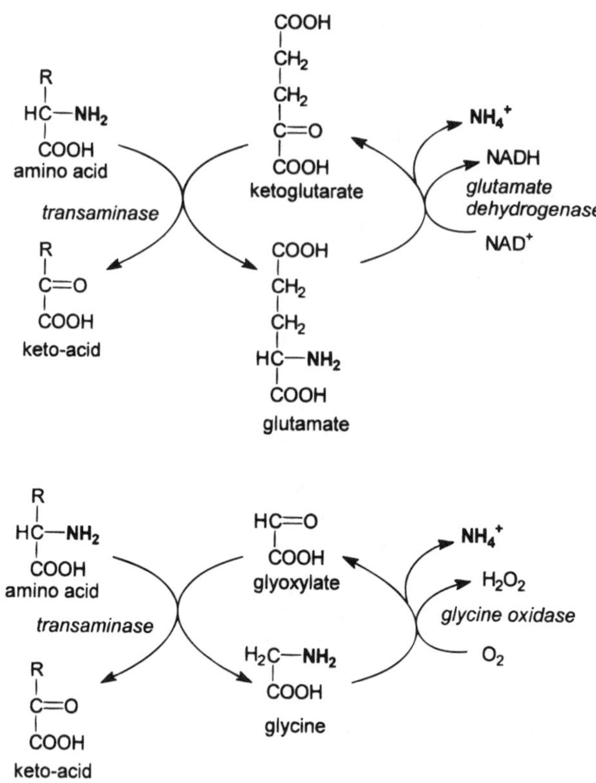

Figure 10.7 Deamination of a variety of amino acids by transamination linked to glutamate dehydrogenase (above) or glycine oxidase (below).

disturbance of consciousness, and in patients whose blood ammonia rises above about 200 μmol per L, ammonia intoxication leads to brain damage and may be fatal.

At any time, the total amount of ammonia to be transported around the body, and eventually excreted, is greatly in excess of the toxic level. What happens is that, as it is formed, ammonia is metabolized, mainly by the formation of glutamate from ketoglutarate, and then glutamine from glutamate, in a reaction catalysed by glutamine synthetase, as shown in Figure 10.8. Glutamine is transported in the bloodstream to the liver and kidneys.

It is the formation of glutamate from ketoglutarate that explains the neurotoxicity of ammonia; as ammonia concentrations in the nervous system rise, the reaction of glutamate dehydrogenase depletes the mitochondrial pool of ketoglutarate, resulting in impairment of the activity of the citric acid cycle (see §7.4.2.3) and so impairing energy-yielding metabolism.

In the kidneys, some glutamine is converted back to glutamate (which remains in the body) and ammonia, which is excreted in the urine to neutralize excess acid excretion. This reaction is a simple hydrolysis.

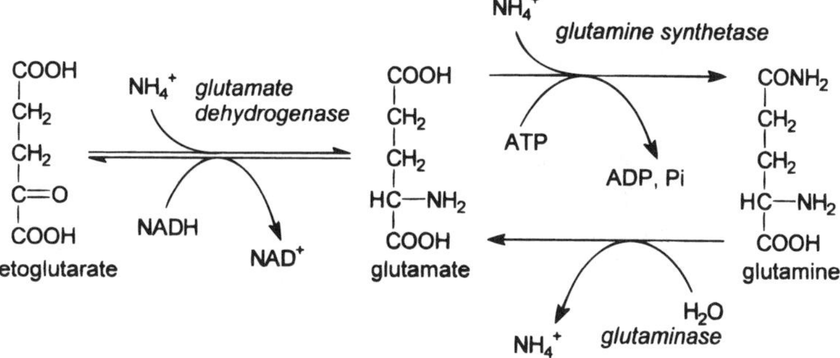

Figure 10.8 The synthesis of glutamine.

10.3.1.4 *The synthesis of urea*

In the liver, glutamine is also hydrolysed to glutamate and ammonia. Here the ammonia is metabolized further, to form urea, which is then transported to the kidneys for excretion. Some urea is retained in the distal renal tubules, where it has an important role in maintaining an osmotic gradient for the resorption of water. The pathway for urea synthesis is shown in Figure 10.9. It is a cyclic pathway. The key compound is ornithine, which acts as a carrier on which the molecule of urea is built up. At the end of the reaction sequence, urea is released by the hydrolysis of arginine, yielding ornithine to begin the cycle again.

The total amount of urea synthesized each day is several-fold higher than the amount that is excreted. Urea diffuses readily from the bloodstream into the large intestine, where it is hydrolysed by bacterial urease to carbon dioxide and ammonia. Much of the ammonia is reabsorbed and used in the liver for the synthesis of glutamate and glutamine, and then for the synthesis of non-essential amino acids, purines and pyrimidines (see §10.3.1.5). However, studies with ^{15}N urea show that a significant amount of label is also found in essential amino acids. This is presumably the result of intestinal bacterial utilization of the ammonia liberated by urease action for amino acid and protein synthesis, followed by digestion of the bacteria and absorption of some of the amino acids from the colon.

The urea synthesis cycle is also the pathway for the synthesis of the amino acid arginine. Ornithine can readily by synthesized from glutamate, and then undergoes the reactions shown in Figure 10.9 to form arginine. Although the whole pathway of urea synthesis occurs only in the liver, the sequence of reactions leading to the formation of arginine occurs in the kidneys, and the kidneys are the main source of arginine in the body.

10.3.1.5 *Incorporation of nitrogen in biosynthesis*

Amino acids are the only significant source of nitrogen for synthesis of nitrogenous compounds such as haem, purines and pyrimidines. Three amino acids are especially important as nitrogen donors:

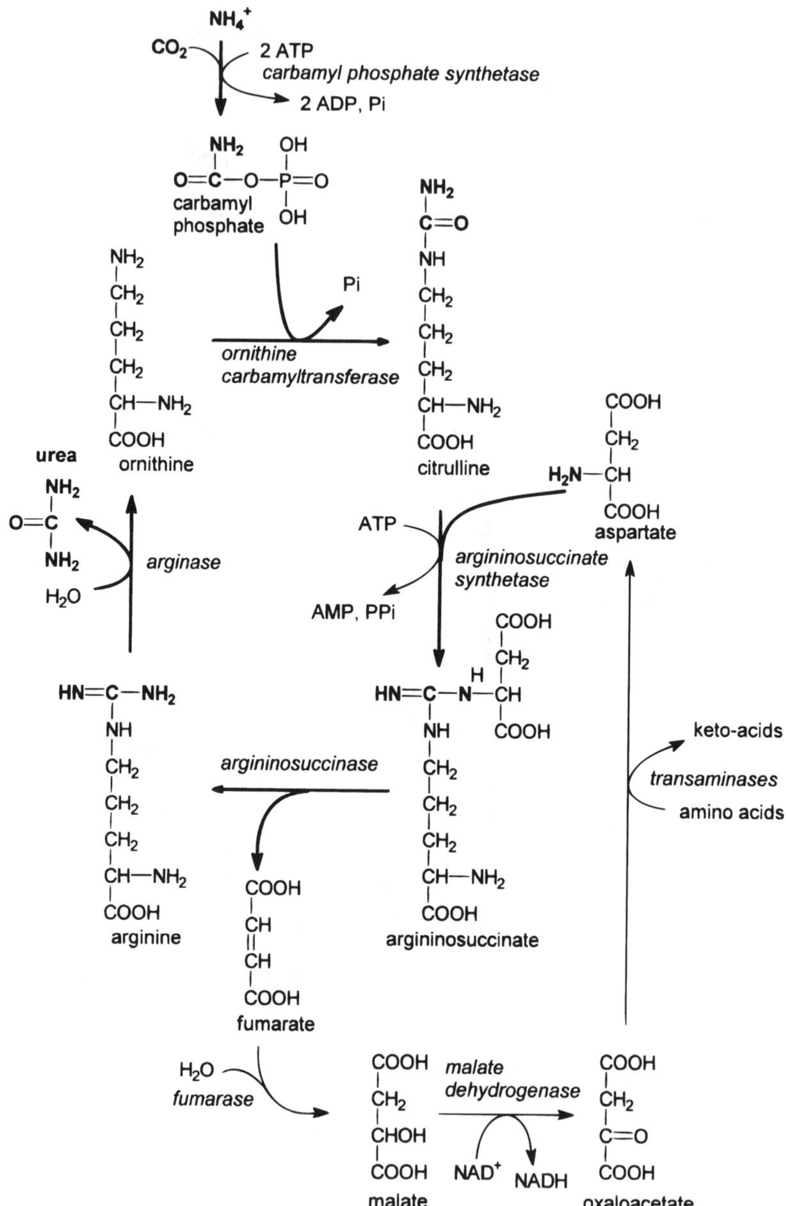

Figure 10.9 The synthesis of urea.

- Glycine is incorporated intact into purines, haem and other porphyrins, and creatine.
- Glutamine; the amide nitrogen is transferred in an ATP-dependent reaction, replacing an oxo group in the acceptor with an amino group.
- Aspartate, which undergoes an ATP- or GTP-dependent condensation reaction with an oxo group, followed by cleavage to release fumarate.

As shown in Figure 10.10, such reactions result in a net gain of ATP, since the fumarate is hydrated to malate, then oxidized to oxaloacetate, which is then available to undergo transamination to aspartate. Adenosine deaminase converts adenosine monophosphate back to inosine monophosphate, liberating ammonia. The sequence of reactions thus provides a pathway for the deamination of a variety of amino acids, linked to transamination, similar to those

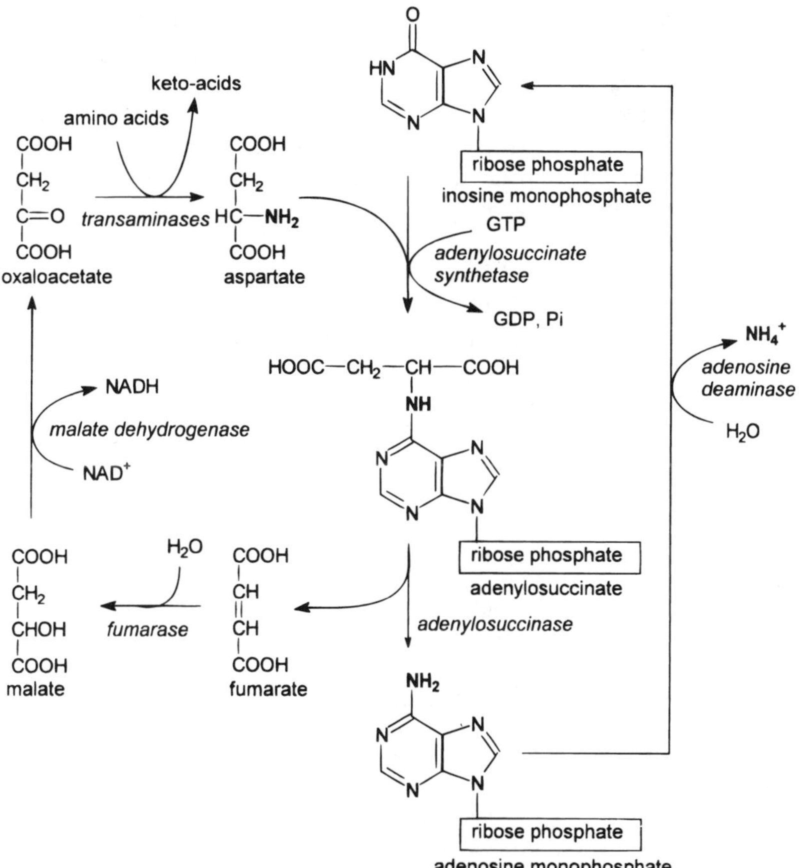

Figure 10.10 The role of aspartate as a nitrogen donor, and of adenosine deaminase as a source of ammonium ions.

shown in Figure 10.7 for transamination linked to glutamate dehydrogenase or glycine oxidase.

10.3.2 The metabolism of amino acid carbon skeletons

Acetyl CoA and acetoacetate arising from the carbon skeletons of amino acids may be used for fatty acid synthesis (see §7.6.1) or may be oxidized as metabolic fuel, but cannot be utilized for the synthesis of glucose (gluconeogenesis, see §7.7). Amino acids that yield acetyl CoA or acetoacetate are termed ketogenic. By contrast, those amino acids that yield intermediates that can be used for gluconeogenesis are termed glucogenic. As shown in Table 10.11, only two amino acids are purely ketogenic: leucine and lysine. Three others yield both glucogenic fragments and either acetyl CoA or acetoacetate: tryptophan, isoleucine and phenylalanine.

The principal substrate for gluconeogenesis is oxaloacetate, which undergoes the reaction catalysed by phosphoenolpyruvate carboxykinase to yield phosphoenolpyruvate, as shown in Figure 7.19. The onward metabolism of phosphoenolpyruvate to glucose is shown in Figure 7.4.

There is obviously a need to ensure that utilization of oxaloacetate for gluconeogenesis does not deplete the pool of oxaloacetate that is essential to maintain citric acid cycle activity. Phosphoenolpyruvate carboxykinase is a mitochondrial enzyme that uses GTP as the phosphate donor; the only source of GTP inside the mitochondrion is the reaction of succinyl CoA synthetase – an enzyme of the citric acid cycle. This means that if too much oxaloacetate was being withdrawn for gluconeogenesis, the rate of citric acid cycle activity,

Table 10.11 Metabolic fates of the carbon skeletons of amino acids

	Glucogenic intermediates	Ketogenic intermediates
Alanine	Pyruvate	—
Glycine → serine	Pyruvate	—
Cysteine	Pyruvate	—
Tryptophan	Pyruvate	Acetyl CoA
Arginine → ornithine	α-Ketoglutarate	—
Glutamine → glutamate	α-Ketoglutarate	—
Proline → glutamate	α-Ketoglutarate	—
Histidine → glutamate	α-Ketoglutarate	—
Methionine	Propionyl CoA	—
Isoleucine	Propionyl CoA	Acetyl CoA
Valine	Succinyl CoA	—
Asparagine → aspartate	Oxaloacetate	—
Aspartate	Oxaloacetate *or* fumarate	—
Phenylalanine → tyrosine	Fumarate	Acetoacetate
Leucine	—	Acetoacetate *and* acetyl CoA
Lysine		Acetyl CoA

and hence of phosphorylation of GDP to GTP, would be reduced, leading to less GTP being available for the withdrawal of oxaloacetate.

The points of entry of amino acid carbon skeletons into central metabolic pathways are shown in Figure 10.11. Those that give rise to ketoglutarate, succinyl CoA, fumarate or oxaloacetate increase the tissue pool of citric acid cycle intermediates, so permitting the withdrawal of oxaloacetate for gluconeogenesis without impairing energy-yielding metabolism.

Those amino acids that give rise to pyruvate also increase the mitochondrial pool of oxaloacetate, since pyruvate is carboxylated to oxaloacetate in the reaction catalysed by pyruvate carboxylase. The control of the metabolic fate of pyruvate, carboxylation to oxaloacetate or oxidative decarboxylation to acetyl CoA, is discussed in §7.4.2.

Gluconeogenesis is an important fate of amino acid carbon skeletons in the fasting state, when the metabolic imperative is to maintain a supply of glucose

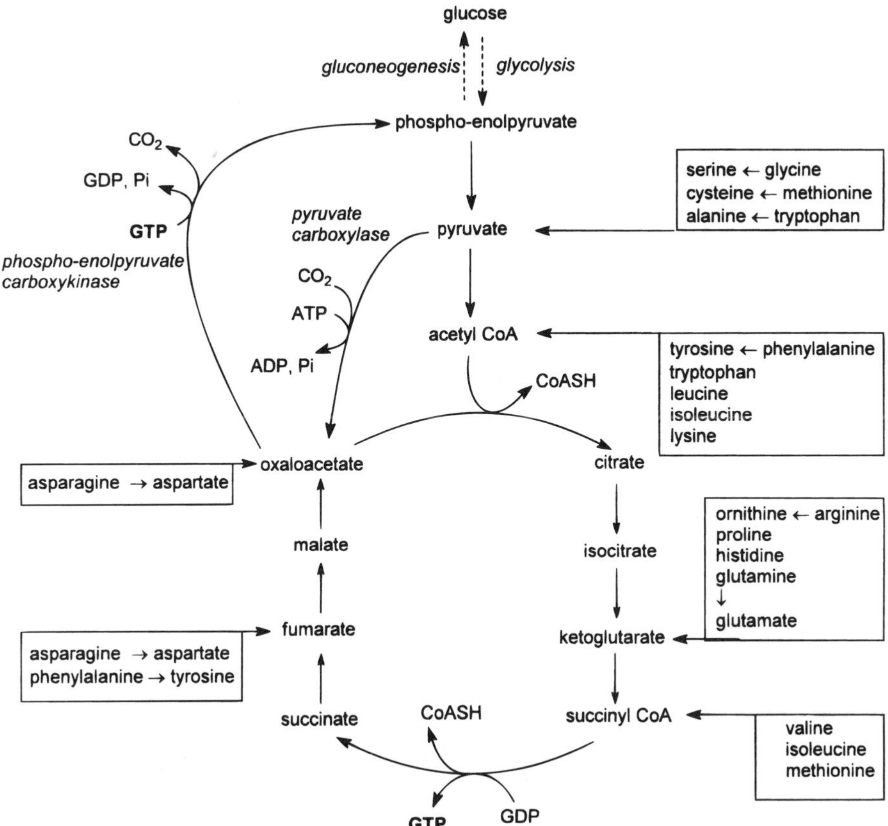

Figure 10.11 Metabolic fates of the carbon skeletons of amino acids; with the exception of those that give rise to acetyl CoA, all can be used for gluconeogenesis.

for the central nervous system and red blood cells. However, in the fed state the carbon skeletons of amino acids in excess of requirements for protein synthesis will mainly be used for formation of acetyl CoA for fatty acid synthesis, and storage as adipose tissue triacylglycerol.

11

The Integration and Control of Metabolism

The rate at which different pathways operate is controlled by changes in the activity of key regulatory enzymes. In general, the first reaction unique to a given pathway or branch of a pathway will be subject to closest regulation, although the activities of other enzymes may also be regulated.

Within any one cell the activities of regulatory enzymes may be controlled by two mechanisms which act instantaneously:

- the availability of substrates
- inhibition or activation by accumulation of precursors, end-products or intermediates of a pathway

On a whole-body basis, metabolic regulation is achieved by the actions of hormones. A hormone is released from the organ in which it is synthesized in response to a stimulus such as the blood concentration of metabolic fuels, circulates in the bloodstream and acts only on target cells that have receptors for that hormone. There are two types of response to hormones:

- Fast responses resulting from changes in the activity of existing enzymes, as a result of covalent modification of the enzyme protein. Fast-acting hormones act by way of cell surface receptors which release a second messenger inside the cell. This second messenger then acts directly or indirectly to activate an enzyme which catalyses the covalent modification of the target enzymes. Many neurotransmitters act in a similar way. The main second messengers released in response to hormone and neurotransmitter binding are: cyclic AMP and cyclic GMP (see §11.2.2), inositol trisphosphate and diacylglycerol (§11.2.3) and calcium ions (§12.3.1).
- Slow responses resulting from changes in the synthesis of enzymes. Slow-acting hormones act by way of intracellular receptors which bind to regulatory regions of DNA and increase or decrease the rate of transcription of one or more genes.

Regardless of the mechanism by which a hormone acts to regulate a metabolic pathway, there are three key features of hormonal regulation:

- Tissue selectivity, determined by whether or not the tissue contains receptors for the hormone.
- Amplification of the hormone signal.
- A mechanism to terminate the hormone action as its secretion decreases. Binding of hormones to receptors is reversible; so, as the secretion of the hormone decreases and its plasma concentration falls as a result of metabolism, bound hormone leaves the receptor and stimulation of the response ceases. In addition to this, there must be a mechanism to reverse the effects of hormone binding: metabolism of the second messenger and reversal of the covalent changes in the case of fast-acting hormones, or gradual turnover of proteins in the case of slow-acting hormones.

11.1 Intracellular regulation of enzyme activity

As discussed in §4.2.1.3, the rate at which an enzyme catalyses a reaction increases with increasing concentration of substrate, until the enzyme is more or less saturated with substrate. This means that an enzyme that has a high K_m, relative to the usual intracellular concentration of its substrate, will be sensitive to changes in substrate availability. By contrast, an enzyme that has a low K_m, relative to the usual intracellular concentration of its substrate, will act at a more or less constant rate regardless of changes in substrate availability.

In most tissues the phosphorylation of glucose to glucose 6-phosphate is catalysed by hexokinase (see Figure 11.1 and §7.4.1). The K_m of hexokinase is 0.15 mmol per L, while plasma and tissue concentrations of glucose rarely, if ever, fall below 2.5–3 mmol per L, even in severe hypoglycaemia. This means that hexokinase always acts at it maximum rate. In the liver there is also an isoenzyme of hexokinase, sometimes called glucokinase, which has a considerably higher K_m, of the order of 20 mmol per L. This enzyme has little or no activity at low concentrations of glucose. However, as the concentration of glucose in the hepatic portal vein rises after a meal, so the activity of glucokinase becomes more important, and the liver is able to trap more glucose as glucose 6-phosphate.

This provides the first step in the control by the liver of the availability of metabolic fuels to the rest of the body. The constant rate of hexokinase activity is adequate to meet the liver's need for glycolysis (see §7.4.1), and the additional glucose 6-phosphate that is formed is used for the synthesis of glycogen (see §7.6.2, and 11.1.1 for a discussion of the hormonal regulation of glycogen metabolism in the liver).

Glucokinase is also found in the β-cells of the pancreas, where its activity is important in initiating the secretion of insulin in response to a rising concentration of glucose in the portal blood. As a result of glucokinase activity, there is an increased rate of formation of glucose 6-phosphate, which results in an

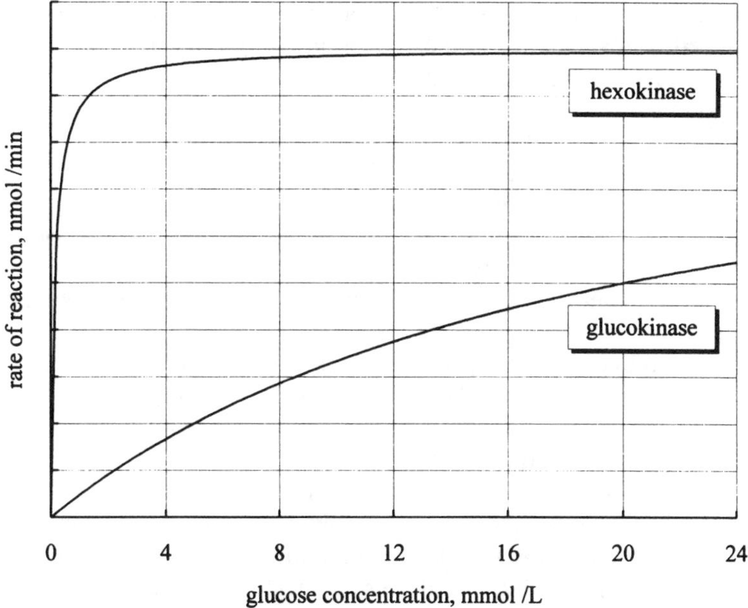

Figure 11.1 The substrate dependence of hexokinase and glucokinase; the concentration of glucose in peripheral blood is between 3.5 and 6 mmol per L; it may rise to 20 mmol per L in the hepatic portal vein in the fed state.

increased rate of glycolysis and synthesis of fatty acids in the pancreas (see §7.6.1). The free fatty acids are believed to act as the stimulus for insulin secretion.

In the same way, the central nervous system is able to respond to changes in the availability of the amino acid tryptophan in the bloodstream. Tryptophan hydroxylase is the first enzyme in the pathway that leads to synthesis of the neurotransmitter serotonin (5-hydroxytryptamine), and has a relatively high K_m – around 50 μmol per L, compared with 20–25 μmol per L free tryptophan in the brain. As the uptake of tryptophan into the brain increases, so the rate at which serotonin is synthesized also increases. This is believed to be one of the mechanisms that activate the hypothalamic centres that control hunger and satiety (see Figure 1.1).

11.1.1 Allosteric modification of the activity of regulatory enzymes

Allosteric regulation of enzyme activity is the result of reversible, non-covalent, binding of compounds other than the substrate to regulatory sites on the enzyme. Binding of the effector to the regulatory site leads to a change in the conformation of the protein, and a change in the conformation of the active site. This may result in either increased catalytic activity (allosteric activation) or decreased catalytic activity (allosteric inhibition). Enzymes that are subject to allosteric regulation are often multiple subunit proteins.

Compounds that act as allosteric inhibitors are commonly products of the pathway, and this type of inhibition is known as end-product inhibition. The decreased rate of enzyme activity results in a lower rate of formation of an end-product that is present is adequate amounts.

Compounds that act as allosteric activators of enzymes are often precursors of the pathway, so this is a mechanism for feed-forward activation, increasing the activity of a controlling enzyme in anticipation of increased availability of substrate.

As discussed in §4.2.1.3, enzymes that consist of multiple subunits frequently display cooperativity between the subunits, so that binding of substrate to the active site of one subunit leads to conformational changes that enhance the binding of substrate to the other active sites of the complex. This again is allosteric activation of the enzyme, in this case by the substrate itself. The activity of allosteric enzymes is more sharply dependent on the concentration of substrate than is the case for enzymes that do not show cooperativity.

As shown in Figure 11.2, an allosteric activator of an enzyme that shows substrate cooperativity acts by increasing that cooperativity, so that the enzyme has a greater activity at a low concentration of the substrate than would otherwise be the case. Conversely, an allosteric inhibitor of a cooperative enzyme acts by decreasing the cooperativity, so that the enzyme has less

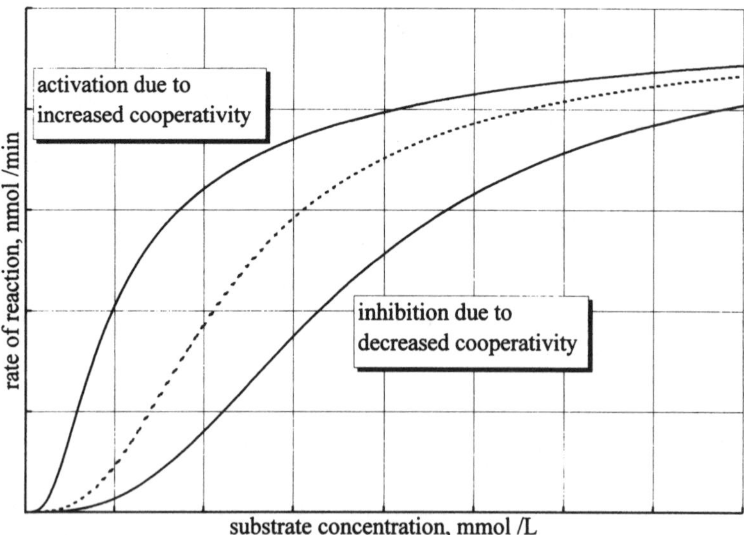

Figure 11.2 Allosteric regulation of enzyme activity: activation arising from increased substrate cooperativity and inhibition from decreased substrate cooperativity.

activity at a low concentration of substrate than it would in the absence of the inhibitor.

11.2 Responses to fast-acting hormones by covalent modification of enzyme proteins

Many regulatory enzymes have a serine or tyrosine residue at either the active site or a regulatory site. This can undergo phosphorylation catalysed by protein kinase, as shown in Figure 11.3. Phosphorylation may increase or decrease the activity of the enzyme. Later, the phosphate group is removed from the enzyme by phosphoprotein phosphatase, thus restoring the enzyme to its original state.

The reduction in activity of pyruvate dehydrogenase in response to increased concentrations of acetyl CoA and NADH (see §11.4.2) is the result of phosphorylation. Pyruvate dehydrogenase kinase is allosterically activated by acetyl CoA and NADH, and catalyses the phosphorylation of pyruvate dehydrogenase to an inactive form. Pyruvate dehydrogenase phosphatase acts constantly to dephosphorylate the inactive enzyme, so restoring its activity, and maintaining sensitivity to changes in the concentrations of acetyl CoA and NADH.

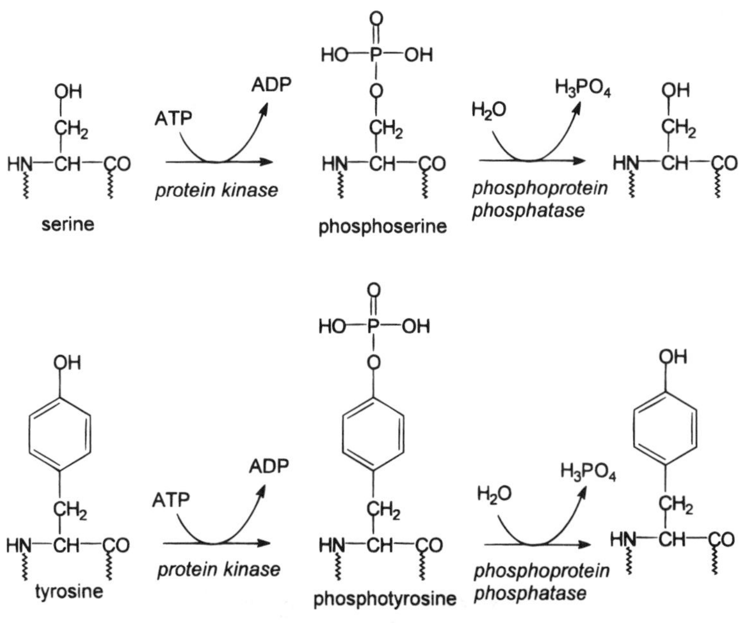

Figure 11.3 Covalent modification of enzymes by phosphorylation of serine (above) or tyrosine (below), and reversal by phosphatase action.

This control of enzyme phosphorylation by substrates is unusual. In most cases, the activities of protein kinases and phosphoprotein phosphatases are regulated by second messengers released intracellularly in response to fast-acting hormones binding to receptors at the cell surface.

The hormonal regulation of glycogen synthesis and utilization is one of the best understood of such mechanisms. Two enzymes are involved, and obviously it is not desirable that both enzymes should be active at the same time:

- Glycogen synthase catalyses the synthesis of glycogen, adding glucose units from UDP-glucose (see §7.6.2 and Figure 7.18).
- Glycogen phosphorylase catalyses the removal of glucose units from glycogen, as glucose 1-phosphate (see §7.4.1 and Figure 7.3).

In response to insulin (secreted in the fed state) there is increased synthesis of glycogen, and inactivation of glycogen phosphorylase. In response to glucagon (secreted in the fasting state) or adrenaline (secreted in response to fear or fright) there is activation of glycogen phosphorylase, permitting utilization of glycogen reserves, and inactivation of glycogen synthase. As shown in Figure 11.4, both effects are mediated by protein phosphorylation and dephosphorylation:

1 Protein kinase is activated in response to glucagon or adrenaline:
   (i) phosphorylation of glycogen synthase results in loss of activity
   (ii) phosphorylation of glycogen phosphorylase results in activation of the inactive enzyme
2 Phosphoprotein phosphatase is activated in response to insulin:
   (i) dephosphorylation of phosphorylated glycogen synthase restores its activity
   (ii) dephosphorylation of phosphorylated glycogen phosphorylase results in loss of activity

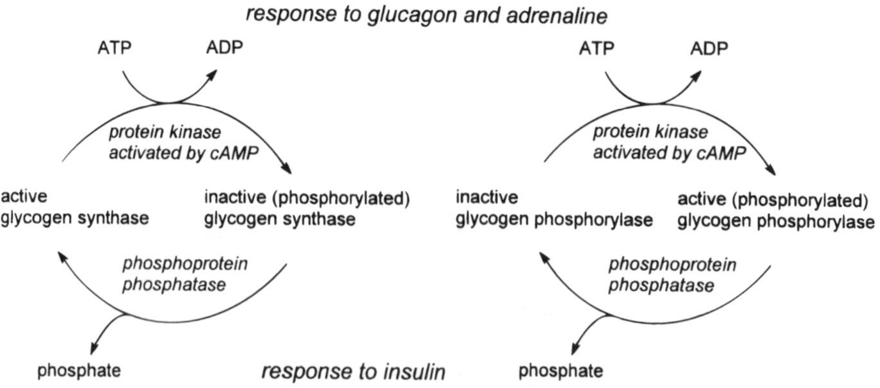

Figure 11.4 The regulation of glycogen synthesis (left) and utilization (right) by phosphorylation and dephosphorylation of enzymes in response to hormones.

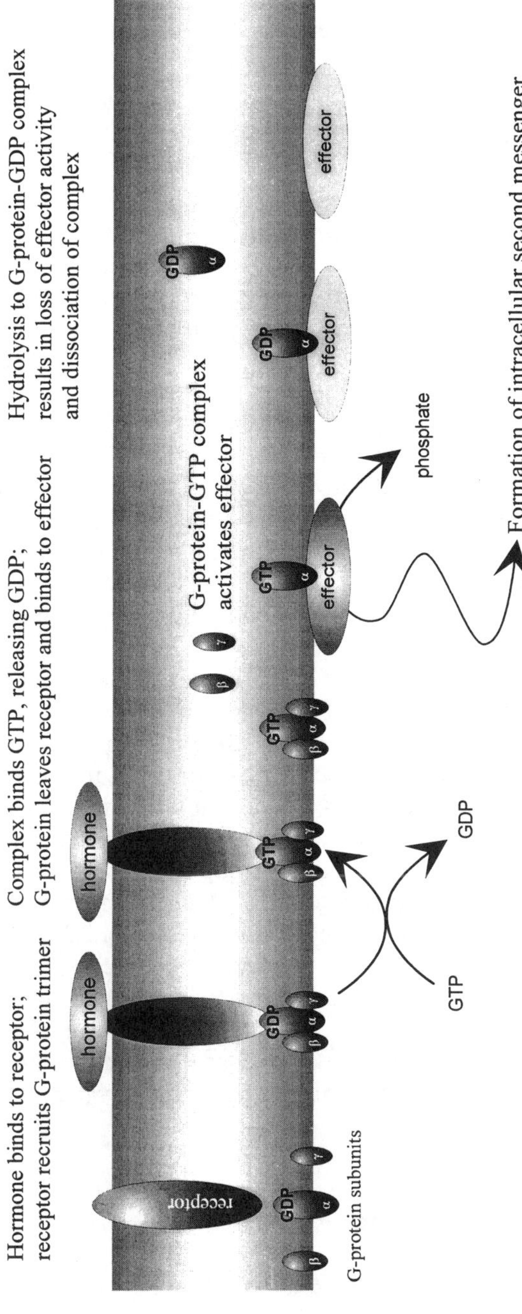

Figure 11.5 The role of G proteins in the response to fast-acting hormones binding to cell surface receptors.

There is a further measure of instantaneous control by intracellular metabolites which can override this hormonal regulation:

- Inactive glycogen synthase is allosterically activated by high concentrations of glucose 6-phosphate.
- Active glycogen phosphorylase is allosterically inhibited by ATP, glucose and glucose 6-phosphate.

11.2.1 Membrane receptors and G-proteins

A cell will respond to a fast-acting hormone only if it has cell-surface receptors that bind the hormone. These receptors are membrane proteins (see Figure 3.9); at the outer face of the membrane they have a site that binds the hormone, in the same way as an enzyme binds its substrate, by non-covalent equilibrium binding.

When the receptor binds the hormone, it undergoes a conformational change that permits it to interact with proteins at the inner face of the membrane. These are known as G-proteins because they bind guanine nucleotides (GDP or GTP, see §5.1). They function to transmit information from an occupied membrane receptor protein to an intracellular effector, which in turn leads to the release into the cytosol of a second messenger, ultimately resulting in the activation of protein kinases.

The G-proteins that are important in hormone responses consist of three subunits, α-, β- and γ-. As shown in Figure 11.5, in the resting state the subunits are separate, and the β-subunit binds GDP. When the receptor at the outer face of the membrane is occupied by its hormone, it undergoes a conformational change and recruits the α-, β- and γ-subunits to form a (G-protein trimer)–receptor complex. The complex then reacts with GTP, which displaces the bound GDP. Once GTP has bound, the complex dissociates.

The α-subunit of the G-protein with GTP bound then binds to, and activates, the effector, which may be adenylyl cyclase (see §11.2.2), phospholipase C (§11.2.3) or an ion transport channel in a cell membrane, resulting in formation of the second messenger. The α-subunit slowly catalyses hydrolysis of its bound GTP to GDP. As this occurs, the α-subunit–effector complex dissociates, and the effector loses its activity. The G-protein subunits are then available to be recruited by another receptor that has been activated by binding the hormone.

11.2.2 Cyclic AMP and cyclic GMP as second messengers

One of the intracellular effectors that is activated by the G-protein α-subunit–GTP complex is adenylyl cyclase. This is an integral membrane protein that catalyses the formation of cyclic AMP (cAMP) from ATP (see Figure 11.6).

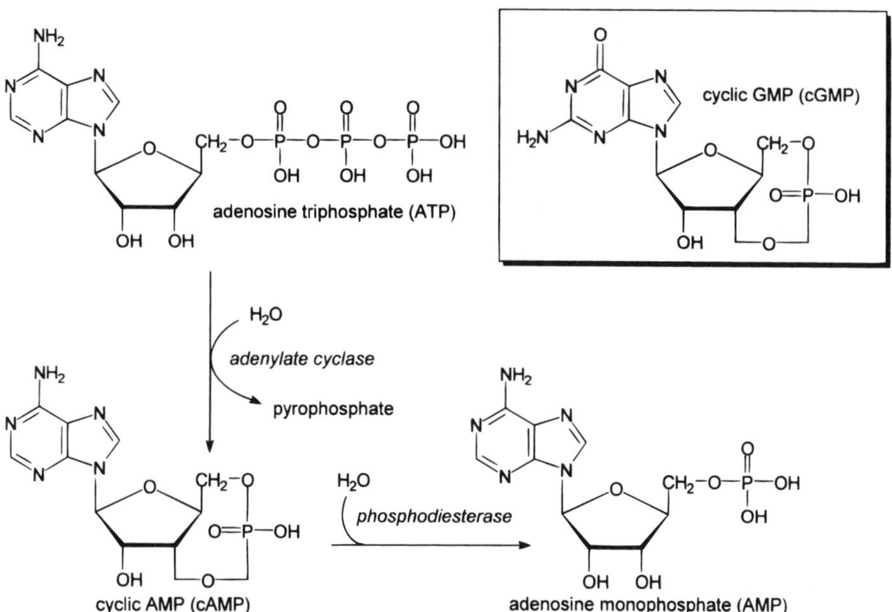

Figure 11.6 The formation of cyclic AMP as a second messenger in response to fast-acting hormones; guanylate cyclase forms cyclic GMP (inset) from GTP.

cAMP then acts as the second messenger in response to hormones such as glucagon and adrenaline. It is an allosteric activator of protein kinases. cAMP is also formed in the same way in response to some neurotransmitters.

As shown in Figure 11.6, phosphodiesterase catalyses the hydrolysis of cAMP to yield AMP, thus providing a mechanism for termination of the intracellular response to the hormone. Phosphodiesterase is activated in response to insulin action (which thus acts to terminate the actions of glucagon and adrenaline), and is inhibited by drugs such as caffeine and theophylline, which therefore potentiate hormone action.

In the same way as cAMP is formed from ATP by adenylyl cyclase, the guanine analogue cGMP can be formed from GTP by guanylyl cyclase. These may either be integral membrane proteins, like adenylyl cyclase, or may be soluble cytosolic proteins. cGMP is produced in response to some neurotransmitters and also nitric oxide, the endothelium-derived relaxation factor that is important in vasodilatation.

The active (G-protein α-subunit)–GTP released in response to binding of 1 mol of hormone to the cell surface receptor will activate adenylyl cyclase or guanylyl cyclase for as long as it contains GTP. The hydrolysis to inactive (G-protein α-subunit)–GDP only occurs relatively slowly. Therefore, a single molecule of (G-protein α-subunit)-GTP will lead to the production of many molecules of cAMP or cGMP as second messenger.

There is an equilibrium between cAMP or cGMP bound to protein kinase and in free solution in the cytosol, and therefore accessible to phosphodiesterase for inactivation. Each molecule of cAMP or cGMP activates a molecule of protein kinase for as long as it remains bound, resulting in the phosphorylation of many molecules of target protein.

Each enzyme molecule that has been activated by protein kinase will catalyse the metabolism of many molecules of substrate before it is dephosphorylated by phosphoprotein phosphatase.

11.2.3 *Inositol trisphosphate and diacylglycerol as second messengers*

The other response to G-protein activation involves phosphatidylinositol, one of the phospholipids in cell membranes (see §6.3.1.2). As shown in Figure 11.7, phosphatidylinositol can undergo two phosphorylations, catalysed by phosphatidylinositol kinase, to yield phosphatidylinositol bisphosphate (PIP_2). PIP_2 is a substrate for phospholipase C, which is activated by the binding of (G-protein α-subunit)–GTP. The products of phospholipase C action are inositol trisphosphate (IP_3) and diacylglycerol, both of which act as intracellular second messengers.

Inositol trisphosphate opens a calcium transport channel in the membrane of the endoplasmic reticulum. This leads to a 10-fold increase in the cytosolic concentration of calcium ions, as a result of influx of calcium from storage in the endoplasmic reticulum. Calmodulin is a small calcium-binding protein found in all cells. Its affinity for calcium is such that at the resting concentration of calcium in the cytosol (of the order of 0.1 μmol per L), little or none is bound to calmodulin. When the cytosolic concentration of calcium rises to about 1 μmol per L, as occurs in response to opening of the endoplasmic reticulum calcium transport channel, calmodulin binds 4 mol of calcium per mole of protein. When this occurs, calmodulin undergoes a conformational change, and calcium–calmodulin binds to, and activates, cytosolic protein kinases.

The diacylglycerol released by phospholipase C action remains in the membrane, where it activates a membrane-bound protein kinase. It may also diffuse into the cytosol, where it enhances the binding of calcium–calmodulin to cytosolic protein kinase.

Inositol trisphosphate is inactivated by further phosphorylation to inositol tetrakisphosphate (IP_4), and the diacylglycerol is inactivated by hydrolysis to glycerol and fatty acids.

The active (G-protein α-subunit)–GTP released in response to binding of 1 mol of hormone to the cell surface receptor will activate phospholipase C for as long as it contains GTP, and therefore, a single molecule of (G-protein α-subunit)–GTP complex will lead to the production of many molecules of IP_3 and diacylglycerol as second messengers.

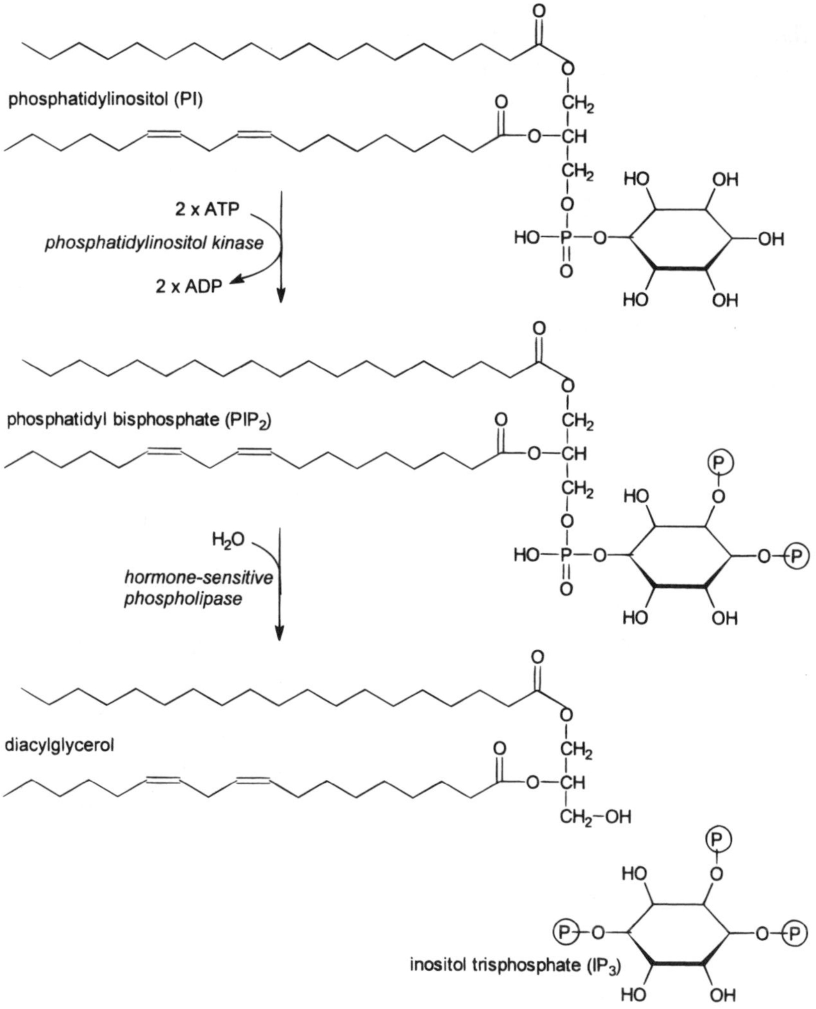

phosphatidylinositol (PI)

2 x ATP
phosphatidylinositol kinase
2 x ADP

phosphatidyl bisphosphate (PIP_2)

H_2O
hormone-sensitive phospholipase

diacylglycerol

inositol trisphosphate (IP_3)

Figure 11.7 The formation of inositol trisphosphate and diacylglycerol as second messengers in response to fast-acting hormones.

Each molecule of diacylglycerol will activate membrane protein kinase until it is hydrolysed (relatively slowly) by lipase, so resulting in the phosphorylation of many molecules of target protein, each of which will catalyse the metabolism of many molecules of substrate before it is dephosphorylated by phosphoprotein phosphatase.

Similarly, each molecule of IP_3 will continue to keep the endoplasmic reticulum calcium channel open until it is metabolized to the inactive form, thus maintaining a flow of calcium ions into the cytosol. Each molecule of calcium–

calmodulin will bind to, and activate, a molecule of protein kinase for as long as the cytosol calcium concentration remains high. It is only as the calcium is pumped back into the endoplasmic reticulum that the cytosolic concentration falls low enough for calmodulin to lose its bound calcium and be inactivated. Again each molecule of phosphorylated enzyme will catalyse the metabolism of many molecules of substrate before it is dephosphorylated by phosphoprotein phosphatase.

11.2.4 The insulin receptor

The insulin receptor is itself a protein kinase, which phosphorylates susceptible tyrosine residues in proteins. When insulin binds to the external part of the receptor complex, there is a conformational change in the whole of the receptor protein, which results in activation of the protein kinase region at the inner face of the membrane. This phosphorylates, and activates, cytosolic protein kinases, which in turn phosphorylate target enzymes, including phosphoprotein phosphatase (see Figure 11.4), cAMP phosphodiesterase (see Figure 11.6) and acetyl CoA carboxylase.

There is amplification of the response to insulin. As long as insulin remains bound to the receptor, the intracellular tyrosine kinase is active, phosphorylating, and therefore activating, many molecules of protein kinase, each of which phosphorylates many molecules of target enzyme.

Some receptors for growth factors have the same type of intracellular tyrosine kinase as does the insulin receptor. A mutant of the receptor for the epidermal growth factor (EGF) is permanently activated, even when not occupied by EGF. This results in continuous signalling for cell division, which is one of the underlying mechanisms in cancer.

11.3 Slow-acting hormones: changes in enzyme synthesis

As discussed in §10.1.1, there is continual turnover of proteins in the cell, and not all proteins are broken down and replaced at the same rate. Some are relatively stable; others, and especially enzymes that are important in metabolic regulation, have short half-lives – of the order of minutes or hours. This rapid turnover means that it is possible to control metabolic pathways by changing the rate at which a key enzyme is synthesized, and hence the total amount of that enzyme in the tissue. An increase in the rate of synthesis of an enzyme is induction, while the reverse, a decrease in the rate of synthesis of the enzyme by a metabolite, is repression. Key enzymes in metabolic pathways are often induced by their substrates, and similarly many are repressed by high concentrations of the end-products of the pathways they control.

Slow-acting hormones, including the steroid hormones such as cortisol and the sex steroids (androgens, oestrogens and progesterone, see §6.3.1.3), vitamin A (see §12.2.1.1), vitamin D (§12.2.2.3) and the thyroid hormones (see §12.3.3.3) act by changing the rate at which the genes for individual enzymes are expressed.

As shown in Figure 11.8, the hormone enters the cell and binds to a receptor protein in the nucleus. On binding the hormone, the receptor forms a dimer, and is activated, so that it will bind to a regulatory region of DNA (the hormone response element). Binding of the hormone–receptor complex to the hormone response element acts as a signal for RNA polymerase to transcribe

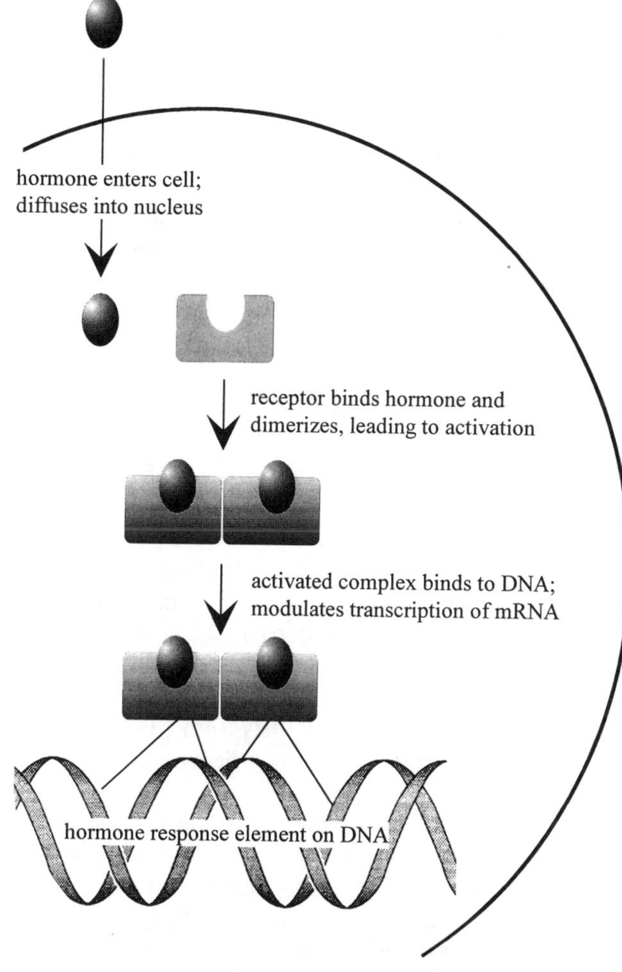

Figure 11.8 The response to slow-acting hormones that bind to intracellular (nuclear) receptors.

the gene that follows, resulting in an increase in the synthesis of the mRNA for that gene. Increased mRNA synthesis results in increased synthesis of the protein (see §10.2).

The amplification of the hormone signal in such cases is the result of increased mRNA, which results in much increased synthesis of the enzyme; again, each molecule of enzyme catalyses the metabolism of many molecules of substrate. The response is considerably slower than for hormones that increase the activity of existing enzyme molecules, because of the need for an adequate amount of new enzyme protein to be synthesized. Similarly, the response is prolonged, since after the hormone has ceased to act there is still an increased amount of enzyme protein in the cell, and the effect will only diminish as the newly synthesized enzyme is catabolized.

Although there is a great deal of information about the molecular mechanisms involved in initiating the responses to nuclear-acting hormones, less is known about the termination of hormone action. It is known that vitamin B_6 (see §12.2.8) has a role, and there is good evidence that the responsiveness of target tissues to slow-acting hormones is increased in vitamin B_6 deficiency.

The control of gene expression by slow-acting hormones is not usually a matter of switching on a gene that is otherwise silent. Rather, the hormone causes an increase in the expression of a gene that is already being transcribed at a low rate. Similarly, the secretion of steroid hormones is not a strictly on/off affair, rather a matter of changes in the amount being secreted.

11.4 Hormonal control in the fed and fasting states

In the fed state, when there is an ample supply of metabolic fuels from the gut, the main processes occurring are synthesis of reserves of triacylglycerol and glycogen; glucose is in plentiful supply, and is the main fuel for most tissues. By contrast, in the fasting state the reserves of triacylglycerol and glycogen are mobilized for use, and glucose, which is now scarce, must be spared for use by the brain and red blood cells. As discussed in §7.3, the principal hormones involved are insulin, in the fed state, and glucagon, in the fasting state. Adrenaline and noradrenaline share many of the actions of glucagon, and act to provide an increased supply of metabolic fuels from triacylglycerol and glycogen reserves in response to fear or fright, regardless of whether or not fuels are being absorbed from the gut.

In the liver, insulin and glucagon act to regulate the synthesis and breakdown of glycogen, as discussed in §11.2. They also regulate glycolysis (stimulated by insulin and inhibited by glucagon) and gluconeogenesis (inhibited by insulin and stimulated by glucagon). The result of this is that in the fed state the liver takes up and utilizes glucose to form either glycogen or triacylglycerols, which are exported to other tissues in very low density lipoproteins. By contrast, in the fasting state the liver exports glucose formed from the breakdown of glycogen and gluconeogenesis. As discussed in §7.5.3, in the fasting state the liver also oxidizes fatty acids and exports ketones for use by other tissues.

11.4.1 Hormonal control of adipose tissue metabolism

As shown in Figure 11.9, insulin has three actions in adipose tissue in the fed state:

- *Stimulation of glucose uptake*: This results in an increased rate of glycolysis (see §7.4.1) and hence an increased availability of acetyl CoA for fatty acid synthesis (§7.6.1). In the fasting state, when insulin secretion is low, little or no glucose is taken up into adipose tissue cells.
- *Activation of lipoprotein lipase at the cell surface*: This permits the adipose tissue cell to take up fatty acids from the triacylglycerol in chylomicrons coming from the small intestine (see §6.3.2.2) and very low-density lipoproteins coming from the liver. These are used for synthesis of triacylglycerol in the adipose tissue.

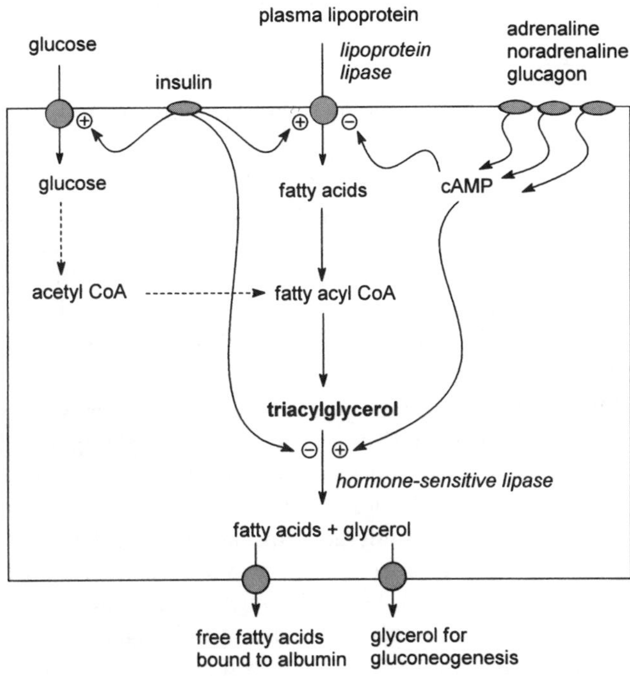

Figure 11.9 Hormonal control of the synthesis and hydrolysis of triacylglycerol in adipose tissue.

- *Inhibition of intracellular lipase* (*hormone-sensitive lipase*): This prevents the hydrolysis of triacylglycerol reserves and the release of free fatty acids and glycerol into the bloodstream.

cAMP, produced in response to glucagon in the fasting state, or in response to adrenaline and noradrenaline in the fed or fasting state, stimulates protein kinase. This has two actions:

- Inactivation of lipoprotein lipase, so that adipose tissue will not take up any fatty acids from plasma lipoproteins.
- Activation of hormone sensitive lipase, which catalyses the hydrolysis of the triacylglycerol stored in adipose tissue cells, leading to release into the bloodstream of free fatty acids (which are transported bound to albumin) and glycerol, which is an important substrate for gluconeogenesis in the liver.

11.4.2 Control of fuel utilization in muscle

Glucose is the main fuel for muscle in the fed state, but in the fasting state glucose is spared for use by the brain and red blood cells; glycogen, fatty acids and ketones are now the main fuels for muscle.

As shown in Figure 11.10, there are five mechanisms involved in this control of glucose utilization:

- The uptake of glucose into muscle is dependent on insulin. This means that in the fasting state, when insulin secretion is low, there will be little uptake of glucose into muscle.
- Hexokinase is subject to inhibition by its product, glucose 6-phosphate. As shown in Figure 7.3, glucose 6-phosphate may arise either as a result of the action of hexokinase on glucose or by isomerization of glucose 1-phosphate from glycogen breakdown. The activity of glycogen phosphorylase is increased in response to glucagon in the fasting state (see Figure 11.4) and the resultant glucose 6-phosphate inhibits utilization of any glucose that has entered the muscle cell.
- The activity of pyruvate dehydrogenase is reduced in response to increasing concentrations of both NADH and acetyl CoA (see §11.2). This means that the oxidation of fatty acids and ketones will inhibit the decarboxylation of pyruvate. Under these conditions the pyruvate that is formed from muscle glycogen by glycolysis will undergo transamination (see §10.3.1.2) to form alanine. Alanine is exported from muscle and used for gluconeogenesis in the liver (see §7.7 and §10.3.2). Thus, although muscle cannot directly release glucose from its glycogen reserves (because it lacks glucose 6-phosphatase), muscle glycogen is an indirect source of blood glucose in the fasting state.
- If alanine accumulates in muscle because it is not being removed by the liver at an adequate rate, then it acts as an allosteric inhibitor of pyruvate kinase,

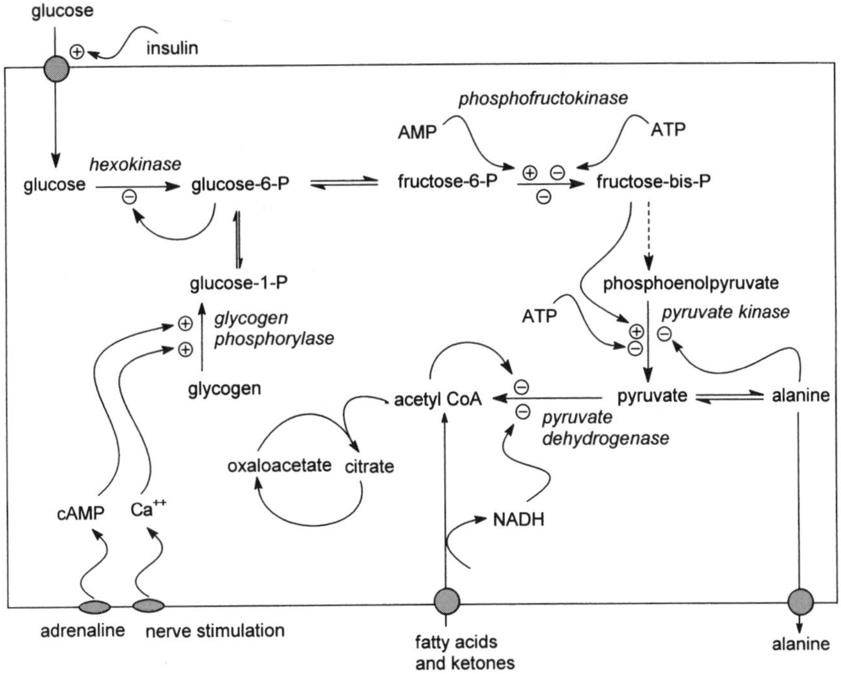

Figure 11.10 Control of the utilization of metabolic fuels in muscle.

so reducing the rate at which pyruvate is formed. This end-product inhibition of pyruvate kinase by alanine is overridden by high concentrations of fructose bisphosphate, which acts as a feed-forward activator of pyruvate kinase if it accumulates unduly.

- ATP is a product inhibitor of pyruvate kinase, and at high concentrations acts to inhibit the enzyme. More importantly, ATP acts as an allosteric inhibitor of phosphofructokinase. This means that under conditions where the supply of ATP (which can be regarded as the end-product of all energy-yielding metabolic pathways) is more than adequate to meet requirements, the metabolism of glucose is inhibited.

In the fed state there is an additional control over the rate of glucose utilization. Phosphofructokinase is inhibited allosterically by citrate, which accumulates in the cytosol when fatty acids are to be synthesized (see §7.6.1). Therefore, when the supply of citrate is more than adequate to meet immediate needs for fatty acid synthesis, there is a reduction in the rate at which glucose is utilized.

There is a need for an increased rate of glycolysis in response to exercise. This is achieved in three ways:

- As ADP begins to accumulate in muscle, it undergoes a reaction catalysed by adenylate kinase: $2 \times ADP \rightleftharpoons ATP + AMP$. This reaction maintains the pool of ATP for muscle contraction and, more importantly, AMP is a potent activator of phosphofructokinase, reversing the inhibition of this key regulatory enzyme by ATP, and so increasing the rate of glycolysis.
- Nerve stimulation of muscle results in an increased cytosolic concentration of calcium ions, and hence activation of calmodulin. Calcium–calmodulin activates glycogen phosphorylase, so increasing the rate of formation of glucose 1-phosphate and providing an increased amount of substrate for glycolysis.
- Adrenaline, released from the adrenal glands in response to fear or fright, acts on cell surface receptors, leading to the formation of cAMP, which leads to increased activity of protein kinase, and increased activity of glycogen phosphorylase (see Figure 11.4).

11.5 Diabetes mellitus: a failure of hormonal regulation

Diabetes mellitus is an impaired ability to regulate the utilization of blood glucose, as a result of a failure of the normal control by insulin. Therefore, the plasma glucose concentration is considerably higher than normal, especially after a meal. When it rises above the capacity of the kidney to resorb it from the glomerular filtrate (the renal threshold), the result is glucosuria – excretion of glucose in the urine. As a result of glucosuria, there is increased excretion of urine; one of the common presenting signs of diabetes is frequent urination, accompanied by excessive thirst.

There are two main types of diabetes mellitus:

- Type I diabetes (insulin-dependent diabetes mellitus, IDDM) is a failure to secrete insulin, as a result of damage to the β-cells of the pancreatic islets caused by viral infection or autoimmune disease. It commonly develops in childhood, and is sometimes known as juvenile-onset diabetes. Injection of insulin and strict control of carbohydrate intake are essential for control of blood glucose.
- Type II diabetes (non-insulin-dependent diabetes mellitus, NIDDM) is impaired responsiveness to insulin, as a result of decreased formation or sensitivity of cell-surface insulin receptors. Insulin secretion in response to glucose is normal or higher than normal. There is a clear genetic susceptibility to type II diabetes, which usually develops in middle age, with a gradual onset, and is sometimes known as maturity-onset diabetes. The condition is more common in obese people (see §8.2.2) and in its early stages the disease can be treated simply by weight reduction and control of carbohydrate intake. Better control of glucose metabolism can be achieved by use

of oral hypoglycaemic agents, which stimulate increased insulin secretion and enhance insulin receptor function. Increasingly, as biosynthetic human insulin has become widely available, treatment of NIDDM includes insulin injection to maintain better control over blood glucose concentration.

Acutely, diabetics are liable to coma as a result of hypo- or hyperglycaemia:

- Hypoglycaemic coma occurs if the plasma concentration of glucose falls below about 2 mmol per L, as a result of administration of insulin or oral hypoglycaemic agents without an adequate intake of carbohydrate. Strenuous exercise without additional food intake can also cause hypoglycaemia. In such cases, oral or intravenous glucose is required.
- Hyperglycaemic coma develops in people with insulin-dependent diabetes because, despite an abnormally high plasma concentration of glucose, tissues are unable to utilize it in the absence of insulin. Therefore, ketones are synthesized in the liver (see §7.5.3). However, when the metabolism of glucose is impaired, there is little or no pyruvate available for synthesis of oxaloacetate to maintain citric acid cycle activity (see §7.4.2.3). The result is severe keto-acidosis together with a very high plasma concentration of glucose. In such cases insulin injection is required.

In the long term, failure of glycaemic control and a persistently high plasma glucose concentration results in damage to capillary blood vessels (especially in the retina, leading to a risk of blindness), kidneys and peripheral nerves (leading to loss of sensation), and the development of cataracts in the lens of the eye and abnormal metabolism of plasma lipoproteins (which increases the risks of atherosclerosis and ischaemic heart disease). Two mechanisms have been proposed to explain these effects:

- At high concentrations, glucose can be reduced to sorbitol by aldose reductase. In tissues such as the lens of the eye and nerves, which cannot metabolize sorbitol, it accumulates, causing osmotic damage.
- Glucose can react non-enzymically with exposed lysine residues on proteins. Such glycated proteins include collagen (which may explain the problems of arthritis experienced by many diabetics), serum albumin, apolipoprotein A (which may explain the increased risk of atherosclerosis and ischaemic heart disease), α-crystallin in the lens (which may explain the development of cataracts), and haemoglobin A. Glycation of haemoglobin A provides a sensitive means of assessing the adequacy of glycaemic control over the preceding 4–6 weeks, and is commonly measured in diabetes clinics.

12

Micronutrients: The Vitamins and Minerals

In addition to an adequate source of metabolic fuels (carbohydrates, fats and proteins, see Chapter 7) and protein (see Chapter 10), there is a requirement for very much smaller amounts of other nutrients: the vitamins and minerals. Collectively these are referred to as micronutrients because of the small amounts that are required.

Vitamins are organic compounds required for the maintenance of normal health and metabolic integrity. They cannot be synthesized in the body and must be provided in the diet. They are required in very small amounts, of the order of milligrams or micrograms per day, and thus can be distinguished from the essential fatty acids (see §6.3.1.1) and the essential amino acids (see §10.1.3), which are required in larger amounts (several grams per day).

The essential minerals are those inorganic elements that have a physiological function in the body. Obviously, since they are elements, they must be provided in the diet, because elements cannot be interconverted. The amounts required vary from grams per day for sodium and calcium, through milligrams per day (e.g. iron) to micrograms per day for the trace elements (so called because they are required in such small amounts).

12.1 The determination of requirements and reference intakes

For any nutrient there is a range of intakes between that which is clearly inadequate, leading to clinical deficiency disease, and that which is so much in excess of the body's metabolic capacity that there may be signs of toxicity. Between these two extremes is a level of intake that is adequate for normal health and the maintenance of metabolic integrity, which is difficult to define, and a series of more precisely definable levels of intake that are adequate to meet specific criteria, and may be used to determine appropriate levels of intake:

- Clinical deficiency disease, with clear anatomical and functional lesions, and severe metabolic disturbances, possibly proving fatal. Prevention of deficiency disease is a minimal goal in determining requirements.

- Covert deficiency, where there are no signs of deficiency under normal conditions, but any trauma or stress reveals the precarious state of the body reserves and may precipitate clinical signs. For example, as discussed in §12.2.13.2, an intake of 10 mg of vitamin C per day is adequate to prevent clinical deficiency, but at least 20 mg per day is required for healing of wounds.
- Metabolic abnormalities under normal conditions, such as impaired carbohydrate metabolism in thiamin deficiency (see §12.2.5.1), or excretion of methylmalonic acid in vitamin B_{12} deficiency.
- Abnormal response to a metabolic load, such as the inability to metabolize a test dose of histidine in folate deficiency, or tryptophan in vitamin B_6 deficiency, although at normal levels of intake there may be no metabolic impairment.
- Inadequate saturation of enzymes with (vitamin-derived) coenzymes. This can be tested for three vitamins, using red blood cell enzymes: thiamin (see §12.2.5), riboflavin (§12.2.6) and vitamin B_6 (§12.2.8).
- Low plasma concentration of the nutrient, indicating that there is an inadequate amount in tissue reserves to permit normal transport between tissues. For some nutrients this may reflect failure to synthesize a transport protein rather than primary deficiency of the nutrient itself.
- Low urinary excretion of the nutrient, reflecting low intake and changes in metabolic turnover.
- Incomplete saturation of body reserves.
- Adequate body reserves and normal metabolic integrity. This is the (untestable) goal.
- Possibly beneficial effects of intakes more than adequate to meet requirements: the promotion of optimum health and life expectancy. There is fairly good evidence that relatively high intakes of vitamin E (see §12.2.3.2) and possibly other antioxidant nutrients (see §2.5.3) may reduce the risk of developing cardiovascular disease and some forms of cancer. High intakes of folate during early pregnancy reduce the risk of neural tube defects in the foetus (see §12.2.10.2).
- Pharmacological (drug-like) actions at very high levels of intake.
- Abnormal accumulation in tissues and overloading of normal metabolic pathways, leading to signs of toxicity and possibly irreversible lesions. Iron (see §12.3.2.3), selenium (§12.3.2.5), niacin (§12.2.7.3), and vitamins A (§12.2.1.5), D (§12.2.2.6) and B_6 (§12.2.8.4), are all known to be toxic in excess.

After an appropriate criterion of adequacy has been decided, requirements are determined by feeding volunteers on an otherwise adequate diet, but lacking the nutrient under investigation, until there is a detectable metabolic or other abnormality. They are then repleted with graded intakes of the nutrient until the abnormality is just corrected.

An alternative approach to determining requirements is to measure the rate at which the body content of the nutrient turns over (e.g. using isotopically labelled nutrients); the requirement is then the amount which is required to replace what is lost each day.

Problems arise in interpreting the results, and therefore defining requirements, when different markers of adequacy respond to different levels of intake. This explains the difference in the tables of reference intakes published by different national and international authorities.

12.1.1 Dietary reference values

Individuals do not all have the same requirement for nutrients, even when expressed relative to body size or energy expenditure. There is a range of individual requirements of up to 25 per cent around the observed average or mean requirement. Therefore, in order to set population goals, and assess the adequacy of diets, it is necessary to set a reference level of intake which is high enough to ensure that no one will either suffer from deficiency or be at risk of toxicity.

As shown in the upper graph in Figure 12.1, if it is assumed that individual requirements are distributed in a statistically normal fashion around the observed mean requirement, then a range of $\pm 2 \times$ the standard deviation (SD) around the mean will include the requirements of 95 per cent of the population. This 95 per cent range is conventionally used as the 'normal' or reference range (e.g. in clinical chemistry to assess the normality or otherwise of a test result), and is used to define three levels of nutrient intake:

- *The estimated average requirement* (*EAR*): This is the observed mean requirement to meet the chosen criterion of adequacy in experimental studies.
- *The reference nutrient intake* (*RNI*): This is $2 \times$ SD above the observed mean requirement, and is therefore more than adequate to meet the individual requirements of 97.5 per cent of the population. This is the goal for planning diets (e.g. in institutional feeding) and the standard against which the intake of a population can be assessed. In the European Union tables (see Table 12.3) this is called the population reference intake (PRI); in the USA it is called the recommended dietary allowance (RDA; Table 12.1).
- *The lower reference nutrient intake* (*LNRI*): This is $2 \times$ SD below the observed mean requirement, and is therefore adequate to meet the requirements of only 2.5 per cent of the population. In The European Union tables this is called the lower threshold intake, to stress that it is a level of intake at or below which it is extremely unlikely that normal metabolic integrity could be maintained.

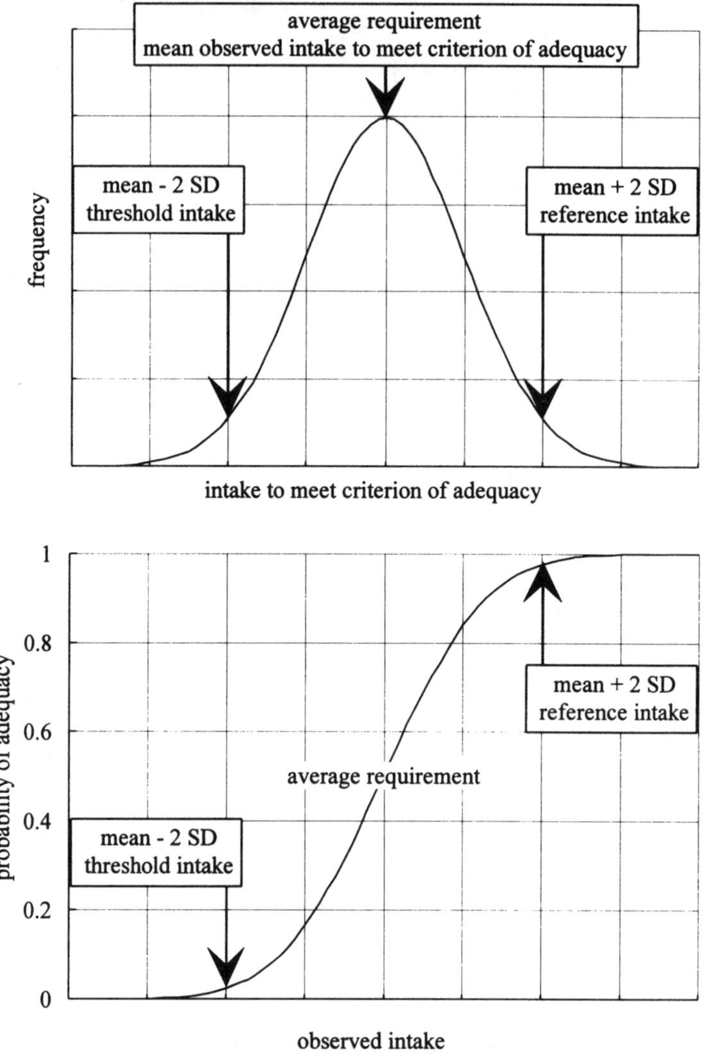

Figure 12.1 The derivation of reference intakes of nutrients from the distribution of requirements around the mean observed requirement; plotted below as a cumulative distribution curve permitting estimation of the probability of adequacy of a given level of intake for an individual.

The lower graph in Figure 12.1 shows the distribution of requirements plotted as the cumulative percentage of the population whose requirements have been met at each level of intake. This can therefore be used to estimate the probability that a given level of intake is adequate to meet an individual's requirements.

Table 12.1 US recommended daily amounts of nutrients

Age	Vit A μg	Vit D μg	Vit E mg	Vit K mg	Vit C mg	Vit B_1 mg	Vit B_2 mg	Niacin mg	Vit B_6 mg	Folate μg	Vit B_{12} μg	Ca mg	P mg	Mg mg	Fe mg	Zn mg	I μg	Se μg
0–6 m	375	7.5	3	5	30	0.3	0.4	5	0.3	25	0.3	400	300	40	6	5	40	10
6–12 m	375	10	4	10	35	0.4	0.5	6	0.6	35	0.5	600	500	60	10	5	50	15
1–3 y	400	10	6	15	40	0.7	0.8	9	1.0	50	0.7	800	800	80	10	10	70	20
4–6 y	500	10	7	20	45	0.9	1.1	12	1.1	75	1.0	800	800	120	10	10	90	20
7–10 y	700	10	7	30	45	1.0	1.2	13	1.4	100	1.4	800	800	170	10	10	120	30
Males																		
11–14 y	1000	10	10	45	50	1.3	1.5	17	1.7	150	2.0	1200	1200	270	12	15	150	40
15–18 y	1000	10	10	65	60	1.5	1.8	20	2.0	200	2.0	1200	1200	400	12	15	150	50
19–24 y	1000	10	10	70	60	1.5	1.7	19	2.0	200	2.0	1200	1200	350	10	15	150	70
25–50 y	1000	5	10	80	60	1.5	1.7	19	2.0	200	2.0	800	800	350	10	15	150	70
51 + y	1000	5	10	80	60	1.2	1.4	15	2.0	200	2.0	800	800	350	10	15	150	70
Females																		
11–14 y	800	10	8	45	50	1.1	1.3	15	1.4	150	2.0	1200	1200	280	15	12	150	45
15–18 y	800	10	8	55	60	1.1	1.3	15	1.5	180	2.0	1200	1200	300	15	12	150	50
19–24 y	800	10	8	60	60	1.1	1.3	15	1.6	180	2.0	1200	1200	280	15	12	150	55
25–50 y	800	5	8	65	60	1.1	1.3	15	1.6	180	2.0	800	800	280	15	12	150	55
51 + y	800	5	8	65	60	1.0	1.2	13	1.6	180	2.0	800	800	280	10	12	150	55
Pregnant	800	10	10	65	70	1.5	1.6	17	2.2	400	2.2	1200	1200	320	30	15	175	65
Lactating	1300	10	10	65	95	1.6	1.8	20	2.1	280	2.6	1200	1200	355	15	19	200	75

Table 12.2 UK reference nutrient intakes

Age	Vit B_1 mg	Vit B_2 mg	Niacin mg	Vit B_6 mg	Vit B_{12} μg	Folate μg	Vit C mg	Vit A μg	Vit D μg	Ca mg	P mg	Mg mg	Fe mg	Zn mg	Cu mg	Se μg	I μg
0–3 m	0.2	0.4	3	0.2	0.3	50	25	350	8.5	525	400	55	1.7	4.0	0.2	10	50
4–6 m	0.2	0.4	3	0.2	0.3	50	25	350	8.5	525	400	60	4.3	4.0	0.3	13	60
7–9 m	0.2	0.4	4	0.3	0.4	50	25	350	7	525	400	75	7.8	5.0	0.3	10	60
10–12 m	0.3	0.4	5	0.4	0.4	50	25	350	7	525	400	80	7.8	5.0	0.3	10	60
1–3 y	0.5	0.6	8	0.7	0.5	70	30	400	7	350	270	85	6.9	5.0	0.4	15	70
4–6 y	0.7	0.8	11	0.9	0.8	100	30	500	—	450	350	120	6.1	6.5	0.6	20	100
7–10 y	0.7	1.0	12	1.0	1.0	150	30	500	—	550	450	200	8.7	7.0	0.7	30	110
Males																	
11–14 y	0.9	1.2	15	1.2	1.2	200	35	600	—	1000	775	280	11.3	9.0	0.8	45	130
15–18 y	1.1	1.3	18	1.5	1.5	200	40	700	—	1000	775	300	11.3	9.5	1.0	70	140
19–50 y	1.0	1.3	17	1.4	1.5	200	40	700	—	700	550	300	8.7	9.5	1.2	75	140
50 + y	0.9	1.3	16	1.4	1.5	200	40	700	10	700	550	300	8.7	9.5	1.2	75	140
Females																	
11–14 y	0.7	1.1	12	1.0	1.2	200	35	600	—	800	625	280	14.8	9.0	0.8	45	130
15–18 y	0.8	1.1	14	1.2	1.5	200	40	600	—	800	6254	300	14.8	7.0	1.0	60	140
19–50 y	0.8	1.1	13	1.2	1.5	200	40	600	—	700	550	270	14.8	7.0	1.2	60	140
50 + y	0.8	1.1	12	1.2	1.5	200	40	600	10	700	550	270	8.7	7.0	1.2	60	140
Pregnant	+0.1	+0.3	—	—	—	+100	+10	+100	10	—	—	—					
Lactating	+0.1	+0.5	+2	—	+0.5	+60	+30	+350	10	+550	+440	+50		+6.0	+0.3	+15	

Table 12.3 EU population reference intakes of nutrients

Age	Vit A	Vit B_1	Vit B_2	Niacin	Vit B_6	Folate	Vit B_{12}	Vit C	Ca	P	Fe	Zn	Cu	Se	I
	μg	mg	mg	mg	mg	μg	μg	mg	mg	mg	mg	mg	mg	μg	μg
6–12 m	350	0.3	0.4	5	0.4	50	0.5	20	400	300	6	4	0.3	8	50
1–3 y	400	0.5	0.8	9	0.7	100	0.7	25	400	300	4	4	0.4	10	70
4–6 y	400	0.7	1.0	11	0.9	130	0.9	25	450	350	4	6	0.6	15	90
7–10 y	500	0.8	1.2	13	1.1	150	1.0	30	550	450	6	7	0.7	25	100
Males															
11–14 y	600	1.0	1.4	15	1.3	180	1.3	35	1000	775	10	9	0.8	35	120
15–17 y	700	1.2	1.6	18	1.5	200	1.4	40	1000	775	13	9	1.0	45	130
18 + y	700	1.1	1.6	18	1.5	200	1.4	45	700	550	9	9.5	1.1	55	130
Females															
11–14 y	600	0.9	1.2	14	1.1	180	1.3	35	800	625	18	9	0.8	35	120
15–17 y	600	0.9	1.3	14	1.1	200	1.4	40	800	625	17	7	1.0	45	130
18 + y	600	0.9	1.3	14	1.1	200	1.4	45	700	550	16	7	1.1	55	130
Pregnant	700	1.0	1.6	14	1.3	400	1.6	55	700	550	16	7	1.1	55	130
Lactating	950	1.1	1.7	16	1.4	350	1.9	70	1200	950	16	12	1.4	70	160

Tables 12.1, 12.2 and 12.3 show the reference intakes of vitamins and minerals published in the USA, UK and European Union.

12.1.1.1 *Safe and adequate levels of intake*

For some nutrients, such as the vitamins pantothenic acid (see §12.2.12) and biotin (§12.2.11) and some trace minerals, deficiency is unknown except under experimental conditions. For these nutrients there are no estimates of average requirements, and therefore no reference intakes. Since deficiency does not occur, it is obvious that average levels of intake are more than adequate to meet requirements, and for these nutrients there is a range of intakes that is defined as safe and adequate, based on the observed range of intakes.

12.1.1.2 *Labelling reference values*

As shown in Tables 12.1–12.3, reference intakes depend on age and gender. For purposes of nutritional labelling of foods it is obviously essential to have a single labelling reference value which will permit the consumer to compare the nutrient yields of different foods. Apart from foods aimed at infants and small children, for which age-related reference intakes are used, there are two ways of determining labelling reference values:

- To use the highest value of reference intake of any group in the population. This is the basis of labelling in the USA and (at present) the European Union. The disadvantage of this is that the highest reference intakes are considerably higher than are appropriate for most groups in the population, and therefore perfectly adequate foods may appear to be poor sources of nutrients, and consumers may be encouraged to take inappropriate and unnecessary nutrient supplements.
- To use the average requirement for adult men, which in most cases equals the reference intake for women. This is the approach favoured by the Scientific Committee for Food of the European Union, but has not yet been adopted in EU labelling legislation.

12.2 The vitamins

A vitamin is defined as an organic compound that is required in small amounts for the maintenance of normal metabolic function. Deficiency causes a specific disease, which is cured or prevented only by restoring the vitamin to the diet. This is important; it is not enough just to show that the compound has effects when added to the diet, since these may be pharmacological actions and may not be related to the maintenance of normal health and metabolic integrity. The metabolic functions of all the vitamins are now known. Therefore, before a new substance could be accepted as a possible vitamin, there must be not only evidence that deprivation caused a specific deficiency disease, which could be cured only with that compound, but also definition of a clear metabolic function.

As can be seen from Table 12.4, the vitamins are named in a curious way. This is an historical accident resulting from the way in which they were discovered. Studies at the beginning of the twentieth century showed that there was something in milk that was essential, in very small amounts, for the growth of animals fed on a diet consisting of purified fat, carbohydrate, protein and mineral salts. Two factors were found to be essential: one was found in the cream and the other in the watery part of milk. Logically, they were called Factor A (fat-soluble, in the cream) and Factor B (water-soluble, in the watery part of the milk). Factor B was identified chemically as an amine, and in 1913 the name 'vitamin' was coined for these 'vital amines'.

Further studies showed that 'vitamin B' was a mixture of several compounds, with different actions in the body, and so they were given numbers as well: vitamin B_1, vitamin B_2, and so on. There are gaps in the numerical order of the B vitamins. When what might have been called vitamin B_3 was discovered, it was found to be a chemical compound that was already known, nicotinic acid. It was therefore not given a number. Other gaps are because compounds assumed to be vitamins and given numbers, such as B_4, B_5, and so on, were later shown either not to be vitamins, or to be vitamins that had already been described by other workers, and given other names.

Vitamins C, D and E were named in the order of their discovery. The name 'vitamin F' was used at one time for what we now call the essential fatty acids (see §6.3.1.1); 'vitamin G' was later found to be what was already known as vitamin B_2. Biotin is still sometimes called vitamin H. Vitamin K was discovered by Henrik Dam, in Denmark, as a result of studies of disorders of blood coagulation, and he named it for its function – *koagulation* in Danish, hence vitamin K.

As the chemistry of the vitamins was elucidated, so they were given names as well, as shown in Table 12.4. Where only one chemical compound has the biological activity of the vitamin, this is quite easy. Thus, vitamin B_1 is thiamin, vitamin B_2 is riboflavin, and so on. With several of the vitamins, several chemically related compounds found in foods can be interconverted in the body, and all show the same biological activity. Such compounds are called vitamers, and a general name (a generic descriptor) is used to include all compounds that display the same biological activity. Thus, niacin is the generic descriptor for two compounds, nicotinic acid and nicotinamide, which have the same biological activity. Vitamin B_6 is used to describe the six compounds that have vitamin B_6 activity.

Correctly, for a compound to be classified as a vitamin, it should be a dietary essential that cannot be synthesized in the body. By this strict definition, two vitamins should not really be included, since they can be made in the body. However, both were discovered as a result of investigations of deficiency diseases, and they are usually considered as vitamins:

Table 12.4 The vitamins

	Vitamin	Principal metabolic functions	Deficiency disease
A	Retinol β-Carotene	Visual pigments in the retina; Cell differentiation; β-carotene is an antioxidant	Night blindness, xerophthalmia; keratinization of skin
D	Calciferol	Maintenance of calcium balance; enhances intestinal absorption of Ca^{2+} and mobilizes bone mineral	Rickets = poor mineralization of bone; osteomalacia = bone demineralization
E	Tocopherols, Tocotrienols	Antioxidant, especially in membranes	Extremely rare – serious neurological dysfunction
K	Phylloquinone, menaquinones	Coenzyme in formation of carboxyglutamate in enzymes of blood clotting and bone matrix	Impaired blood clotting, haemorrhagic disease
B_1	Thiamin	Coenzyme in pyruvate and 2-oxo-glutarate dehydrogenases, and transketolase; poorly defined function in nerve conduction	Peripheral nerve damage (beriberi) or CNS lesions (Wernicke–Korsakoff syndrome); acidosis
B_2	Riboflavin	Coenzyme in oxidation and reduction reactions; prosthetic group of flavoproteins	Lesions of corner of mouth, lips and tongue, sebhorroeic dermatitis
Niacin	Nicotinic acid, nicotinamide	Coenzyme in oxidation and reduction reactions, functional part of NAD and NADP	Pellagra – photosensitive dermatitis, depressive psychosis, fatal
B_6	Pyridoxine, pyridoxal, pyridoxamine	Coenzyme in transamination and decarboxylation of amino acids and glycogen phosphorylase; role in steroid hormone action	Disorders of amino acid metabolism, convulsions
	Folic acid	Coenzyme in transfer of one-carbon fragments	Megaloblastic anaemia
B_{12}	Cobalamin	Coenzyme in transfer of one-carbon fragments and metabolism of folic acid	Pernicious anaemia = megaloblastic anaemia with degeneration of the spinal cord
	Pantothenic acid	Functional part of CoA and acyl carrier protein	Peripheral nerve damage (burning foot syndrome)
	Biotin	Coenzyme in carboxylation reactions in gluconeogenesis and fatty acid synthesis	Impaired fat and carbohydrate metabolism, dermatitis
C	Ascorbic acid	Coenzyme in hydroxylation of proline and lysine in collagen synthesis; antioxidant; enhances absorption of iron	Scurvy – impaired wound healing, loss of dental cement, subcutaneous haemorrhage

- Vitamin D is made in the skin after exposure to sunlight (see §12.2.2.1), and should really be regarded as a steroid hormone rather than a vitamin. It is only when sunlight exposure is inadequate that a dietary source is required.
- Niacin (see §12.2.7) can be formed from the essential amino acid tryptophan. Indeed, synthesis from tryptophan is probably more important than a dietary intake of preformed niacin.

12.2.1 Vitamin A

Two groups of compounds shown in Figure 12.2 have vitamin A activity: retinol, retinaldehyde and retinoic acid (preformed vitamin A), which are found only in animal foods; and a variety of carotenes, which are found in

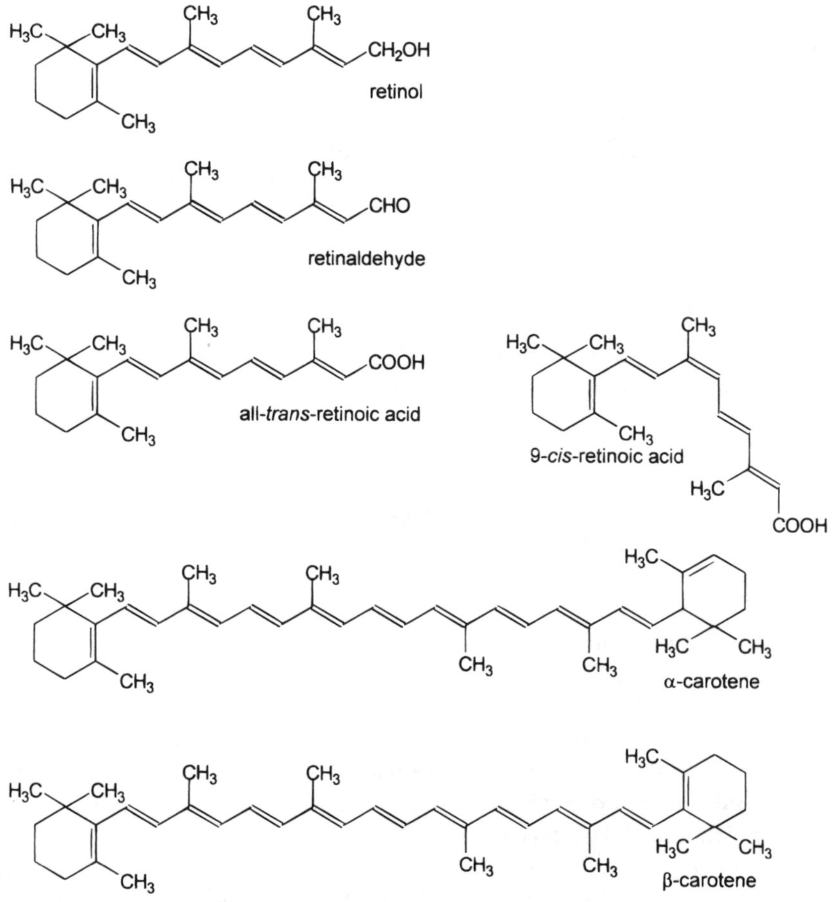

retinol

retinaldehyde

all-*trans*-retinoic acid

9-*cis*-retinoic acid

α-carotene

β-carotene

Figure 12.2 Vitamin A vitamers and the major vitamin A carotenoids.

yellow, red and green vegetables, as well as in meat and dairy produce. The main sources of preformed vitamin A are meat (and especially liver), milk and milk products, and eggs.

Many, but not all, of the carotenes can be metabolized in the intestinal mucosa to give rise to retinol. These are known as provitamin A carotenoids. The most important of the carotenes with vitamin A activity is β-carotene. Although it would appear from its structure that one molecule of β-carotene will yield two of retinol, this is not so in practice, because the intestinal mucosal enzyme is readily saturated, and a considerable amount is absorbed as carotene. Nutritionally, 6 μg of β-carotene is equivalent to 1 μg of preformed retinol. For other carotenes with vitamin A activity, 12 μg is equivalent to 1 mg of preformed retinol.

The total amount of vitamin A in foods is expressed as micrograms of retinol equivalents, calculated from the sum of:

μg preformed vitamin A + 1/6 × μg β—carotene + 1/12 × μg other provitamin A carotenoids.

Before pure vitamin A was available for chemical analysis, the vitamin A content of foods was determined by biological assays, and the results expressed in standardized international units (iu): 1 iu = 0.3 μg retinol, or 1 μg of retinol = 3.33 iu. Although now obsolete, iu are sometimes still used in nutritional labelling.

12.2.1.1 *Metabolic functions of vitamin A*

The best known, and best defined, function of vitamin A is in vision. Retinol undergoes a conformational change to the *cis*-isomer, which is then oxidized to *cis*-retinaldehyde. In the rod cells of the retina, *cis*-retinaldehyde condenses with a lysine residue in the opsin, forming the pigment rhodopsin, as shown in Figure 12.3. In the cone cells, the equivalent pigments are the iodopsins, with sensitivity to red, green or blue light, depending on the cell type. The sequence of events involved in detection of light is the same for rhodopsin and the iodopsins.

When rhodopsin is exposed to light, it undergoes a conformational change that results in the release of the retinaldehyde, which undergoes isomerization to the all-*trans*-form. The altered form of opsin interacts with other proteins, activating a second messenger system which results in the transmission of a nerve impulse, and the perception of light. *Trans*-retinaldehyde is oxidized to retinol, then slowly converted to *cis*-retinaldehyde for the formation of rhodopsin. Under conditions where there is little retinol or retinaldehyde in the eye (i.e. in deficiency), vision is impaired (see below).

Although this is the best understood function of vitamin A, its main function in the body is in the control of cell differentiation and turnover. All-*trans*-retinoic, acid and 9-*cis*-retinoic acid are active in the regulation of growth,

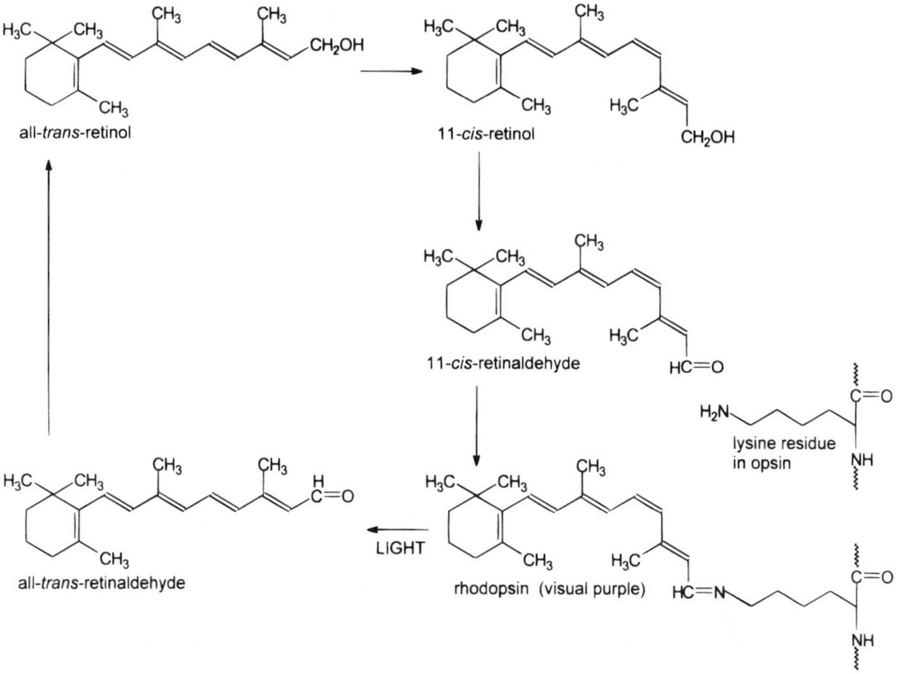

Figure 12.3 The role of vitamin A in vision.

development and tissue differentiation; they have different actions in different tissues. Like the steroid hormones (see §11.3) and vitamin D (§12.2.2.3), retinol and retinoic acid bind to nuclear receptors, and regulate the transcription of genes.

Many genes are sensitive to control by retinol and retinoic acid in different tissues, and at different stages in development. In some cases both 9-*cis* and all-*trans*-retinoic acids are required together for nuclear action, and in others retinoic acid receptors require to interact with receptors for vitamin D (see §12.2.2.3) or thyroid hormone before binding to DNA to modulate gene expression.

12.2.1.2 *Metabolic functions of carotene*

In addition to their role as precursors of vitamin A, carotenes may be important in their own right. As discussed in §2.5.2, free radical damage to tissues can have a variety of serious effects, including damage to DNA, which may result in the development of cancer. Carotene is one of a group of micronutrients collectively known as the antioxidant nutrients, because they can prevent oxidative damage to cells. Carotenes can react with radicals to form relatively stable unreactive radicals because the unpaired electron can be delocalized through the conjugated double-bond system of carotene.

There is epidemiological evidence that high intakes of carotene are associated with a lower risk of developing some forms of cancer, or at least that some forms of cancer are associated with low intakes of fruits and vegetables rich in carotene, and with low plasma and tissue concentrations of carotene. However, studies using supplements of carotene have not yielded any evidence of protection against cancer or other diseases, and there is no evidence on which to base reference intakes of carotene other than as a precursor of retinol.

12.2.1.3 *Vitamin A deficiency: night blindness and xerophthalmia*

Worldwide, vitamin A deficiency is a major problem of public health, and the most important preventable cause of blindness. Table 12.5 shows the numbers of millions of people at risk of deficiency.

The earliest signs of deficiency are connected with vision. Initially, there is a loss of sensitivity to green light; this is followed by impairment of the ability to adapt to dim light, followed by inability to see at all in dim light: night blindness. More prolonged or severe deficiency leads to the condition called xerophthalmia: keratinization of the cornea, followed by ulceration – irreversible damage to the eye, which causes blindness. At the same time there are changes in the skin, again with considerable excessive formation of keratinized tissue.

Vitamin A also has an important role in the function of the immune system, and mild deficiency, not severe enough to cause any disturbance of vision, leads to increased susceptibility to a variety of infectious diseases.

As discussed in §9.2, signs of vitamin A deficiency also occur in protein-energy malnutrition, regardless of whether or not the intake of vitamin A is adequate. This is because of impairment of the synthesis of the plasma retinol-binding protein that is required to transport retinol from liver reserves to its sites of action. Hence, functional vitamin A deficiency can occur secondary to protein-energy malnutrition. In this case there is severely impaired immunity to infection, as a result of both the functional vitamin A deficiency and also the impairment of immune responses associated with undernutrition.

Table 12.5 Millions of people at risk of vitamin A deficiency

Region	At risk	Children with xerophthalmia
South-East Asia	138	10.0
Western Pacific	19	1.4
Africa	18	1.3
Eastern Mediterranean	13	1.0
Americas	2	0.1
Europe	—	—

12.2.1.4 *Vitamin A requirements*

Vitamin A requirements are based on the intakes required to maintain a concentration of 20 μg retinol per g in the liver. This concentration is adequate to maintain normal plasma concentrations of the vitamin, and people with this level of liver reserves can be maintained on a diet free of vitamin A for many months before they develop any detectable signs of deficiency. As the concentration of retinol in the liver increases above about 20 μg per g, so there is an increased rate of metabolism and excretion of the vitamin. The average requirement to maintain a concentration of 20 μg per gram of liver is 6.7 μg retinol equivalents per kilogram body weight.

12.2.1.5 *Toxicity of preformed vitamin A*

Although there is an increase in the rate of metabolism and excretion of retinol as the concentration in the liver rises above 20 μg per g, there is only a limited capacity to metabolize the vitamin. Excessively high intakes lead to accumulation in the liver and other tissues, beyond the capacity of normal binding proteins, so that free, unbound, vitamin A is present. This leads to liver and bone damage, hair loss, vomiting and headaches. Although large single doses can be acutely toxic, the main concern is with the chronic toxicity of habitually high intakes. The recommended upper limits of habitual intake of retinol, compared with reference intakes, are shown in Table 12.6.

Although it is required for normal foetal limb development, vitamin A can be teratogenic in excess, causing a variety of foetal abnormalities. Pregnant women are recommended to consume no more than 3300 μg per day. Indeed, because of the high vitamin A content of some liver on sale, pregnant women have been advised to avoid eating liver and liver products.

High levels of carotene intake are not known to have any adverse effects, apart from giving an orange-yellow colour to the skin.

Table 12.6 Recommended upper limits of habitual intakes of preformed retinol

	Upper limit of intake μg per day	RNI μg per day
Infants	900	350
1–3 years	1800	400
4–6 years	3000	500
6–12 years	4500	500
13–20 years	6000	600–700
Adult men	9000	700
Adult women	7500	600
Pregnant women	3300	700

RNI, reference nutrient intake.

12.2.2 *Vitamin D*

The normal dietary form of vitamin D is cholecalciferol. This is also the compound formed in the skin in sunlight. Some foods are enriched or fortified with the synthetic compound ergocalciferol, which is synthesized by ultraviolet irradiation of the steroid ergosterol. Ergocalciferol undergoes the same metabolism as cholecalciferol, and has the same biological activity. Early studies assigned the name vitamin D_1 to an impure mixture of products derived from the irradiation of ergosterol; when ergocalciferol was identified it was called vitamin D_2, and when the physiological vitamin was identified as cholecalciferol it was called vitamin D_3.

Like vitamin A, vitamin D was originally measured in international units of biological activity before the pure compound was isolated: 1 iu = 25 ng of cholecalciferol; 1 μg of cholecalciferol = 40 iu.

12.2.2.1 *Synthesis of vitamin D in the skin*

As shown in Figure 12.4, the steroid 7-dehydrocholesterol (which is an intermediate in the synthesis of cholesterol), can undergo a non-enzymic reaction in the dermis on exposure to ultraviolet light, yielding previtamin D, which slowly undergoes a further reaction (over a period of many hours) to form cholecalciferol, which is absorbed into the bloodstream.

There are very few rich dietary sources of vitamin D: oily fish such as herring and mackerel, eggs, butter and margarine. In temperate climates there is a marked seasonal variation in the plasma concentration of vitamin D; it is highest at the end of summer and lowest at the end of winter. Although there may be bright sunlight in winter, even in the south of England there is very little ultraviolet radiation of the appropriate wavelength for cholecalciferol synthesis when the sun is low in the sky. By contrast, in summer, when the sun is more or less overhead, there is a considerable amount of ultraviolet light, even on a slightly cloudy day, and enough can penetrate thin clothes to result in significant formation of vitamin D.

In northerly climates, and especially in polluted industrial cities with little sunlight, people may well not be exposed to enough ultraviolet light to meet their vitamin D needs, and they will be reliant on the few dietary sources of the vitamin.

12.2.2.2 *The metabolism of vitamin D*

Cholecalciferol, either synthesized in the skin or taken in from foods, is metabolized as shown in Figure 12.4. In the liver it is hydroxylated to form calcidiol, then in the kidney this is converted to either calcitriol, which is the active hormone, or to 24-hydroxycalcidiol, which has no biological activity, but is metabolized further, then excreted in the bile.

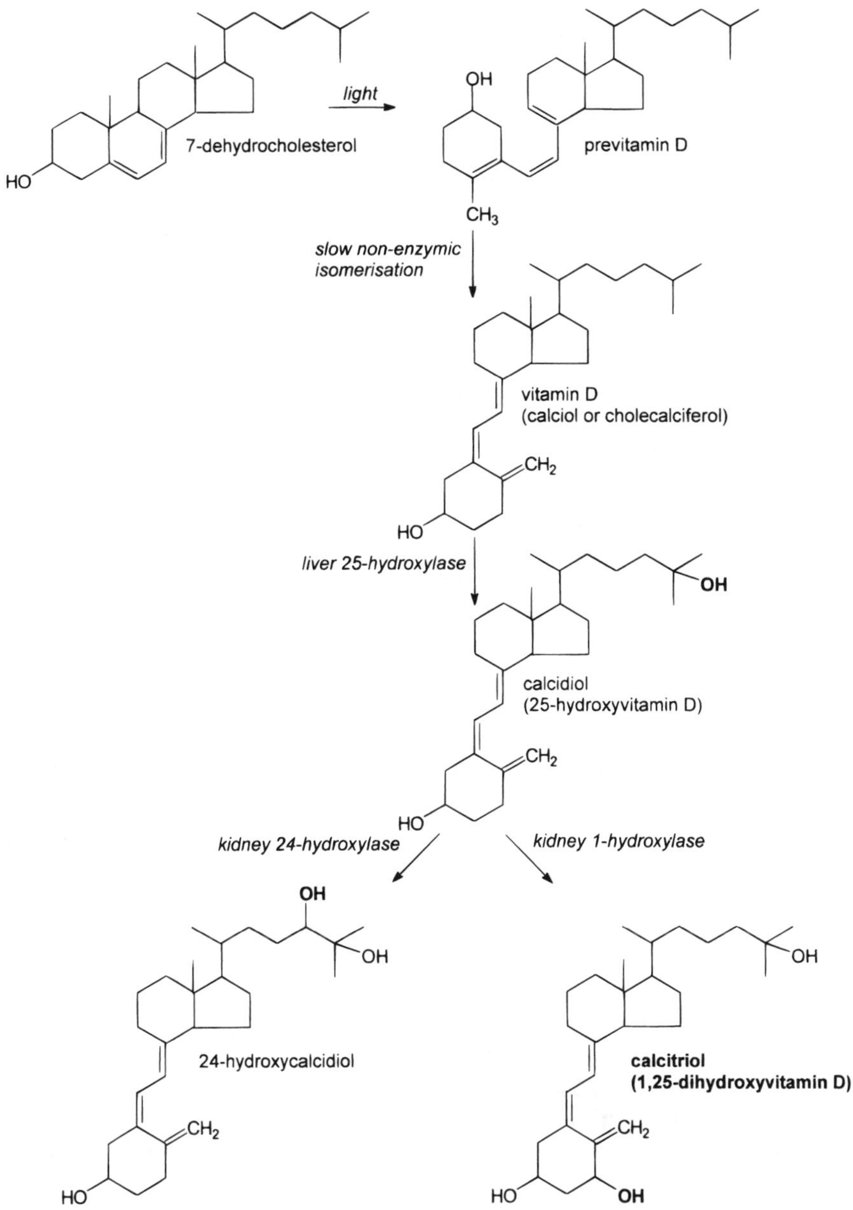

Figure 12.4 The metabolism of vitamin D.

The metabolic role of vitamin D is in the control of calcium homeostasis (see §12.3.1). In turn, the activities of the two enzymes that metabolize calcidiol to either (active) calcitriol or (inactive) 24-hydroxycalcidiol are controlled by the state of calcium balance. As serum calcium falls, parathyroid hormone is secreted from the parathyroid gland. Parathyroid hormone both stimulates the enzyme that forms calcitriol and inhibits the enzyme that forms 24-hydroxycalcidiol. Thus, as serum calcium falls, so there is increased formation of the active metabolite of vitamin D, which acts to raise serum calcium.

12.2.2.3 *Metabolic functions of vitamin D*

Calcitriol acts like a steroid hormone (see §11.3), binding to a nuclear receptor protein. The calcitriol–receptor complex then binds to the enhancer site of the gene coding for a calcium-binding protein, increasing its transcription and so increasing the amount of calcium-binding protein in the cell.

The best studied actions of vitamin D are in the intestinal mucosa, where the intracellular calcium-binding protein is essential for the absorption of calcium from the diet. Here the vitamin has another action as well, to increase the transport of calcium across the mucosal membrane. This increase in transport of calcium is seen immediately after feeding vitamin D, whereas the increase in absorption is a slower response, since it depends on new synthesis of the binding protein.

Calcitriol also acts to raise the plasma concentration of calcium by stimulating the mobilization of calcium from bone. It achieves this by activating osteoclast cells. However, it later acts to stimulate the laying down of new bone to replace the loss, by stimulating the differentiation and recruitment of osteoblast cells.

In addition to these actions, calcidiol is involved in a wide range of regulatory functions, all associated with changes in intracellular calcium-binding proteins, and hence intracellular concentrations of calcium. The synthesis of some regulatory enzymes, and the secretion of some hormones, including insulin, is regulated by calcitriol, although in most cases it does not act alone, but together with vitamin A, or another steroid hormone. Calcitriol receptors have also been identified in the immune system, so, like vitamin A, vitamin D is also required for resistance to infection.

12.2.2.4 *Vitamin D deficiency: rickets and osteomalacia*

Historically, rickets is a disease of toddlers, especially in industrial cities in the northern hemisphere. The bones are undermineralized, as a result of poor absorption of calcium in the absence of adequate amounts of calcitriol. When the child begins to walk, the long bones of the legs are deformed, leading to bow legs or knock knees. More seriously, rickets can also lead to collapse of the rib cage, and deformities of the bones of the pelvis. Similar problems may also occur in adolescents who are deficient in vitamin D during the adolescent growth spurt, when there is again a high demand for calcium for new bone formation.

Osteomalacia is the adult equivalent of rickets. It results from the demineralization of bone, rather than the failure to mineralize it in the first place, as is the case with rickets. Women who have little exposure to sunlight are especially at risk from osteomalacia after several pregnancies, because of the strain that pregnancy places on their marginal reserve of calcium. Osteomalacia also occurs fairly commonly in the elderly. Here again the problem may be inadequate exposure to sunlight, but there is also evidence that the capacity to form 7-dehydrocholesterol in the skin decreases with advancing age, so that the elderly are more reliant on the few dietary sources of vitamin D.

See §12.3.1.1 for a discussion of osteoporosis in the elderly, a degenerative bone disease, not due to vitamin D deficiency.

12.2.2.5 *Vitamin D requirements*

It is difficult to determine requirements for vitamin D, since the major source is synthesis in the skin. For this reason, there are no RNI for children over 4 years of age, or for adults aged under 65. For the elderly, the RNI is 10 μg per day, a level of intake that maintains a plasma concentration of calcidiol above 20 nmol per L, the lower end of the reference range in younger people who have adequate sunlight exposure. This will almost certainly require either fortification of foods with the vitamin or the use of vitamin D supplements – the average intake of vitamin D from the few foods that are rich sources is less than 4 μg per day.

12.2.2.6 *Vitamin D toxicity*

During the 1950s, rickets was more or less totally eradicated in Britain. This was the result of enrichment of many infant foods with vitamin D. However, a few infants suffered from vitamin D poisoning, the most serious effect of which is an elevated plasma concentration of calcium. This can lead to contraction of blood vessels, and hence dangerously high blood pressure. It can also lead to calcinosis – the calcification of soft tissues, including the kidney, heart, lungs and blood vessel walls.

Some infants are sensitive to intakes of vitamin D as low as 50 μg per day (compared with an RNI of 8.5 μg for infants). In order to avoid the serious problem of vitamin D poisoning in these susceptible infants, the extent to which infant foods are fortified with vitamin D has been reduced considerably. Unfortunately, this means that a small proportion, who have relatively high requirements, are now at risk of developing rickets. The problem is to identify those who have high requirements, and provide them with supplements.

The toxic threshold in adults is not known, but all those patients suffering from vitamin D intoxication who have been investigated were taking more than 250 μg of vitamin D per day. Although excess dietary vitamin D is toxic, excessive exposure to sunlight does not lead to vitamin D poisoning. There is a limited capacity to form the precursor, 7-dehydrocholesterol, in the skin, and a limited capacity to take up cholecalciferol from the skin. Furthermore, prolonged exposure of previtamin D to ultraviolet light results in further reactions to yield biologically inactive compounds.

12.2.3 *Vitamin E*

Vitamin E is the generic descriptor for two families of compounds, the tocopherols and the tocotrienols (see Figure 12.5). The different vitamers have different biological potency. The most active is α-tocopherol, and it is usual to express vitamin E intake in terms of milligrams of α-tocopherol equivalents. This is the sum of:

$$\text{mg } \alpha\text{—tocopherol} + 0.5 \times \text{mg } \beta\text{—tocopherol} + 0.1 \times \text{mg } \gamma\text{—tocopherol} + 0.3 \times \text{mg } \alpha\text{—tocotrienol}$$

The other vitamers either occur in negligible amounts in foods or have negligible vitamin activity. The obsolete international unit of vitamin E activity is

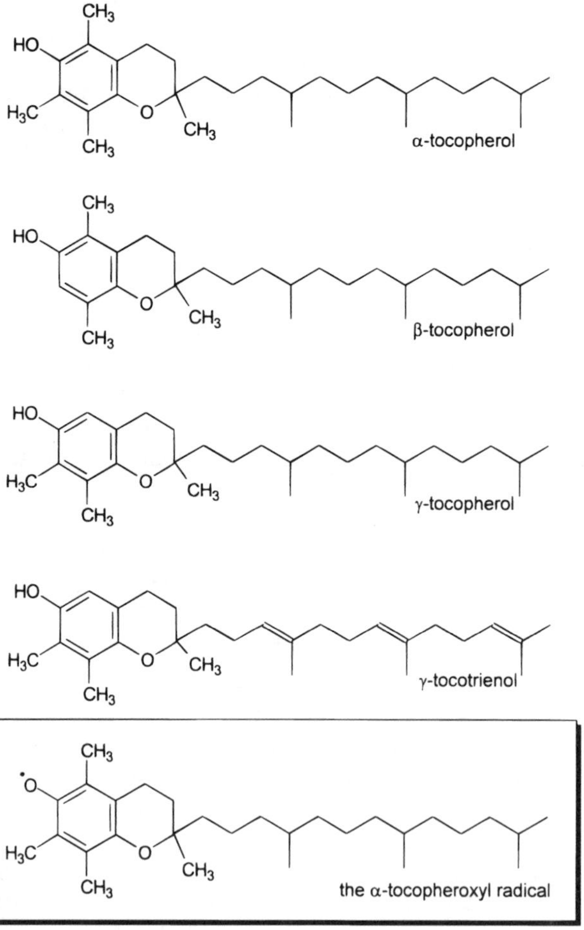

Figure 12.5 The major vitamin E vitamers.

still sometimes used: 1 iu = 0.67 mg α-tocopherol equivalent; 1 mg α-tocopherol = 1.49 iu.

Synthetic α-tocopherol does not have the same biological potency as the naturally occurring compound. This is because the side chain of tocopherol has three centres of asymmetry and, when it is synthesized chemically, the result is a mixture of the various isomers. In the naturally occurring compound all three centres of asymmetry have the *R*-configuration (see §3.7.1.2). Therefore, naturally occurring α-tocopherol is sometimes called (all-*R*)-, or (*RRR*)-α-tocopherol.

12.2.3.1 *Metabolic functions and deficiency of vitamin E*

The function of vitamin E is as a radical-trapping antioxidant (see §2.5.3) in cell membranes. It is especially important in limiting oxidative radical damage to polyunsaturated fatty acids before they can establish a chain reaction in the membrane. The radical formed from vitamin E is relatively unreactive and quenches radical chain reactions. The vitamin E radical is inactivated, and the active vitamin reformed, by reaction with vitamin C, as shown in Figure 12.6.

Dietary deficiency of vitamin E in human beings is unknown, although patients with severe fat malabsorption, cystic fibrosis, some forms of chronic liver disease and (very rarely) congenital lack of plasma β-lipoprotein, suffer deficiency because they are unable to absorb the vitamin or transport it around the body. They suffer from severe damage to nerve and muscle membranes.

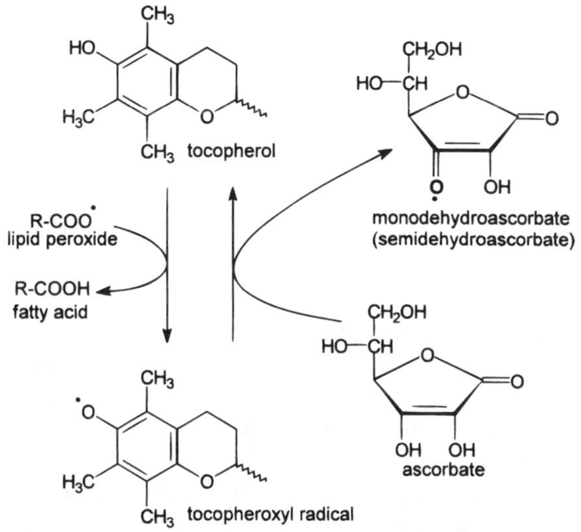

Figure 12.6 Reduction of lipid peroxides in membranes by vitamin E and reduction of the tocopheroxyl radical by interaction with vitamin C at the membrane surface.

Premature infants are at risk of vitamin E deficiency, since they are often born with inadequate reserves of the vitamin. The red blood cell membranes of deficient infants are abnormally fragile, as a result of unchecked oxidative radical attack. This may lead to haemolytic anaemia if they are not given supplements of the vitamin.

Experimental animals that are depleted of vitamin E become sterile. However, there is no evidence that vitamin E nutritional status is in any way associated with human fertility, and there is certainly no evidence that vitamin E supplements increase sexual potency, prowess or vigour.

12.2.3.2 *Vitamin E requirements and desirable levels of intake*

It is difficult to establish vitamin E requirements, partly because deficiency is more or less unknown, and also because the requirement depends on the intake of polyunsaturated fatty acids. It is generally accepted that the intake of vitamin E should be 0.4 mg α-tocopherol equivalent per gram of dietary polyunsaturated fatty acid. This does not present any problem, since foods that are rich sources of polyunsaturated fatty acids (the plant oils, see Table 2.6) are also rich sources of vitamin E.

There is some evidence that higher intakes of vitamin E may have a useful protective effect against the development of ischaemic heart disease. This is because high concentrations of vitamin E inhibit the oxidation of polyunsaturated fatty acids in plasma lipoproteins, and it is this oxidation that is responsible for the initiation of atherosclerosis. The levels that appear to be beneficial are of the order of 17–40 mg α-tocopherol per day, which is above what could be achieved by eating ordinary foods. There is no known hazard from consuming even considerably higher amounts of vitamin E.

12.2.4 Vitamin K

Vitamin K was discovered as a result of investigations into the cause of a bleeding disorder (haemorrhagic disease) of cattle fed on silage made from sweet clover and chickens fed on a fat-free diet. The missing factor in the diet of the chickens was identified as vitamin K; the problem in the cattle was that the feed contained an antagonist of the vitamin.

Since the effect of either deficiency of the vitamin or an excessive intake of the antagonist was severely impaired blood clotting, the antagonist was isolated and tested in smaller amounts as an anticoagulant, for use in patients at risk of thrombosis. Although it was effective, the naturally occurring antagonist had unwanted side effects, and synthetic vitamin K antagonists were developed for clinical use as anticoagulants. The most commonly used of these is Warfarin. Warfarin is also used as a poison to kill rats and mice. In small doses it causes a slight impairment of blood clotting, which is what is required in patients at risk of thrombosis. In excess, it causes a very severe impairment of blood clotting, and the victims suffer from haemorrhage.

Three compounds have the biological activity of vitamin K (see Figure 12.7):

- Phylloquinone, which is the normal dietary source, found in green leafy vegetables.
- Menaquinones, which are a family of closely related compounds synthesized by intestinal bacteria, with differing lengths of the side chain; it is not known to what extent bacterial menaquinones are utilized by the body.
- Menadione and menadiol diacetate, synthetic compounds which can be metabolized to yield phylloquinone.

12.2.4.1 *Metabolic functions of vitamin K*

Although it has been known since the 1920s that vitamin K was required for blood clotting, it was not until the 1970s that its precise function was established. It is the cofactor for the carboxylation of glutamate residues in the post-synthetic modification of proteins to form the unusual amino acid γ-carboxyglutamate (see Figure 12.8).

Prothrombin and several other proteins of the blood clotting system contain between four and six γ-carboxyglutamate residues. This amino acid chelates calcium ions, and so permits the binding of the blood clotting proteins to lipid membranes. In vitamin K deficiency, or in the presence of an

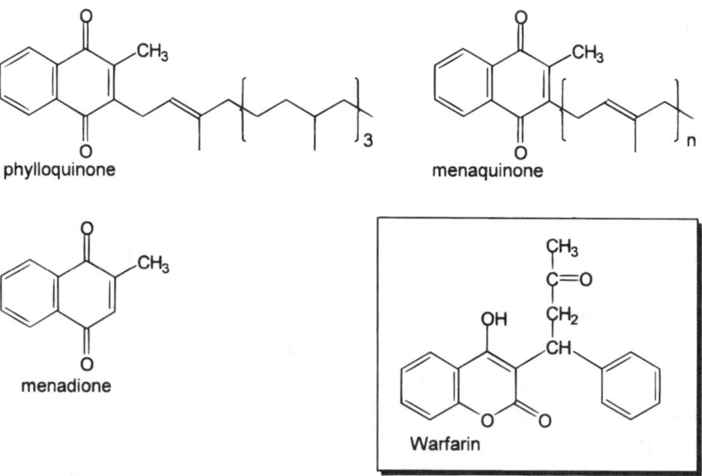

Figure 12.7 The vitamin K vitamers and the vitamin K antagonist Warfarin, used as an anticoagulant. Phylloquinone is found in plant foods, and menaquinone is synthesized by intestinal bacteria; menadione is a synthetic compound which is metabolized to active vitamin K in the liver.

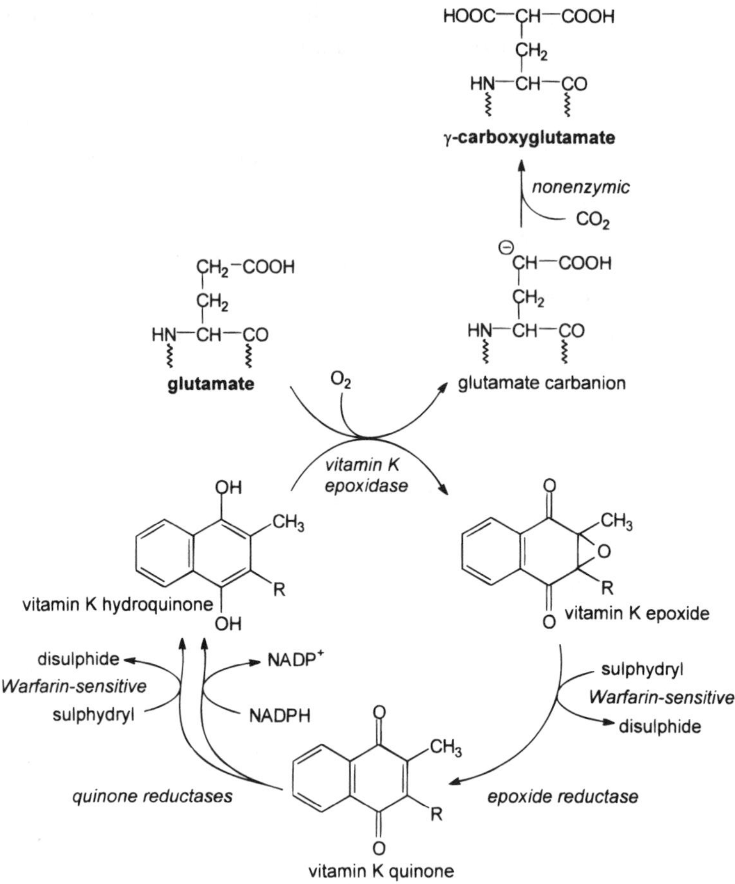

Figure 12.8 The role of vitamin K in the formation of γ-carboxyglutamate.

antagonist such as Warfarin, an abnormal precursor of prothrombin containing little or no γ-carboxyglutamate is released into the circulation. This abnormal protein cannot chelate calcium or bind to phospholipid membranes, and so is unable to initiate blood clotting.

Another protein also contains γ-carboxyglutamate, and is dependent on vitamin K for its formation. This is osteocalcin, one of the calcium binding proteins of bone matrix. Infants born to mothers treated with Warfarin are at risk of severe bone deformities (the foetal Warfarin syndrome) as a result of impaired synthesis of osteocalcin.

It can be seen from Figure 12.8 that vitamin K is oxidized to the epoxide during the carboxylation of glutamate. Normally the epoxide is reduced back to the active form of the vitamin. It is this reduction that is inhibited by Warfarin. Even in the presence of Warfarin, glutamate carboxylation can proceed more or less normally if there is enough vitamin K available to be used just once, then excreted as the epoxide and its metabolites. High doses of vitamin K are used to treat patients who have received an overdose of Warfarin.

It is possible that patients who are being treated with Warfarin could overcome the beneficial effects of their medication if they took supplements of vitamin K. The danger is that, if their dose of Warfarin is increased to counteract the effects of the vitamin supplements and they then stop taking the supplements, they would be receiving considerably too much Warfarin and would be at risk of haemorrhage. It is most unlikely that a normal diet could provide such an excess of vitamin K; it would need an habitual intake of 250 g a day of broccoli or other vegetables rich in vitamin K to have any significant effect on Warfarin action.

12.2.4.2 *Vitamin K requirements*

Determination of vitamin K requirements is complicated by a lack of data on the importance of menaquinones synthesized by intestinal bacteria. However, a prolonged blood-clotting time is observed in volunteers maintained on diets deficient in vitamin K, even without the use of antibiotics to inhibit intestinal bacterial synthesis of menaquinone, so there is clearly a need for a dietary intake.

Because of the lack of data, there is no RNI for vitamin K. An intake of 1 mg per kilogram body weight per day is considered safe and adequate, since at this level of intake there is no evidence of any impairment of blood clotting.

A few newborn infants have very low reserves of vitamin K and are at risk of haemorrhagic disease of the newborn. It is therefore generally recommended that all newborn infants should be given a single prophylactic dose of vitamin K. This should preferably be given by mouth, rather than by injection, since there is some evidence to suggest a link between injection of synthetic vitamin K (menadione or menadiol diacetate) at birth and an increased risk of leukaemia.

12.2.5 *Vitamin B_1 (thiamin)*

Thiamin, as the diphosphate (see Figure 12.9), is the coenzyme for oxidative decarboxylation reactions. The most important of these are pyruvate dehydrogenase (see Figure 7.7) and transketolase (Figure 7.5) in carbohydrate metabolism and ketoglutarate dehydrogenase in the citric acid cycle (Figure 7.9). This means that thiamin has a central role in metabolism. In addition, thiamin triphosphate has a role in the conduction of nerve impulses; it activates the chloride ion channel in nerve membranes.

12.2.5.1 *Thiamin deficiency: beriberi and the Wernicke–Korsakoff syndrome*

Two different diseases are associated with thiamin deficiency: beriberi and the Wernicke–Korsakoff syndrome.

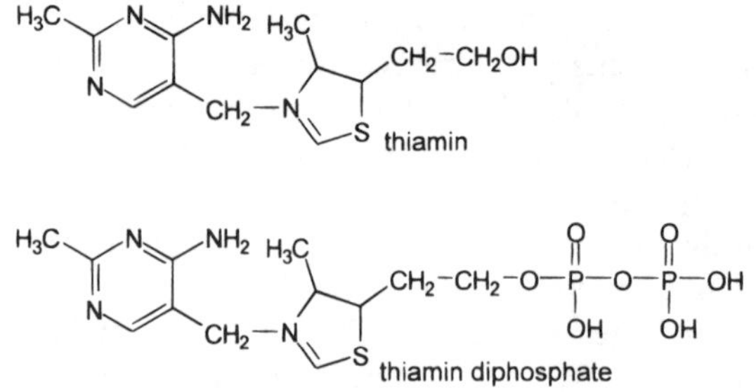

Figure 12.9 Vitamin B_1: thiamin and the coenzyme thiamin diphosphate.

Beriberi is associated with long-term thiamin deficiency, with a generally low food intake but a relatively high intake of carbohydrate. It is mainly a problem in South-East Asia. There is damage to the peripheral nervous system, with ascending neuritis, which causes muscle weakness and atrophy. This begins with weakness, pain and stiffness in the legs, and spreads upwards; the ankle jerk reflex is lost, then the muscles of the calf are affected, and the patient is unable to keep either the toes or the whole foot off the ground. The hands and arms may also be affected. Although there is loss of sensation in the affected regions, there is also deep muscle pain.

The heart can also be affected in beriberi, especially in people whose diet is high in carbohydrate. There is right-sided heart failure, leading to oedema. In some patients, the oedema and heart failure may occur without the nerve damage being apparent.

In Western countries, thiamin deficiency is seen mainly in alcoholics. Here the problem of a possibly low intake of thiamin is confounded by the inhibition of thiamin absorption and metabolism by alcohol. As in beriberi, the heart may be affected, and cardiac enlargement leading to heart failure as a result of thiamin deficiency is a problem among heavy drinkers.

Thiamin deficiency may develop relatively rapidly, within a week or so, as a result of prolonged heavy binge drinking with little food intake. In such cases the main effect is severe impairment of the activity of pyruvate dehydrogenase (see Figure 7.7), leading to abnormally high blood concentrations of pyruvate and lactate, and potentially life-threatening acidosis.

More prolonged alcohol abuse leads to damage to the central nervous system, again because of thiamin deficiency. Patients develop Korsakoff's psychosis, which is characterized by loss of recent memory, although memory for distant events is normally unimpaired, and what is called confabulation: the making up of wondrous stories. Later there are physical signs of damage to the central nervous system: Wernicke's encephalopathy.

12.2.5.2 *Thiamin requirements*

The requirement for thiamin depends on energy expenditure, and more precisely on the proportion of energy from carbohydrate. Reference intakes are based on 95 μg thiamin per MJ energy expenditure. The main sources of thiamin in the diet are cereals (it is added to flour and breakfast cereals to replace losses in milling), vegetables and meat. Pork and ham are especially rich sources of thiamin.

12.2.6 *Vitamin B_2 (riboflavin)*

Like thiamin, riboflavin is involved in the metabolism of metabolic fuels, as the coenzyme of a wide variety of enzymes involved in oxidation and reduction reactions (the flavoproteins, see Figure 4.7). Riboflavin and the flavin coenzymes are shown in Figure 12.10. Flavoproteins are important in the metabolism of carbohydrates, fatty acids and amino acids, as well as in the mitochondrial electron transport chain.

12.2.6.1 *Riboflavin deficiency*

Although riboflavin is involved in all areas of metabolism, and deficiency is widespread on a global scale, deficiency is not fatal. The clinical signs of deficiency are cracking at the edges of the lips (cheilosis) and corners of the mouth (angular stomatitis), painful loss of the normal epithelium of the tongue (glossitis), and skin lesions resembling sebhorroea.

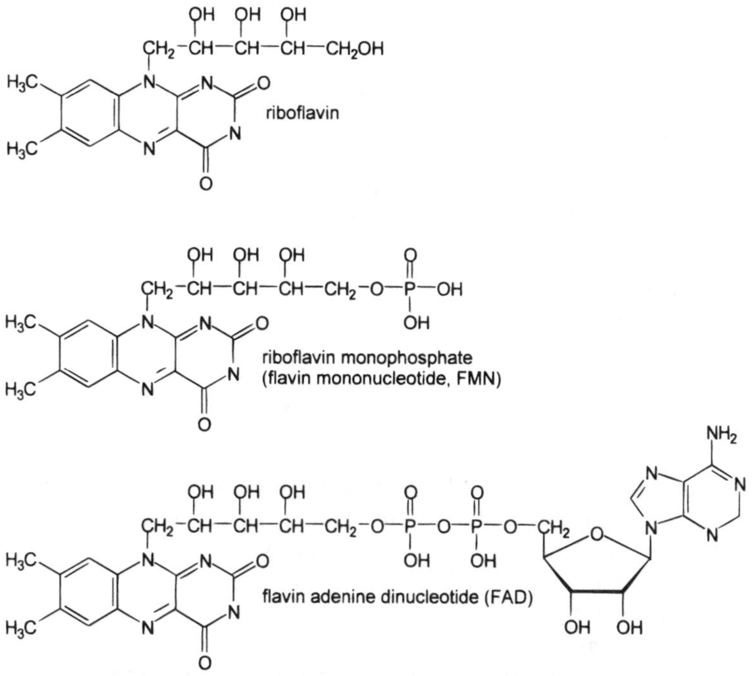

riboflavin

riboflavin monophosphate
(flavin mononucleotide, FMN)

flavin adenine dinucleotide (FAD)

Figure 12.10 Vitamin B_2 : riboflavin and the flavin coenzymes (see also Figure 4.7).

There seem to be two reasons why deficiency is not fatal. One is that although deficiency is common, the vitamin is widespread in foods, and most diets will provide minimally adequate amounts of the vitamin to permit maintenance of central metabolic pathways. The second, more important, reason is that in deficiency there is extremely efficient re-utilization of the riboflavin that is released by the turnover of flavoproteins, so that only a very small amount is metabolized or excreted.

12.2.6.2 *Riboflavin requirements*

Estimates of riboflavin requirements are based on depletion/repletion studies to determine the minimum intake at which there is significant excretion of the vitamin. In deficiency there is virtually no excretion of the vitamin; as requirements are met, so any excess is excreted in the urine. Although estimates of riboflavin requirements were at one time based on energy expenditure, there is no sound basis for this given the wide range of flavin-dependent enzymes.

A more generous estimate of requirements, and the basis of RNI, is the level of intake at which there is normalization of the activity of the red cell enzyme, glutathione reductase, which is a flavoprotein whose activity is especially sensitive to riboflavin nutritional status.

The main sources of riboflavin are milk and milk products, meat (especially liver and kidney) and eggs.

12.2.7 *Niacin*

Two compounds, nicotinic acid and nicotinamide, have the biological activity of niacin (see Figure 12.11). As discussed below, it can also be synthesized in the body from the essential amino acid tryptophan.

The best defined role of niacin is in the metabolism of metabolic fuels as the functional nicotinamide part of the coenzymes NAD and NADP (see Figure 4.8). NAD also has a role in activating the DNA repair mechanism, and in regulating the activity of some enzymes; here it is the ADP-ribose of the coenzyme that is important, and free nicotinamide is released. Cyclic-ADP-ribose formed from NAD has a role in controlling intracellular concentrations of calcium.

12.2.7.1 *Pellagra – tryptophan and niacin deficiency*

Deficiency of niacin results in the disease pellagra. This is characterized by a sunburn-like rash in areas of the skin exposed to sunlight, and a depressive psychosis. Untreated pellagra is fatal and was a major cause of death in the southern USA throughout the first half of the twentieth century. It is still a problem in parts of Africa and India.

Death from pellagra is presumably the result of lack of NAD(P) for energy-yielding metabolism, and the depressive psychosis is assumed to be because of inadequate formation of the neurotransmitter serotonin, as a result of tryp-

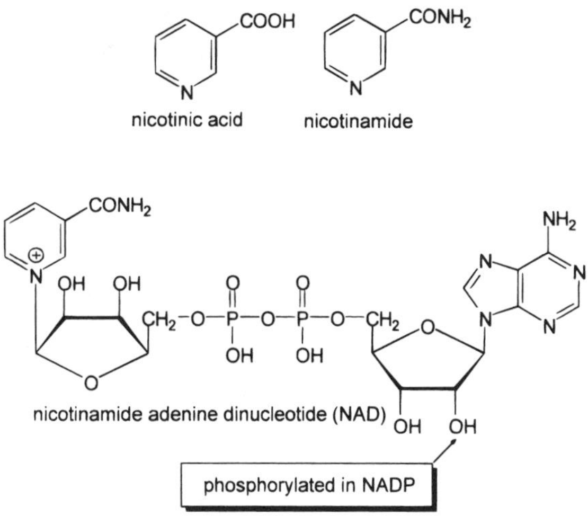

Figure 12.11 Niacin and the nicotinamide nucleotide coenzymes NAD and NADP (see also Figure 4.8).

tophan deficiency; no satisfactory mechanism has been described to explain the extreme sensitivity to sunlight.

12.2.7.2 *Niacin requirements*

Determination of requirements for niacin is complicated by the fact that the nicotinamide part of NAD(P) can be formed from either preformed niacin or by the metabolism of the essential amino acid tryptophan. On average, 60 mg of dietary tryptophan is equivalent to 1 mg of preformed niacin in the diet. It is usual to express niacin intake as milligrams of niacin equivalents. This is calculated by adding mg preformed niacin $+1/60$ mg tryptophan. The niacin in cereals is usually excluded from the calculation of intake because much of it is present in a chemically bound form which is not released during digestion, so that the vitamin is not biologically available.

The average requirement for niacin is 1.3 mg niacin equivalents per MJ energy expenditure, and reference intakes are based on 1.6 mg per MJ.

The metabolic pathway that leads to NAD formation from tryptophan is also the main pathway of tryptophan metabolism. This means that, for an adult in nitrogen balance (see §10.1), an amount of tryptophan equal to the whole of the dietary intake is available for NAD synthesis. Average intakes of tryptophan in Western countries are adequate to meet niacin requirements without any need for preformed niacin in the diet.

12.2.7.3 *Niacin toxicity*

Nicotinic acid has been used to lower blood triacylglycerol and cholesterol in patients with hyperlipidaemia. However, relatively large amounts are required (of the order of 1–6 g per day, compared with RNI of 18–20 mg per day). At this level of intake, nicotinic acid causes dilatation of blood vessels and flushing, with skin irritation, itching and a burning sensation. This effect wears off after a few days.

High intakes of both nicotinic acid and nicotinamide, in excess of 500 mg per day, also cause liver damage, and prolonged use can result in liver failure. This is especially a problem with sustained release preparations of niacin, which permit a high blood level to be maintained for a relatively long time.

Supplements of tryptophan have been associated with the development of an apparently autoimmune disease, the fatal eosinophilia–myalgia syndrome. All the reported cases have been traced to a single batch of tryptophan, and the problem is assumed to have been caused by a trace contaminant in that batch. Nevertheless, in most countries there is strict control over the conditions under which tryptophan supplements may be used.

12.2.8 Vitamin B_6

Six related compounds have the biological activity of vitamin B_6 ; they are all converted in the body to the metabolically active form, pyridoxal phosphate (see Figure 12.12).

Pyridoxal phosphate is a coenzyme in three main areas of metabolism:

- In a wide variety of reactions of amino acids, and especially transamination, in which it functions as the intermediate carrier of the amino group (see §10.3.1.2), and decarboxylation reactions to form amines.
- As the cofactor of glycogen phosphorylase in muscle and liver (see §7.4.1).
- In the regulation of the action of steroid hormones (see §11.3). Pyridoxal phosphate acts to remove the hormone–receptor complex from DNA binding, and so terminate the action of the hormones. In vitamin B_6 deficiency there is increased sensitivity of target tissues to the actions of low concentrations of such hormones as the oestrogens, androgens, cortisol and vitamin D.

12.2.8.1 Vitamin B_6 deficiency

Deficiency of vitamin B_6 severe enough to lead to clinical signs is extremely rare, and clear deficiency has been reported in only one outbreak, during the 1950s, when babies were fed on a milk preparation that had been severely overheated during manufacture. Many of the affected infants suffered convulsions, which ceased rapidly following the administration of vitamin B_6.

The cause of the convulsions was severe impairment of the activity of the enzyme glutamate decarboxylase, which is a pyridoxal phosphate dependent enzyme. The product of glutamate decarboxylase is GABA (γ-amino-butyric acid), which is a regulatory neurotransmitter in the central nervous system.

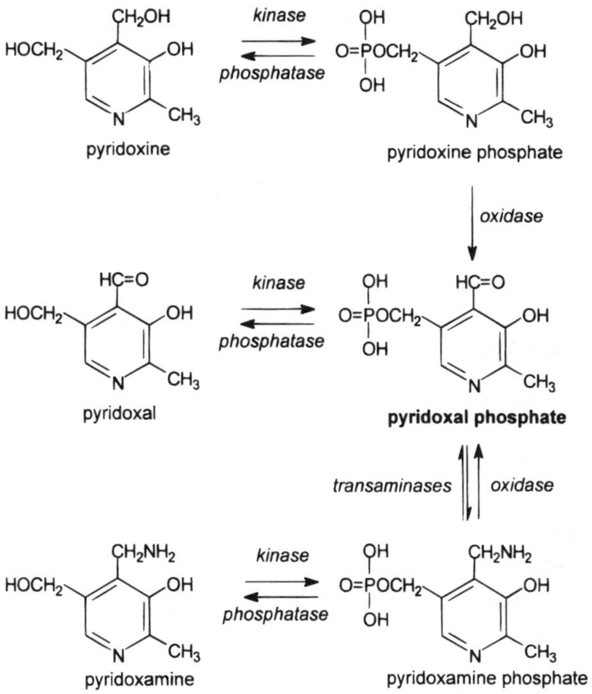

Figure 12.12 The metabolism of vitamin B_6 (see Figure 10.6 for the role of vitamin B_6 in transamination of amino acids).

Moderate vitamin B_6 deficiency results in abnormalities of amino acid metabolism. The metabolism of tryptophan and methionine is especially severely affected, and tests of tryptophan and methionine metabolism are widely used to assess vitamin B_6 nutritional status. The activity of transaminases is also impaired in vitamin B_6 deficiency, and measurement of red blood cell transaminase activity provides an additional way of assessing vitamin B_6 nutritional status. There is evidence that moderate vitamin B_6 deficiency or inadequacy, as detected by such biochemical abnormalities, may be relatively common.

12.2.8.2 *Vitamin B_6 requirements*

Although most of the body's vitamin B_6 is associated with glycogen phosphorylase in muscle, this is relatively stable and well conserved, and it is the smaller pool (about 20% of the total) involved in amino acid metabolism and steroid hormone action that shows rapid turnover and responds to deficiency.

Depletion/repletion studies to determine requirements showed that depletion occurred faster, and the requirement for repletion was higher, when the subjects were fed a high protein diet. Therefore, requirements are based on protein intake; the average requirement is 13 μg per gram dietary protein;

reference intakes are calculated on the basis of 15 μg per gram protein, and the observed intake of protein, which is 15 per cent of energy intake in Western countries.

The main sources of vitamin B_6 are meat, whole grain cereals, vegetables and nuts.

12.2.8.3 *Vitamin B_6, oral contraceptives and the premenstrual syndrome*

Some studies have suggested that oral contraceptives cause vitamin B_6 deficiency. As a result of this, supplements of vitamin B_6 of between 50 and 100 mg per day, and sometimes higher, have been used to overcome the side effects of oral contraceptives. Similar supplements have also been recommended for the treatment of the premenstrual syndrome.

All of the studies that have suggested that oral contraceptives cause vitamin B_6 deficiency have used the metabolism of tryptophan as a means of assessing vitamin B_6 nutritional status. When other biochemical markers of status have also been assessed, they are not affected by oral contraceptive use. Furthermore, all of these studies were performed using the now obsolete high-dose contraceptive pills.

Oral contraceptives do not cause vitamin B_6 deficiency. The problem is that both the oestrogens and the progestagens in the contraceptives inhibit the metabolism of tryptophan. This results in the excretion of abnormal amounts of tryptophan metabolites, similar to what is seen in vitamin B_6 deficiency, but for quite a different reason. There is no evidence that supplements have any beneficial effect in overcoming the side effects of oral contraceptive use, and very little that vitamin B_6 supplements have any beneficial effect in the premenstrual syndrome.

12.2.8.4 *Vitamin B_6 toxicity*

Very high intakes of vitamin B_6 (several hundred milligrams per day) over a period of several weeks or months cause severe damage to peripheral nerves, resulting in partial paralysis. This is only partially cured by ceasing the supplements. More modest doses (of the order of 50–100 mg per day, still vastly in excess of requirements) may cause less serious nerve damage, and result in a tingling sensation in the fingers and toes. This is reversed on cessation of the supplements.

12.2.9 ***Vitamin B_{12}***

Vitamin B_{12} (see Figure 12.13) functions in the transfer of methyl groups. Its metabolic function is closely linked with that of folic acid (see §12.2.10), and indeed the megaloblastic anaemia of vitamin B_{12} deficiency results from derangement of folic acid metabolism.

Vitamin B_{12} is found only in foods of animal origin, although it is also formed by some bacteria. There are no plant sources of this vitamin. This

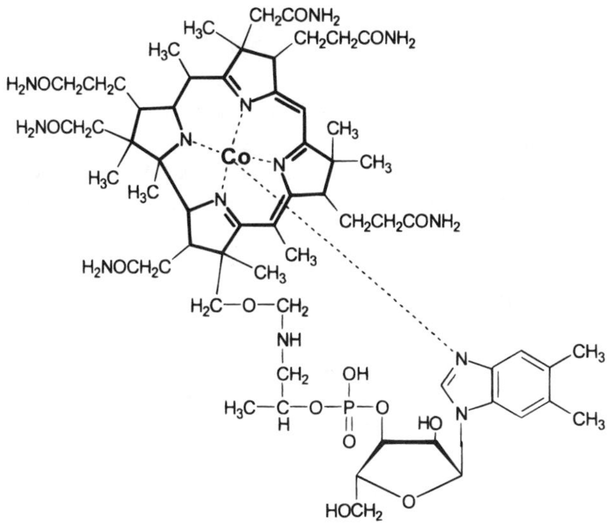

Figure 12.13 Vitamin B_{12}.

means that strict vegetarians (vegans), who eat no foods of animal origin, are at risk of developing dietary vitamin B_{12} deficiency. Preparations of vitamin B_{12} made by bacterial fermentation which are ethically acceptable to vegans are readily available.

Interestingly, there are claims that yeasts and some plants (especially some algae) contain vitamin B_{12}. This seems to be incorrect. The problem is that the officially recognized, and legally required, method of determining vitamin B_{12} in food analysis depends on the growth of microorganisms for which vitamin B_{12} is an essential growth factor. However, these organisms can also use some compounds that are chemically related to vitamin B_{12} but have no vitamin activity in man. Therefore, analysis reveals the presence of something that appears to be vitamin B_{12} but in fact is not the active vitamin, and is useless in human nutrition.

12.2.9.1 *Vitamin B_{12} deficiency: pernicious anaemia*

Vitamin B_{12} deficiency causes what is known as pernicious anaemia. The anaemia is because of the release into the bloodstream of immature precursors of red blood cells: megaloblastic anaemia. As shown in Figure 12.15, folic acid is required for the synthesis of thymidine for DNA synthesis, and vitamin B_{12} deficiency interferes with the metabolism of folic acid. As a result, the rapid multiplication of red blood cells is disturbed, and immature precursors are released into the circulation.

The other clinical feature of vitamin B_{12} deficiency, which is very rarely seen in folic acid deficiency, is degeneration of the spinal cord; hence the name 'pernicious' for the anaemia of vitamin B_{12} deficiency. The spinal cord degeneration is the result of a failure of the methylation of one arginine residue on myelin basic protein; it occurs in about one-third of patients with pernicious anaemia caused by vitamin B_{12} deficiency, and in about one-third of patients who do not show signs of anaemia.

The commonest cause of pernicious anaemia is failure of the absorption of vitamin B_{12} (see §6.5), rather than dietary deficiency, although dietary deficiency does occur in strict vegetarians.

At an early stage in vitamin B_{12} depletion, before there is any evidence of anaemia, there is impairment of the activity of methylmalonyl CoA mutase, the enzyme that catalyses the conversion of methylmalonyl CoA, arising from propionyl CoA, itself a product of the metabolism of isoleucine, valine, methionine and the side chain of cholesterol, to succinyl CoA (see Figure 10.11). As a result, methylmalonic acid is excreted in the urine; this provides a sensitive way of monitoring the treatment of patients with pernicious anaemia and of detecting people at risk of deficiency.

12.2.9.2 *Vitamin B_{12} requirements*

Early estimates of vitamin B_{12} requirements were based on the amounts required to maintain normal red blood cell maturation in patients with pernicious anaemia due to failure of absorption of the vitamin. However, there is a considerable enterohepatic circulation of vitamin B_{12}. It is secreted in the bile and reabsorbed in the small intestine. In patients with defective secretion of intrinsic factor, or those secreting anti-intrinsic factor antibodies, the vitamin cannot be reabsorbed, and is excreted in the faeces. They therefore have a very much higher requirement for vitamin B_{12} than normal. The reference intakes for vitamin B_{12} is 1 μg per day. The average intake of adults who eat meat and meat products is of the order of 5 μg per day.

12.2.10 **Folic acid**

Folic acid is involved in a wide variety of metabolic reactions, as a carrier of methyl groups and other one-carbon fragments. As shown in Figure 12.14, there are several different forms of folic acid found in foods, with different numbers of glutamate residues attached and carrying different one-carbon fragments. The extent to which the different forms of folate acid can be absorbed varies; on average only about half of the folic acid in the diet is available.

The metabolism of folic acid is closely linked to that of vitamin B_{12}. Methyl-folic acid is a normal intermediate of folic acid metabolism; it can only be converted back to free folic acid by the methylation of homocysteine to methionine. This is catalysed by a vitamin B_{12} dependent enzyme, and in vitamin B_{12} deficiency much of the body's folic acid accumulates as methyl-

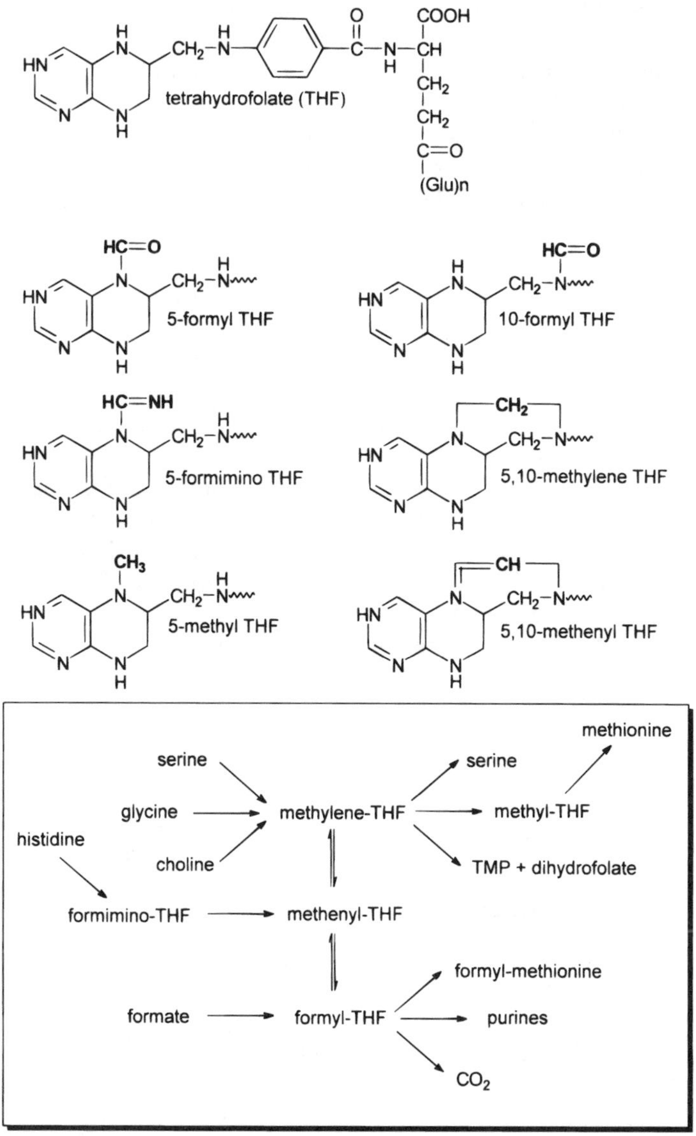

Figure 12.14 Folic acid and the major one-carbon substituted folates. The box shows the sources, interconversion and routes of utilization of one-carbon substituted folates.

folate, which cannot now be utilized. Thus, vitamin B_{12} deficiency results in secondary folic acid deficiency, despite an apparently adequate intake of this vitamin.

The administration of folic acid supplements to patients with megaloblastic anaemia caused by vitamin B_{12} deficiency can precipitate degeneration of the spinal cord, so it is important to eliminate vitamin B_{12} deficiency as a cause of megaloblastic anaemia before treating with folic acid.

The other folic acid dependent reaction that is important to an understanding of the basis of the effects of folic acid and vitamin B_{12} deficiency is the formation of thymidine for DNA synthesis. As shown in Figure 12.15, this reaction involves the transfer of a methylene ($=CH_2$) fragment from methylene-folic acid onto dUTP, associated with reduction of the methylene group to a methyl group ($-CH_3$). In the process, folic acid is oxidized to dihydrofolic acid. The second step in the reaction involves the reduction of dihydrofolate back to the active form, tetrahydrofolate.

12.2.10.1 *Folate deficiency: megaloblastic anaemia*

Dietary deficiency of folic acid is not uncommon and, as noted above, deficiency of vitamin B_{12} also leads to functional folic acid deficiency. In either case, it is cells that are dividing rapidly, and which therefore have a large requirement for thymidine for DNA synthesis, that are most severely affected. These are the cells of the bone marrow that form red blood cells, the cells of the intestinal mucosa which turn over in about 48 hours, and the hair follicles. Clinically, folic acid deficiency leads to megaloblastic anaemia, the release into the circulation of immature precursors of red blood cells.

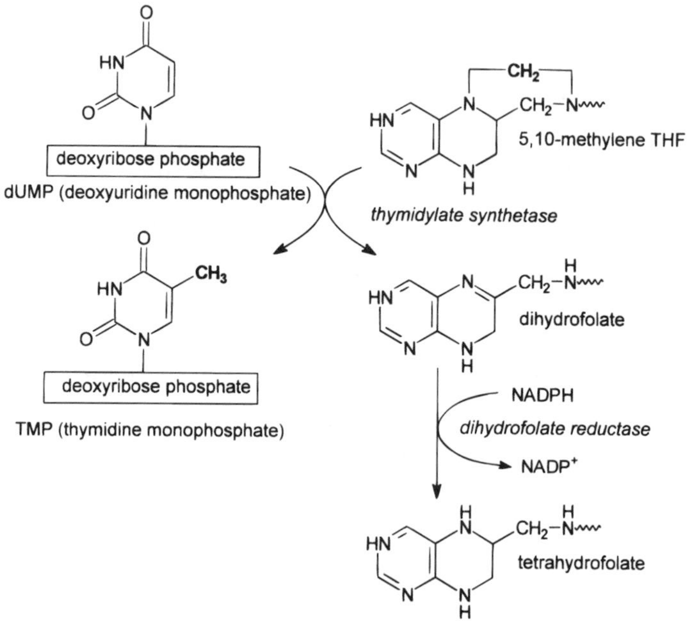

Figure 12.15 The reactions of thymidylate synthetase and dihydrofolate reductase.

12.2.10.2 *Folate requirements and pregnancy*

Folic acid requirements have been estimated in depletion and repletion studies, in which biochemical markers of folic acid deficiency are followed in response to graded intakes of the free vitamin. Allowing for the incomplete absorption of the mixed derivatives of folic acid in foods, the RNI for adults is 200 μg per day. Rich sources of folic acid are mainly green leafy vegetables, liver and kidney, nuts and whole grain cereals.

One factor in the development of spina bifida and other congenital neural tube defects is inadequate folic acid nutrition of the expectant mother. Folate supplements of 400 μg per day, begun before conception, have a significant effect in reducing the incidence of neural tube defects. Closure of the neural tube occurs early in embryological development, at about day 28 of pregnancy, before the mother knows that she is pregnant. Folate supplements after this will have no effect on the risk of neural tube defect. It is obviously desirable that all women who may become pregnant should have an adequate intake of folic acid; it is not known whether the amount that would be provided by a good diet is adequate to provide protection against neural tube defect in women who are at risk. An intake of 400 μg of free folic acid per day is considerably higher than can be obtained from foods, and there is controversy as to whether or not fortification of foods with folic acid, to ensure high intakes for women of child-bearing age, is desirable, in view of the potential risks associated with excessive intakes of the vitamin, discussed below.

12.2.10.3 *Folate toxicity*

There is no evidence that moderately large supplements of folic acid have any adverse effects. However, there are two potential problems:

- Folic acid supplements will mask the megaloblastic anaemia of vitamin B_{12} deficiency, and may hasten the development of the (irreversible) nerve damage. This is especially a problem of the elderly, who may suffer impaired absorption of vitamin B_{12} as a result of gastric atrophy with increasing age.
- Some people with epilepsy controlled by anticonvulsants show signs of mild folic acid deficiency. This is the result of an increased rate of metabolism of folic acid caused by the anticonvulsants. However, antagonism between folic acid and the anticonvulsants is part of the mechanism of action of these drugs. Relatively large supplements of folic acid (in excess of 1000 μg per day) may antagonize the beneficial effects of the anticonvulsants, and lead to an increase in the frequency of epileptic attacks.

12.2.10.4 *Folic acid antagonists in chemotherapy*

Since folic acid is required for the synthesis of thymidine for DNA synthesis, rapidly dividing cells are the most susceptible to folic acid deficiency: the bone marrow and intestinal mucosal cells and hair follicles. Cancer cells also have a very high requirement for DNA synthesis and are especially sensitive to folic acid deficiency. Folic acid antagonists, such as methotrexate, are used in the chemotherapy of cancer.

Bacteria and parasites also have a rapid rate of reproduction, and hence are again sensitive to the folic acid status of the host. Some bacteria, and parasites such as the malarial parasite, have a dihydrofolate reductase (see Figure 12.15) which differs from the human enzyme and can be inhibited by drugs such as trimethoprim, which have little or no effect on human dihydrofolate reductase.

12.2.11 Biotin

Biotin is required as the cofactor for carboxylation reactions; it acts as the carrier for carbon dioxide, as shown in Figure 12.16. The most important such reactions are the formation of malonyl CoA from acetyl CoA in fatty acid synthesis (see Figure 7.16) and the carboxylation of pyruvate to oxaloacetate for gluconeogenesis (see Figure 7.19).

Biotin is widely distributed in foods, and deficiency is unknown, except among people maintained for many months on total parenteral (intravenous) nutrition, and a very few people who eat abnormally large amounts of uncooked egg. There is a protein in egg white (avidin) which binds biotin

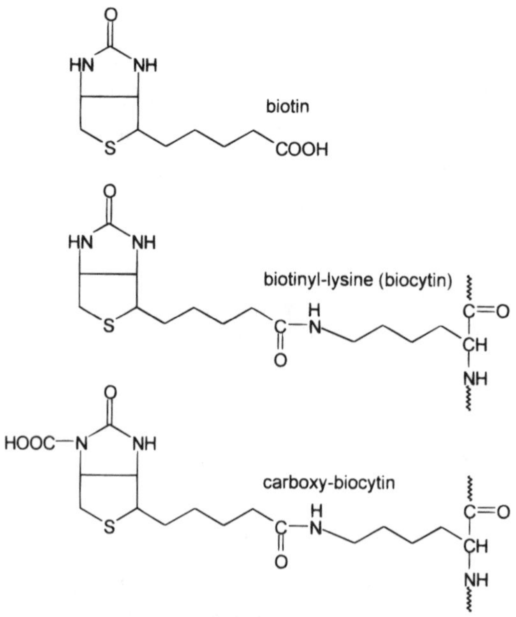

Figure 12.16 Biotin.

extremely tightly and renders it unavailable for absorption. Avidin is denatured by cooking and then loses its ability to bind biotin. The amount of avidin in uncooked egg white is relatively small, and problems of biotin deficiency have occurred only in people eating abnormally large amounts, such as a dozen or more raw eggs a day, for many years.

There is no evidence on which to estimate requirements for biotin. Average intakes are 10–200 μg per day. Since dietary deficiency does not occur, such intakes are obviously more than adequate to meet requirements.

12.2.12 *Pantothenic acid*

Pantothenic acid is part of CoA and the prosthetic group of the acyl carrier protein of fatty acid synthesis (see Figure 12.17). It is widely distributed in foods; indeed, the name pantothenic acid is derived from the Greek for 'from everywhere'. There is no good evidence of a specific pantothenic acid deficiency disease, although metabolic abnormalities have been observed in experimental subjects maintained on pantothenic acid-free diets. Prisoners of war in the Far East at the end of the Second World War suffered from neurological disease involving severe burning pain in the feet (the so-called burning foot syndrome). It was assumed that this was due to pantothenic acid deficiency. However, they were suffering from general malnutrition, and deficiency of a variety of vitamins. Rather than conducting unethical experiments in order to determine whether or not the burning foot syndrome was the result of pantothenic acid deficiency, these patients were treated with rich sources of all the B vitamins (commonly yeast extract).

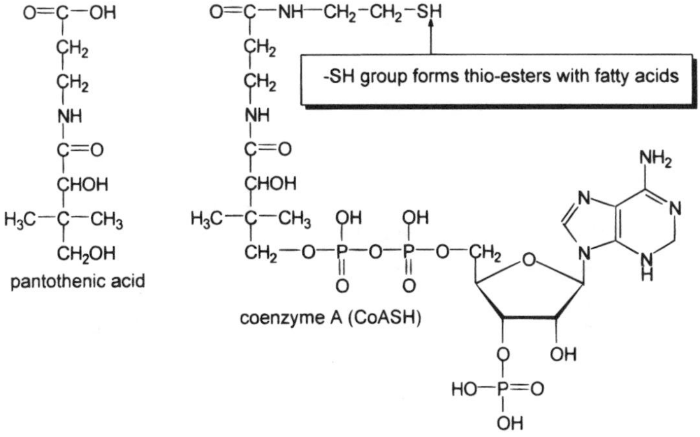

Figure 12.17 Pantothenic acid and coenzyme A.

There is no evidence on which to estimate pantothenic acid requirements. Average intakes are 3–7 mg per day, and since deficiency does not occur, such intakes are obviously more than adequate to meet requirements.

12.2.13 *Vitamin C (ascorbic acid)*

Vitamin C is required as the cofactor for a few hydroxylation reactions. The most important of these are the hydroxylation of proline and lysine in the post-synthetic modification of collagen and the hydroxylation of dopamine to noradrenaline. It also has a general antioxidant role, especially in the reduction of oxidized vitamin E in membranes (see Figure 12.6). The oxidation and reduction of vitamin C is shown in Figure 12.18.

12.2.13.1 *Vitamin C deficiency: scurvy*

The vitamin C deficiency disease, scurvy, was formerly a common problem at the end of winter, when there had been no fresh fruits and vegetables (the dietary sources of the vitamin) for many months. Sailors on long voyages similarly suffered from scurvy before the protective effect of fresh fruit and vegetables, or fruit juice, was discovered. On some of the voyages of exploration during the sixteenth and seventeenth centuries up to 90 per cent of the crew died from scurvy.

Almost all of the clinical signs of scurvy can be attributed to impairment of collagen formation, and hence defects of connective tissue. The earliest sign is the development of petechial haemorrhages around hair follicles. This is followed by inflammation of the gums between the teeth, with loss of dental cement, so that the teeth become loose and fall out. Because of the impairment of collagen synthesis, wound healing is much delayed in vitamin C deficiency. In advanced deficiency, the collagen of bones is affected, leading to severe bone pain. The impaired synthesis of adrenaline and noradrenaline leads to depression and irritability.

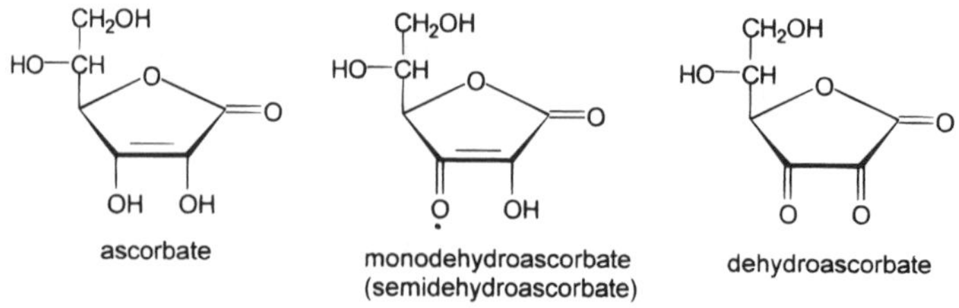

ascorbate

monodehydroascorbate (semidehydroascorbate)

dehydroascorbate

Figure 12.18 Vitamin C.

12.2.13.2 *Vitamin C requirements*

Vitamin C illustrates extremely well how different criteria of adequacy, and different interpretations of experimental evidence, can lead to different estimates of requirements, and to reference intakes ranging between 30 and 80 mg per day for adults.

The requirement for vitamin C to prevent clinical scurvy is less than 10 mg per day. However, at this level of intake, wounds do not heal properly, because of the requirement for vitamin C for the synthesis of collagen in connective tissue. An intake of 20 mg per day is required for optimum wound healing. Allowing for individual variation in requirements, this leads to reference intake for adults of 30 mg per day, which was the British RDA until 1991, and is the UN Food and Agriculture Organization/World Health Organization RDA.

The 1991 British RNI for vitamin C is based on the level of intake at which the plasma concentration rises sharply, showing that requirements have now been met, tissues are saturated, and there is spare vitamin C being transported between tissues, available for excretion. This criterion of adequacy gives an RNI of 40 mg per day for adults.

The alternative approach to determining requirements is to estimate the total body content of vitamin C, then measure the rate at which it is metabolized, by giving a test dose of radioactive vitamin. This is the basis of both the US RDA of 60 mg per day for adults and the Netherlands RDA of 80 mg per day. Indeed, it also provides an alternative basis for the RNI of 40 mg per day adopted in Britain in 1991.

The problem lies in deciding what is an appropriate total body content of vitamin C. The US studies were performed on subjects whose total body vitamin C was estimated to be 1500 mg at the beginning of a depletion study. However, there is no evidence that this is a necessary, or even a desirable, body content of the vitamin. It is simply the body content of the vitamin among a small group of young people eating a self-selected diet rich in fruit. There is good evidence that a total body content of 900 mg is more than adequate. It is three times larger than the body content at which the first signs of deficiency are observed, and will protect against the development of any signs of deficiency for several months on a diet completely free from vitamin C.

There is a further problem in interpreting the results of this kind of study. The rate at which vitamin C is metabolized varies with the amount consumed. This means that, as the experimental subjects become depleted, so the rate at which they metabolize the vitamin decreases. Thus, calculation of the amount required to maintain the body content depends on the way in which results obtained during depletion studies are extrapolated to the rate in subjects consuming a normal diet, and on the amount of vitamin C in that diet.

An intake of 40 mg per day (the same as the British RNI) is more than adequate to maintain a total body content of 900 mg of vitamin C. At a higher level of habitual intake, 60 mg per day is adequate to maintain a total body content of 1500 mg (the US RDA). Making allowances for changes in the rate of metabolism with different levels of intake, and allowing for incomplete absorption of the vitamin, gives the Netherlands RDA of 80 mg per day.

12.2.13.3 *High intakes of vitamin C*

At intakes above about 100 mg per day the body's capacity to metabolize vitamin C is saturated, and any further intake is excreted in the urine unchanged. Therefore, it would not seem justifiable to recommend higher levels of intake.

There are those who argue that intakes of vitamin C of the order of 1–5 g per day may confer some benefits. However, there is no good evidence that high intakes of vitamin C either protect against cancer or provide any benefit to patients suffering from cancer. Equally, there is no evidence from several large studies that vitamin C has any useful effect in treating or preventing the common cold or influenza.

The one benefit of a high intake of vitamin C is in aiding the absorption of iron. As discussed in §6.6, the absorption of inorganic iron is enhanced by vitamin C present in the gut together with the iron. This means that taking foods rich in vitamin C together with iron rich foods will increase the absorption of the iron. The best estimate is that optimum iron absorption is achieved with an intake of about 25–50 mg of vitamin C with each meal. Certainly, people who are taking iron supplements to treat iron deficiency anaemia should either take vitamin C tablets with them, or should swallow the iron tablets with a glass of fruit juice.

12.3 Minerals

Those inorganic mineral elements that have a function in the body must obviously be provided in the diet, since elements cannot be interconverted. Many of the essential minerals are of little practical nutritional importance, since they are widely distributed in foods, and most people eating a normal mixed diet are likely to receive adequate intakes.

In general, mineral deficiencies are a problem when people live largely on foods grown in one small region, where the soil may be deficient in some minerals. Iodine deficiency is a major problem in many areas of the world (see §12.3.3.3). For people whose diet consists of foods grown in a variety of different regions, mineral deficiencies are unlikely. However, as discussed in §12.3.2.3, iron deficiency is a problem in most parts of the world, because if iron losses from the body are relatively high (e.g. from heavy menstrual blood loss), it is difficult to achieve an adequate intake to replace the losses.

Mineral deficiency is unlikely among people eating an adequate mixed diet. More importantly, many of the minerals, including those that are dietary essentials, are toxic in even fairly modest excess. This is unlikely to be a problem with high mineral content of foods, although crops grown in regions where the soil content of selenium is especially high may provide dangerously high levels of intake of this mineral (see §12.3.2.5). The problem arises when people take inappropriate supplements of minerals or are exposed to contamination of food and water supplies.

12.3.1 Calcium

The most obvious requirement for calcium in the body is in the mineral of bones and teeth, which is a complex mixture of calcium carbonates and phosphates (hydroxyapatite) together with magnesium salts and fluorides. An adult has about 1.2 kg of calcium in the body, 99 per cent of which is in the skeleton and teeth. This means that calcium requirements are especially high in times of rapid growth: during infancy and adolescence, and in pregnancy and lactation.

Although the major part of the body's calcium is in bones, the most important functions of calcium are in the maintenance of muscle contractility, cell structure and responses to hormones and neurotransmitters (see §11.2). To maintain these essential regulatory functions, bone calcium is mobilized in deficiency, so as to ensure that the plasma and intracellular concentrations are kept within a strictly controlled range. If the plasma concentration of calcium falls, neuromuscular regulation is lost, leading to tetany.

The main sources of calcium are milk and cheese; dietary calcium is absorbed by an active process in the mucosal cells of the small intestine, and is dependent on vitamin D. As discussed in §12.2.2.3, the active metabolite of vitamin D, calcitriol, induces the synthesis of a calcium-binding protein that permits the mucosal cells to accumulate calcium from the intestinal lumen, and in vitamin D deficiency the absorption of calcium is seriously impaired.

Although the effect of vitamin D deficiency is impairment of the absorption and utilization of calcium, rickets (see §12.2.2.4) does not seem to be simply the result of calcium deficiency. Calcium deficient children with adequate vitamin D nutritional status do not develop rickets but have a much reduced rate of growth. Nevertheless, calcium deficiency may be a contributory factor in the development of rickets when vitamin D status is marginal.

12.3.1.1 Osteoporosis

Osteoporosis is a progressive loss of bone mass with increasing age, after the peak bone mass is achieved at the age of about 30. The cause is the normal process of bone turnover, with reduced replacement of the tissue that has been broken down. Both mineral and the organic matrix of bone are lost in osteoporosis, unlike osteomalacia (see §12.2.2.4) where there is loss of bone mineral but the organic matrix is unaffected.

Osteoporosis can occur in relatively young people, as a result of prolonged bedrest: bone continues to be degraded, but without physical activity there is less stimulus for replacement of the lost tissue. More importantly, it occurs as an apparently unavoidable part of the ageing process. Here the main problem is the reduced secretion of oestrogens (in women) and androgens (in men) with increasing age; among other actions, the sex steroids are involved in the stimulation of new bone formation. The problem is especially serious in women, since there is a much more abrupt fall in oestrogen secretion at the menopause than the more gradual (and less severe) fall in androgen secretion in men with increasing age. As a result, very many more elderly women than men suffer from osteoporosis. Post-menopausal hormone replacement therapy with oestrogens has a protective effect against the development of osteoporosis.

Because there is a net breakdown of bone in osteoporosis, there is excretion of considerable amounts of calcium in the urine. This shows as negative calcium balance: excretion is greater than the dietary intake. This has led to suggestions that a high intake of calcium may slow or reverse the process of osteoporosis. However, the negative calcium balance is the result of osteoporosis, not the cause. There is no evidence that higher intakes of calcium post-menopausally have any effect on the development of osteoporosis.

People with higher peak bone mass are less at risk from osteoporosis, since they can tolerate more loss of bone before there are serious effects. Therefore, adequate calcium and vitamin D nutrition through adolescence and young adulthood is likely to provide protection against osteoporosis in old age. High intakes of calcium have no beneficial effect once peak bone mass has been achieved. However, there are no adverse effects either, because of the close regulation of calcium homeostasis; problems of hypercalcaemia and calcinosis (the calcification of soft tissues) occur as a result of vitamin D intoxication (see §12.2.2.6), or other disturbances of calcium homeostasis, not as a result of high intakes of calcium.

High intakes of vitamin D have no beneficial effect on the progression of osteoporosis, although the vitamin will prevent the development of osteomalacia, which can occur together with osteoporosis in the elderly.

12.3.2 Minerals that function as prosthetic groups in enzymes

12.3.2.1 Cobalt

In addition to the role of cobalt in vitamin B_{12} (see §12.2.9), it provides the prosthetic group in a few enzymes. It is therefore a dietary essential, despite the fact that vitamin B_{12} cannot be synthesized in the body. However, no clinical signs of cobalt deficiency are known, except in ruminant animals, whose intestinal bacteria synthesize vitamin B_{12}.

12.3.2.2 Copper

Copper provides the essential functional part of enzymes involved in oxidation and reduction reactions, including dopamine β-hydroxylase in the synthesis of noradrenaline and adrenaline, cytochrome oxidase in the electron transport chain (see §5.3.1.2), and superoxide dismutase, one of the enzymes involved in protection against oxygen radicals (see §2.5). Copper is also important in the oxidation of lysine to form the cross-links in collagen and elastin. In copper deficiency, the bones are abnormally fragile, because the abnormal collagen does not permit the normal flexibility of the bone matrix. More importantly, elastin is less elastic than normal, and copper deficiency can lead to death following rupture of the aorta.

12.3.2.3 *Iron*

The most obvious function of iron is in the haem of haemoglobin, the oxygen-carrying protein in red blood cells, and myoglobin in muscles. Haem is also important in a variety of enzymes, including the cytochromes (see §5.3.1.2), where it is the coenzyme in oxidation and reduction reactions. Some enzymes also contain non-haem iron (i.e. iron bound to the enzyme other than in haem), which is essential to their function.

Deficiency of iron leads to reduced synthesis of haemoglobin, and hence a lower than normal amount of haemoglobin in red blood cells. Iron deficiency anaemia is a major problem worldwide, especially among women. The problem is caused by a loss of blood greater than can be replaced by absorption of dietary iron. In developing countries intestinal parasites (especially hookworm), which cause large losses of blood in the faeces, are a common cause of iron depletion, and hence anaemia, in both men and women. In developed countries it is mainly women who are at risk of iron deficiency anaemia, as a result of heavy menstrual losses of blood. Probably 10–15 per cent of women have menstrual losses of iron greater than can be met from a normal dietary intake, and are therefore at risk of developing anaemia unless they take iron supplements.

Iron in foods occurs in two forms: haem in meat and meat products, and inorganic iron salts in plant foods. The absorption of haem iron is considerably better than that of inorganic iron salts; as discussed in §6.6, only about 10 per cent of the inorganic iron of the diet is absorbed.

12.3.2.4 *Molybdenum*

Molybdenum functions as the prosthetic group of a few enzymes, including xanthine oxidase (which is involved in the metabolism of purines to uric acid for excretion) and pyridoxal oxidase (which metabolizes vitamin B_6 to the inactive excretory product pyridoxic acid). It occurs in an organic complex, molybdopterin, which is chemically similar to folic acid (see §12.2.10) but can be synthesized in the body as long as adequate amounts of molybdenum are available.

Molybdenum deficiency has been associated with increased incidence of cancer of the oesophagus, but this seems to be an indirect association. The problem occurs among people living largely on maize grown on soil poor in molybdenum. For reasons that are not altogether clear, the resultant molybdenum deficient maize is more susceptible to attack by fungi that produce carcinogenic toxins. Thus, although the people living on this diet are at risk of molybdenum deficiency, the main problem is not one of molybdenum deficiency in the people but rather of fungal spoilage of their food.

12.3.2.5 Selenium

Selenium functions in at least two enzymes: glutathione peroxidase and thyroxine deiodinase, which forms the active thyroid hormone, tri-iodothyronine, from thyroxine secreted by the thyroid gland (see Figure 12.19). In both cases it is present as the selenium analogue of the amino acid cysteine, selenocysteine (see §6.4.1).

Glutathione peroxidase acts to reduce the oxygen radicals that would otherwise attack polyunsaturated fatty acids, and also to reduce the products of oxidative damage to polyunsaturated fatty acids. Selenium thus has an important role in the body's overall antioxidant status, to a great extent in conjunction with vitamin E (see §12.2.3.1).

Deficiency is widespread in parts of China, and in some parts of the USA and Finland, the soil is so poor in selenium that it is added to fertilizers, in order to increase the selenium intake of the population, and so prevent deficiency. In New Zealand, despite the low selenium content of the soil, it was decided not to use selenium-rich fertilizers, because of the hazards of selenium toxicity.

Selenium is extremely toxic even in modest excess. The RNI for selenium for adults is 75 μg per day; signs of poisoning can be seen at intakes above 450 μg per day, and the World Health Organization recommends that selenium intakes should not exceed 200 μg per day. In some parts of the world the soil is so rich in selenium that locally grown crops would provide more than this recommended upper limit of selenium intake if they were the main source of food, and it is not possible to graze cattle safely on the pastures in these regions.

12.3.2.6 Zinc

Zinc is the prosthetic group of more than a hundred enzymes, with a wide variety of functions. It is also involved in the receptor proteins for steroid and thyroid hormones, calcitriol and vitamin A. In these proteins, zinc forms an integral part of the region of the protein that interacts with the promoter site on DNA to initiate gene transcription in response to hormone action (see §11.3).

Zinc deficiency occurs only among people living in tropical or subtropical areas, whose diet is very largely based on unleavened wholemeal bread. The problem is seen mainly as delayed puberty, so that young men of 18–20 are still prepubertal. This is a result of reduced sensitivity of target tissues to androgens, because of the role of zinc in steroid hormone receptors. Two separate factors contribute to the deficiency:

- Wheat flour provides very little zinc, and in unleavened wholemeal bread much of the zinc that is present is not available for absorption because it is bound to phytate and dietary fibre.
- Sweat contains a relatively high concentration of zinc, and in tropical conditions there can be a considerable loss of zinc in sweat.

Marginal zinc deficiency in developed countries may be associated with poor wound healing, and impairment of the senses of taste and smell.

12.3.3 *Minerals that have a regulatory role (in neurotransmission, as enzyme activators or in hormones)*

12.3.3.1 Calcium

In addition to its role in bone mineral, calcium has a major function in metabolic regulation (see §11.2), nerve conduction and muscle contraction. Calcium nutrition is discussed in §12.3.1.

12.3.3.2 Chromium

Chromium is involved as an organic complex (the glucose tolerance factor) in the interaction between insulin and cell surface insulin receptors. The precise chemical nature of the glucose tolerance factor has not been elucidated. Chromium deficiency is associated with impaired glucose tolerance, similar to that seen in diabetes mellitus (see §11.5). However, there is no evidence that increased intakes of chromium have any beneficial effect in diabetes and, although there is no evidence of harm from organic chromium complexes, inorganic chromium salts are highly toxic.

12.3.3.3 Iodine

Iodine is required for the synthesis of the thyroid hormones, thyroxine and tri-iodothyronine. Deficiency, leading to goitre (a visible enlargement of the thyroid gland), is widespread in inland upland areas over limestone soil. This is because the soil over limestone is thin, and minerals, including iodine, readily leach out, so that locally grown plants are deficient in iodine. Near the coast, sea spray contains enough iodine to replace these losses. Worldwide, many millions of people are at risk of deficiency, and in parts of central Brazil, the Himalayas and central Africa goitre may affect more than 90 per cent of the population.

Thyroid hormone regulates metabolic activity, and people with thyroid deficiency have a low metabolic rate (see §7.1.3.1), and hence gain weight readily. They tend to be lethargic, and have a dull mental apathy. Children born to iodine deficient mothers are especially at risk, and more so if they are then weaned onto an iodine deficient diet. They may suffer from very severe mental retardation (goitrous cretinism) and congenital deafness.

By contrast, overactivity of the thyroid gland, and hence overproduction of thyroid hormones, leads to a greatly increased metabolic rate, possibly leading to very considerable weight loss, despite an apparently adequate intake of food. People with hyperthyroidism are lean, and have a tense nervous energy.

Iodide is accumulated in the thyroid gland, where specific tyrosine residues in the protein thyroglobulin are iodinated to yield di-iodotyrosine. As shown in Figure 12.19, the next stage is the transfer of the di-iodophenol residue of one di-iodotyrosine onto another, yielding protein-bound thyroxine, which is stored in the colloid of the thyroid gland. In response to stimulation by thyrotropin, thyroglobulin is hydrolysed, releasing thyroxine into the circulation. The active hormone is tri-iodothyronine, which is formed from thyroxine by a selenium-dependent de-iodinase, both in the thyroid gland and, more impor-

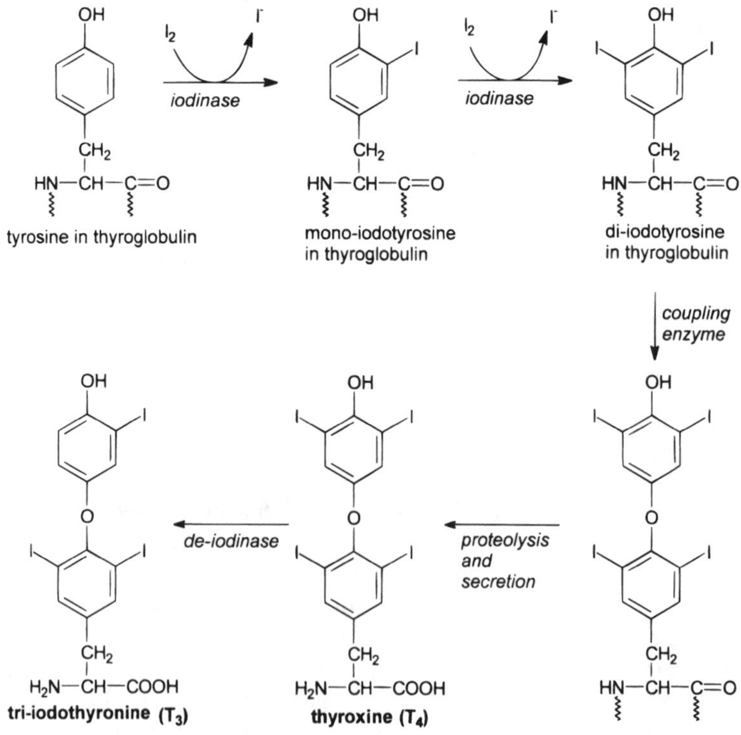

Figure 12.19 The synthesis of the thyroid hormones.

tantly, in target tissues. Because of the role of selenium in the metabolism of the thyroid hormones, the effects of iodine deficiency will be exacerbated by selenium deficiency.

In developed countries where there is a risk of iodine deficiency, supplementation of foods is common. Iodized salt may be available, or bread may be baked using iodized salt. In developing countries, such enrichment of foods is not generally possible, and the treatment and prevention of iodine deficiency generally depends on periodic visits to areas at risk by medical teams who give relatively large doses of iodized oil by intramuscular injection.

The problem of widespread iodization of foods in areas of deficiency is that adults whose thyroid glands have enlarged, in an attempt to secrete an adequate amount of thyroid hormone despite iodine deficiency, now become hyperthyroid. This is considered an acceptable risk to prevent the much more serious problems of goitrous cretinism among the young.

12.3.3.4 *Magnesium*

Magnesium is a cofactor for enzymes that utilize ATP and also several of the enzymes involved in DNA replication and transcription (see §10.2.1.2 and §10.2.2.1). It is not clear whether or not magnesium deficiency is an important nutritional problem, since there are no clear signs of deficiency. However, it has been clearly established that intravenous administration of magnesium salts is beneficial in the short period immediately after a heart attack.

12.3.3.5 *Manganese*

Manganese functions as the prosthetic group of a variety of enzymes, including superoxide dismutase, a part of the body's antioxidant defence system (see §2.5.3), pyruvate carboxylase in gluconeogenesis (see §7.7) and arginase in urea synthesis (see §10.3.1.4). Deficiency has been observed only in deliberate depletion studies.

12.3.3.6 *Sodium and potassium*

The maintenance of the normal composition of intracellular and extracellular fluids, and osmotic homeostasis, depend largely on the maintenance of relatively high concentrations of potassium inside cells and sodium outside. The gradient of sodium and potassium across cell membranes is maintained by active (ATP-dependent) pumping (see §5.2.2.3). Nerve conduction depends on the rapid reversal of this transmembrane gradient to create and propagate the electrical impulse, followed by a more gradual restoration of the normal ion gradient.

There is little or no problem in meeting sodium requirements; indeed, as discussed in §2.4.4, the main problem with sodium nutrition is an excessive intake, rather than deficiency.

12.3.4 Minerals known to be essential, but whose function is not known

12.3.4.1 Silicon

Silicon is known to be essential for the development of connective tissue and the bones, although its function in these processes is not known. The silicon content of blood vessel walls decreases with age and with the development of atherosclerosis. It has been suggested, although the evidence is not convincing, that silicon deficiency may be a factor in the development of atherosclerosis.

12.3.4.2 Vanadium

Experimental animals maintained under very strictly controlled conditions show a requirement for vanadium for normal growth. There is some evidence that vanadium has a role in regulation of the activity of sodium/potassium pumps (see §5.2.2.3), although this has not been proven.

12.3.4.3 Nickel and tin

There is some evidence, from experimental animals maintained under strictly controlled conditions, that a dietary intake of nickel and tin is required for optimum growth and development, although this remains to be demonstrated conclusively. No metabolic function has been established for either mineral.

12.3.5 Minerals that have effects in the body, but whose essentiality is not established

12.3.5.1 Fluoride

Fluoride has clear beneficial effects in modifying the structure of bone mineral and dental enamel. This strengthens the bones and protects teeth against decay. The use of fluoride toothpaste, and the addition of fluoride to drinking water in many regions, has resulted in a very dramatic decrease in the incidence of dental decay, despite high consumption of sucrose and other extrinsic sugars (see §2.4.3.1). These benefits are seen at levels of fluoride of the order of 1 part per million in drinking water. Such concentrations occur naturally in many parts of the world, and this is the concentration at which fluoride is added to water in many areas.

Excessive intake of fluoride leads to brown discoloration of the teeth (dental fluorosis). A concentration above about 12 ppm in drinking water, as occurs naturally in some parts of the world, is associated with excessive deposition of fluoride in the bones, leading to increased fragility (skeletal fluorosis).

Although fluoride has beneficial effects, there is no evidence that it is a dietary essential. Fluoride prevents dental decay, but it is probably not correct to call dental decay a fluoride deficiency disease.

12.3.5.2 *Lithium*

Lithium salts are used in the treatment of manic-depressive disease; they act by altering the responsiveness of some nerves to stimulation. However, this seems to be a purely pharmacological effect, and there is no evidence that lithium has any essential function in the body, nor that it provides any benefits for healthy people.

12.3.5.3 *Other minerals*

In addition to minerals that are known to be dietary essentials, there are some that may be consumed in relatively large amounts, but which have, as far as is known, no function in the body. Indeed, excessive accumulation of these minerals may be dangerous, and some of them are well known as poisons. Such elements include: aluminium, arsenic, antimony, boron, cadmium, caesium, germanium, lead, mercury, silver and strontium.

Appendix One

Units of physical quantities

Physical quantity	Unit	Symbol	Definition
Amount of substance	mole	mol	SI base unit
Electric current	ampere	A	SI base unit
Electric potential difference	volt	V	$J\ A^{-1}\ s^{-1}$
Energy	joule	J	$m^2\ kg\ s^{-1}$
	calorie	cal	4.186 J
Force	newton	N	$J\ m^{-1}$
Frequency	hertz	Hz	s^{-1}
Length	metre	m	SI base unit
Length	ångstrom	Å	10^{-10} m
Mass	kilogram	kg	SI base unit
Power	watt	W	$J\ s^{-1}$
Pressure	pascal	Pa	$N\ m^{-2}$
	bar	bar	10^5 Pa
Radiation dose absorbed	gray	Gy	$J\ kg^{-1}$
Radioactivity	becquerel	Bq	s^{-1}
Temperature	degree Celsius	°C	− 273.15 K
	kelvin	K	SI base unit
Time	second	s	SI base unit
Volume	litre	L (dm^3)	$10^{-3}\ m^3$

Multiples and submultiples of units

Multiple	Name	Symbol
$\times 10^{21}$	zetta	Z
$\times 10^{18}$	exa	E
$\times 10^{15}$	peta	P
$\times 10^{12}$	tera	T
$\times 10^{9}$	giga	G
$\times 10^{6}$	mega	M
$\times 10^{3}$	kilo	k
$\times 10^{2}$	centa	ca
$\times 10$	deca	da
$\times 10^{-1}$	deci	d
$\times 10^{-2}$	centi	c
$\times 10^{-3}$	milli	m
$\times 10^{-6}$	micro	μ (or mc)
$\times 10^{-9}$	nano	n
$\times 10^{-12}$	pico	p
$\times 10^{-15}$	femto	f
$\times 10^{-18}$	atto	a
$\times 10^{-21}$	zepto	z

Appendix Two

The nutrient yields of some common foods (per 100 g)

Breakfast cereals

	kcal	kJ	Prot g	Fat g	Carb g	Na mg	Ca mg	Fe mg	Vit B_1 mg	Vit B_2 mg	Fibre g
All-bran	258	1079	13	2.5	46	1700	85	9	1	1.5	30
Cornflakes	364	1523	8	0.5	82	1200	negl	7	1	1.5	11
Muesli	383	1603	13	7.5	66	180	200	4.5	0.3	0.3	8
Porridge	47	197	1.5	1	8	600	negl	0.5	0.1	0.01	0.7
Puffed Wheat	341	1427	14	1.3	69	negl	25	4.6	negl	0.06	9
Ready Brek	409	1712	12	9	70	25	65	5	1.5	0.1	7
Rice Krispies	382	1600	6	0.7	88	1300	negl	7	1	1.5	1
Shredded Wheat	341	1427	10.5	3	68	negl	40	4	0.3	0.05	10
Special K	377	1578	19	1	73	1000	50	13	1.2	1.7	3
Sugar Puffs	367	1540	6	0.8	84	negl	15	2.1	negl	0.03	6
Weetabix	357	1494	11.5	3.5	70	360	30	7.6	1	1.5	12

Baked goods

(Baked goods containing butter or margarine will be a modest source of vitamin A)

	kcal	kJ	Prot g	Fat g	Carb g	Na mg	Ca mg	Fe mg	Vit B_1 mg	Vit B_2 mg	Fibre g
Biscuits, chocolate	535	2239	6	27	67	160	110	1.7	0.5	0.15	3
cream crackers	454	1900	9.5	16	68	600	100	1.7	0.15	0.1	6
digestive	484	2026	10	20	66	440	110	2	0.15	0.1	5
semi-sweet	481	2013	7	17	75	400	120	2	0.15	0.1	3
shortbread	520	2176	6	26	66	270	100	1.5	0.15	negl	3
wafer	554	2319	5	30	66	70	70	1.6	0.1	0.1	2
water	460	1925	11	12.5	76	470	120	1.6	0.1	0.03	3
Bread, brown	235	984	9	2.2	45	550	100	2.5	0.25	0.05	5
malt	255	1067	8	3	49	280	90	3.5	negl	negl	3
white	246	1030	7.8	1.7	50	540	100	1.7	0.2	0.03	3
wholemeal	227	950	8.8	2.7	42	540	25	2.5	0.3	0.08	7.5
Currant buns	320	1339	7	8	55	100	90	2.5	0.2	0.03	3
Cake, fruit	347	1452	4	11	58	170	75	1.8	0.1	0.1	3
madeira	405	1695	5	17	58	400	40	1	0.05	0.1	2
sponge	481	2013	6.5	27	53	350	140	1.4	negl	0.1	1
iced	427	1787	4	15	69	250	45	1.5	negl	0.05	2
Chapattis	349	1461	8	13	50	130	70	2.3	0.25	0.05	7
Crispbread, rye	340	1423	9.5	2	71	220	50	4	0.3	0.15	12
wheat	395	1653	45	7.5	37	600	60	5.5	0.15	0.1	5
Pastry, flaky	572	2394	6	40	47	500	90	1.5	0.1	negl	2
shortcrust	540	2260	7	32	56	500	100	2	0.2	negl	1
Scones	389	1628	7.5	15	56	800	600	1.5	negl	0.1	2

Sweets and desserts

	kcal	kJ	Prot g	Fat g	Carb g	Na mg	Ca mg	Fe mg	Vit B_1 mg	Vit B_2 mg	Fibre mg
Chocolate, milk	538	2252	8	30	59	120	220	1.6	negl	0.1	0.2
plain	541	2265	5	29	65	negl	40	2.5	negl	0.1	0.1
Custard	120	502	4	4	17	80	140	negl	40	0.05	0.2
Ice cream, dairy	179	749	4	7	25	80	140	0.2	negl	0.04	0.2
non-dairy	168	703	3	8	21	70	120	0.3	negl	0.04	0.15
Egg custard	122	510	6	6	11	80	130	0.5	60	0.05	0.3
Fruit pie	384	1607	4	16	56	200	50	1	negl	0.05	negl
Pancakes	312	1306	6	16	36	50	120	1	40	0.1	0.2
Rice pudding	96	402	3.5	2.5	15	50	100	0.2	30	0.03	0.15

Fruit

The fat content of fruits is negligible, apart from bananas (0.3 g per 100 g); the sodium content is also negligible

	kcal	kJ	Prot g	Carb g	Fe mg	Ca mg	Vit A μg	Vit B_1 mg	Vit B_2 mg	Vit C mg	Fibre g
Apples	36	150	0.2	9	negl	0.2	negl	0.03	0.02	2	2
Apricots	30	125	0.6	7	negl	0.4	250	0.04	0.05	10	2
Bananas	86	360	1	20	negl	0.4	200	0.04	0.07	10	3
Bilberries	58	243	0.5	14	negl	0.7	15	0.02	0.02	20	7
Blackberries	30	125	1.5	6	60	1	15	0.03	0.04	20	7
Blackcurrants	32	134	1	7	60	1.5	30	0.03	0.06	200	9
Cherries	42	176	0.5	10	negl	0.3	15	0.04	0.06	5	2
Cranberries	18	75	0.5	4	15	1	negl	0.03	0.02	10	4
Gooseberries	16	67	1	3	30	0.3	30	0.04	0.03	40	3
Grapefruit	22	92	0.5	5	negl	0.3	negl	0.05	0.02	40	0.5
canned in syrup	66	276	0.5	16	negl	0.7	negl	0.04	0.01	30	0.3
Grapes, black	54	226	0.5	13	negl	0.3	negl	0.04	0.02	negl	0.5
white	62	260	0.6	15	20	0.3	negl	0.04	0.02	negl	0.5
Lemons	16	67	1	3	100	0.4	negl	0.05	0.04	80	0.5
Loganberries	18	75	1	3.5	40	1.5	negl	0.02	0.03	0	6
Mangoes	62	260	0.5	15	negl	0.5	1000	0.03	0.04	0	2
Melon	22	92	0.5	5	negl	0.5	1000	0.05	0.03	5	1
Nectarines	48	200	1	11	negl	0.4	500	0.02	0.05	10	2
Oranges	40	167	1	9	40	0.3	50	0.1	0.03	50	2
juice	38	159	0.6	9	negl	0.3	50	0.08	0.02	50	2
Peaches	34	142	0.5	8	negl	0.3	70	0.02	0.04	10	1
Pears	32	134	0.2	8	negl	negl	negl	0.02	0.02	0	2
Pineapple	50	210	0.5	12	negl	0.4	negl	0.08	0.02	5	1
canned in syrup	81	339	0.3	20	negl	0.4	negl	0.05	0.02	0	1
Plums	42	176	0.5	10	negl	0.4	30	0.05	0.03	negl	2
Prunes	84	352	1	20	negl	1.5	80	0.04	0.08	negl	8
Raspberries	28	117	1	6	40	1.2	15	0.02	0.03	25	8
Rhubarb	42	176	0.5	10	80	0.3	negl	negl	0.03	5	2
Satsumas	36	150	1	8	40	0.3	15	0.07	0.02	30	2
Strawberries	26	109	0.5	6	20	0.7	5	0.02	0.03	60	2
Tangerines	36	150	1	8	40	0.3	15	0.07	0.02	30	2

Nuts

Note that although the sodium content of nuts is negligible, salted nuts are high in sodium

	kcal	kJ	Prot g	Fat g	Carb g	Ca mg	Fe mg	Vit B_1 mg	Vit B_2 mg	Fibre g
Almonds	570	2386	17	54	4	250	4	0.2	1	14
Barcelona nuts	640	2679	11	64	5	170	3	0.1	0.1	10
Brazil nuts	604	2528	12	60	4	180	2.8	1	0.12	9
Chestnuts	180	753	2	2.7	37	50	1	0.2	0.2	7
Coconut	352	1473	3	36	4	negl	2	negl	negl	14
Peanuts	582	2436	24	50	9	60	2	1	0.1	8
Walnuts	532	2227	11	52	5	60	2.5	0.3	0.15	5

Vegetables

	kcal	kJ	Prot g	Fat g	Carb g	Na mg	Ca mg	Fe mg	Vit A μg	Vit B_1 mg	Vit B_2 mg	Vit C mg	Fibre g
Asparagus	8	33	1.7	negl	0.5	negl	negl	0.5	50	0.05	0.04	negl	1
Aubergine	14	57	0.7	negl	3	negl	negl	0.4	negl	0.05	0.03	5	2
Avocados	204	854	4	20	2	negl	15	1.5	15	0.1	0.1	5	2
Beans, baked	64	268	5	0.5	10	480	45	1.4	negl	0.07	0.05	negl	7
broad	49	205	4	0.6	7	20	20	1	40	0.1	0.04	15	4
butter	98	410	7	0.3	17	negl	20	1.7	negl	0.1	negl	negl	5
french	7	29	0.8	negl	1	negl	40	0.6	80	0.04	0.07	5	3
haricot	98	410	6.6	0.5	17	negl	70	2.5	negl	0.2	0.05	negl	7
mung (dahl)	104	435	6	4	11	820	35	2.6	negl	0.1	0.04	negl	5
red kidney	283	1185	22	1.7	45	40	140	6.7	negl	0.5	0.2	negl	25
runner	21	88	2	0.2	3	negl	25	0.7	60	0.03	0.07	5	3
Beetroot	47	197	1.8	negl	10	65	30	0.4	negl	0.02	0.04	5	4
Broccoli	18	75	3	negl	1.6	negl	80	1	500	0.06	0.2	35	4
Brussels sprouts	18	75	3	negl	1.7	negl	25	0.5	60	0.06	0.1	40	3
Cabbage	8	33	1	negl	1	negl	30	0.5	100	0.03	0.03	25	2
white	22	92	2	negl	3.5	negl	45	0.4	negl	0.06	0.05	40	3
Carrots	22	92	0.7	negl	5	100	50	0.6	12 000	0.06	0.05	5	3
Cauliflower	14	59	2	negl	1.5	negl	negl	0.5	5	0.1	0.1	60	2
Celery	9	38	1	negl	1.3	140	50	0.6	negl	0.03	0.03	7	2
Chickpeas	149	624	8	3.3	22	850	65	3.1	90	0.1	0.05	3	5
Chicory	9	38	0.8	negl	1.5	negl	negl	0.7	negl	0.05	0.05	4	2
Cucumber	10	42	0.6	negl	2	negl	25	0.3	negl	0.04	0.04	8	0.5

Vegetables—*Continued*

	kcal	kJ	Prot g	Fat g	Carb g	Na mg	Ca mg	Fe mg	Vit A μg	Vit B_1 mg	Vit B_2 mg	Vit C mg	Fibre g
Leeks	27	113	1.8	negl	5	negl	60	2	negl	0.07	0.03	15	2.5
Lentils	104	435	8	0.5	17	negl	negl	2.4	negl	0.1	0.04	negl	4
Lettuce	8	33	1	negl	1	negl	25	0.9	200	0.07	0.08	15	1.5
Marrow	7	29	0.4	negl	1.4	negl	negl	0.2	5	negl	negl	2	1
Mushrooms	13	54	2	0.6	negl	negl	negl	1	negl	0.1	0.4	3	negl
Onions	24	100	1	negl	5	negl	30	0.3	negl	0.03	0.05	10	1
Parsnips	52	218	2	negl	11	negl	60	0.6	negl	0.1	0.08	4	2.5
Peas	71	297	6	0.4	11	negl	negl	2	50	0.3	0.2	25	5
Peppers	15	63	1	0.4	2	negl	negl	0.4	40	negl	0.03	100	1
Potato	88	368	2	negl	20	negl	negl	0.6	negl	0.1	0.03	10	2
boiled	85	356	1.4	negl	20	negl	negl	0.3	negl	0.1	0.03	10	2
chips	263	1100	4	11	37	negl	negl	0.9	negl	0.1	0.04	10	2
Radishes	16	67	1	negl	3	60	45	1.9	negl	0.04	0.02	25	1
Rice	130	544	2	0.3	30	negl	negl	negl	negl	0.01	0.01	negl	0.8
Spaghetti	122	511	4	0.3	26	negl	negl	0.4	negl	0.01	0.01	negl	2
Spinach	30	126	5	0.5	1.5	120	600	4	1000	0.1	0.15	25	6
Swede	20	84	1	negl	4	negl	40	0.3	negl	0.04	0.03	20	3
Tomatoes	16	67	1	negl	3	negl	negl	0.4	15	0.1	0.05	20	1.5
Turnips	10	42	0.7	negl	2	30	60	0.4	negl	0.03	0.04	20	2
Watercress	14	59	3	negl	0.7	60	220	1.6	500	0.1	0.1	60	3

Milk and dairy produce

	kcal	kJ	Prot g	Fat g	Carb g	Na mg	Ca mg	Fe mg	Vit A μg	Vit B_1 mg	Vit B_2 mg
Butter	740	3097	0.5	82	negl	870	15	0.2	1000	negl	negl
Cheese, soft	299	1252	23	23	negl	1400	400	1	250	0.05	0.6
Cheddar	410	1716	26	34	negl	600	800	0.4	400	0.04	0.5
cottage	66	276	14	0.5	1.5	450	60	0.1	30	0.02	0.2
cream	435	1821	3	47	negl	300	100	0.1	450	0.02	0.15
Danish blue	353	1478	23	29	negl	1400	580	0.2	300	0.03	0.6
Edam	303	1268	24	23	negl	1000	750	0.2	300	0.04	0.4
Parmesan	410	1716	35	30	negl	750	1200	0.4	400	0.02	0.5
processed	313	1310	22	25	negl	1400	700	0.5	250	0.02	0.3
Stilton	464	1942	26	40	negl	1200	350	0.5	450	0.07	0.3
Cream, double	446	1867	1.5	48	2	30	50	0.2	400	0.02	0.1
single	212	887	2.4	21	3	40	80	0.3	250	0.03	0.1
sterilized	229	959	2.6	23	3	60	80	0.3	200	0.01	0.1
whipping	332	1389	1.9	35	2.5	30	60	0.3	300	0.02	0.1
Egg	147	615	12.3	11	negl	140	50	2	140	0.1	0.5
Margarine	729	3051	negl	81	negl	800	negl	negl	1000	negl	negl
Milk, full cream	66	276	3.3	3.8	4.7	50	120	negl	50	0.05	0.2
skimmed	34	142	3.4	0.1	5	50	130	negl	negl	0.04	0.2
evaporated	160	670	8.6	9	11.3	180	280	negl	100	0.06	0.5
Yogurt, flavoured	85	356	5	1	14	60	170	negl	negl	0.05	0.25
plain	53	222	5	1	6	80	180	negl	negl	0.05	0.3

Meat and meat products

	kcal	kJ	Prot g	Fat g	Carb g	Na mg	Ca mg	Fe mg	Vit A μg	Vit B_1 mg	Vit B_2 mg
Bacon rashers	420	1758	15	40	negl	1500	negl	1	negl	0.4	0.15
Beef	248	1038	17	20	negl	70	negl	1.5	negl	0.05	0.15
corned	216	904	27	12	negl	1000	negl	3	negl	negl	0.2
sausages	304	1272	10	24	12	800	50	1.4	negl	0.03	0.1
steak	202	845	19	14	negl	50	negl	2.3	negl	0.08	0.26
stewing	170	712	20	10	negl	70	negl	2.1	negl	0.06	0.23
Black pudding	310	1298	13	22	15	1200	35	20	negl	0.1	0.1
Chicken	145	607	25	5	negl	80	negl	0.8	negl	0.1	0.2
Cornish pastie	336	1406	8	20	31	600	60	1.5	negl	0.1	0.1
Duck	190	795	25	10	negl	100	negl	2.7	negl	0.3	0.5
Gammon	271	1134	25	19	negl	1000	negl	1.3	negl	0.4	0.15
Goose	314	1314	29	22	negl	150	negl	4.6	negl	negl	negl
Haggis	318	1331	11	22	19	800	30	5	2000	0.2	0.2
Ham	117	490	18	5	negl	1200	negl	1.2	negl	0.5	0.3
Hamburger	269	1126	15	21	5	600	25	2.5	negl	0.04	0.2
Heart	112	469	19	4	negl	100	negl	5	negl	0.5	1
Kidney	95	398	17	3	negl	220	negl	7	100	0.5	1.8
Lamb, breast	383	1603	17	35	negl	100	negl	1.3	negl	0.08	0.17
chops	375	1569	15	35	negl	60	negl	1.2	negl	0.1	0.15
cutlets	384	1607	15	36	negl	60	negl	1.2	negl	0.1	0.15
leg	243	1017	18	19	negl	50	negl	1.7	negl	0.14	0.25
shoulder	316	1323	16	28	negl	70	negl	1.2	negl	0.1	0.2
Liver	151	632	20	7	2	90	negl	8	1500	0.2	3.1
Pork, pie	383	1603	10	27	25	700	50	1.4	negl	0.2	0.1
chops	334	1398	16	30	negl	50	negl	0.8	negl	0.6	0.15
luncheon meat	315	1319	13	27	5	1000	15	1	negl	0.07	0.1
leg	275	1151	17	23	negl	60	negl	0.8	negl	0.7	0.2
sausages	372	1557	11	32	10	750	40	1.1	negl	0.04	0.1
Salami	489	2047	19	45	2	2000	negl	1	negl	0.2	0.2
Turkey	106	444	22	2	negl	50	negl	0.8	negl	0.1	0.15
Veal	111	465	21	3	negl	110	negl	1.2	negl	0.1	0.25

Fish and seafoods

	kcal	kJ	Prot g	Fat g	Na mg	Ca mg	Fe mg	Vit A μg	Vit B_1 mg	Vit B_2 mg
Cod	74	310	17	1	80	20	0.3	negl	0.1	0.1
Crab	125	523	20	5	400	30	1.3	negl	0.1	0.2
Fish fingers	183	766	13	7.5	320	45	0.7	negl	0.1	0.1
Halibut	94	393	18	2.5	85	85	negl	0.5	negl	0.1
Herring	239	1000	17	19	70	35	0.8	50	negl	0.2
Kipper	203	849	26	11	1000	70	1.4	50	negl	0.2
Lemon sole	80	335	17	1.4	100	negl	0.5	negl	0.1	0.1
Lobster	120	502	22	3.5	330	60	0.8	negl	0.1	0.1
Mackerel	220	921	19	16	130	25	1	45	0.1	0.35
Mussels	66	276	12	2	300	100	6	negl	negl	negl
Plaice	91	381	18	2	120	50	0.3	negl	0.3	0.1
Prawns	110	460	23	2	1600	150	1.1	negl	negl	negl
Salmon	180	753	18	12	100	30	0.7	negl	0.2	0.15
canned	152	636	20	8	600	100	1.4	100	0.04	0.2
smoked	145	607	25	5	2000	negl	0.6	negl	0.2	0.2
Sardines, in oil	222	929	24	14	650	550	2.9	negl	0.04	0.4
in tomato	182	762	18	12	700	460	4.6	negl	0.02	0.3
Shrimps	118	493	24	2.5	4000	300	1.8	negl	0.03	0.03
Trout	136	569	24	4.5	90	40	1	negl	negl	negl
Tuna, in oil	290	1214	23	22	400	negl	1.1	negl	0.04	0.1

Glossary

In addition to the brief glossary here, the following small and reasonably priced reference books will be useful:

Concise Dictionary of Biology (1990) Oxford University Press.
Concise Dictionary of Chemistry (1990) Oxford University Press.
Penguin Dictionary of Biology (1990). London: Penguin Books.
Penguin Dictionary of Chemistry (1990). London: Penguin Books.
BENDER, A.E. and BENDER, D.A. (1995) *Dictionary of Food and Nutrition.* Oxford University Press.

Acid: A compound that when dissolved in water, dissociates to yield hydrogen ions (H^+).

Acidosis: A condition in which the pH of blood plasma falls below the normal value of 7.4; a fall to pH 7.2 is life-threatening.

Acyl group: In an ester or other compound, the part derived from a fatty acid is called an acyl group.

ADP: Adenosine diphosphate.

Alcohol: A compound with an -OH group attached to an aliphatic carbon chain. Also used generally to mean ethanol (ethyl alcohol), the commonly consumed alcohol in beverages.

Aldehyde: A compound with an HC=O group attached to a carbon atom.

Aliphatic: A compound with chains of carbon atoms (straight or branched), rather than rings. Aliphatic compounds may be saturated or unsaturated.

Alkali: A compound that, when dissolved in water, gives an alkaline solution – one with a pH above 7.

Alkalosis: A condition in which the pH of blood plasma rises above the normal value of 7.4.

Alkane: A saturated hydrocarbon, of general formula $C_nH_{(2n+2)}$.

Alkene: An unsaturated hydrocarbon with a carbon–carbon double bond (C=C), of the general formula C_nH_{2n}.

Alkyne: An unsaturated hydrocarbon with a carbon–carbon triple bond (C≡C), of general formula $C_nH_{(2n-2)}$.

Amide: The product of a condensation reaction between a carboxylic acid and ammonia, a -$CONH_2$ group.

Amine: A compound with an amino (-NH_2) group attached to a carbon atom.

Amino acid: A compound with both an amino (-NH_2) and a carboxylic acid (-COOH) group attached to the α-carbon.

AMP: Adenosine monophosphate.

Amylopectin: The branched chain structure of starch.

Amylose: The straight-chain structure of starch.

Anabolism: Metabolic reactions resulting in the synthesis of more complex compounds from simple precursors. Commonly linked to the hydrolysis of ATP to ADP and phosphate.

Anaerobic: Occurring in the absence of oxygen.

Anion: An ion that has a negative electric charge and therefore migrates to the anode (positive pole) in an electric field. The ions of non-metallic elements are anions.

Anticodon: The three-base region of transfer RNA which recognizes and binds to the codon on messenger RNA.

Aromatic: A cyclic compound in which the ring consists of alternating single and double bonds.

Atom: The smallest particle of an element that can exist as an entity. The atom consists of a nucleus containing protons, neutrons and other uncharged particles, surrounded by a cloud of electrons.

Atomic mass: The mass of the atom of any element, relative to that of carbon = 12; 1 unit of atomic mass = 1.660×10^{-27} kg.

Atomic number: The number of protons in the nucleus of an atom (and hence the number of electrons surrounding the nucleus) determines the atomic number of that element.

ATP: Adenosine triphosphate.

Basal metabolic rate: The energy expenditure by the body at complete rest, but not asleep, in the post-prandial state.

Base: Chemically, an alkali. Also used as a general term for the purines and pyrimidines in DNA and RNA.

Body mass index (BMI): The ratio of body weight (in kg) to height^2 (in m). BMI over 25 is considered to be overweight, and over 30 is obesity.

Buffer: A solution of a weak acid and its salt, which can prevent changes in pH as the concentration of H^+ ions changes, by shifting the equilibrium between the dissociated and undissociated acid. Any buffer system only acts around the pH at which the acid is half dissociated.

Calorie: An (obsolete) unit of heat or energy. The amount of heat required to raise 1 g of water through 1°C. Nutritionally the kcal is sometime used; 1 kcal = 1000 cal. 1 cal = 4.186 joules, 1 joule = 0.239 cal.

Calorimetry: The measurement of energy expenditure by heat output; indirect calorimetry estimates heat output from oxygen consumption.

Carbohydrate: Compounds of carbon, hydrogen and oxygen in the ratio $C_nH_{2n}O_n$ The dietary carbohydrates are sugars, starches and non-starch polysaccharides.

Carboxylic acid: A compound with a -COOH group attached to a carbon atom.

Catabolism: Metabolic reactions resulting in the breakdown of complex molecules to simpler products, commonly oxidation to carbon dioxide and water, linked to the phosphorylation of ADP to ATP.

Catalyst: Something that increases the rate at which a chemical reaction achieves equilibrium, without itself being consumed in, or altered by, the reaction.

Cation: A positively charged ion that migrates to the cathode (negative pole) in an electric field. The ions of metallic elements are cations.

Cellulose: A polymer of glucose, linked by β 1–4-glycoside links, which are not digested by human enzymes.

Codon: A sequence of three nucleic acid bases in DNA or mRNA which specify an individual amino acid.

Coenzyme: A non-protein organic compound which is required for an enzyme reaction. Coenzymes may be loosely or tightly associated with the enzyme protein, and may be covalently bound to the enzyme, in which case they are known as prosthetic groups.

Condensation: A chemical reaction in which water is eliminated from two compounds to result in the formation of a new compound. The formation of esters, peptides and amides are condensation reactions.

Covalent bond: A bond between two atoms in which electrons are shared between the atoms.

Deoxyribose: A pentose (five-carbon) sugar in which one hydroxyl (-OH) group has been replaced by hydrogen. The sugar of DNA.

Dietary fibre: The residue of plant cell walls after extraction and treatment with digestive enzymes. Chemically a mixture of lignin and a variety of non-starch polysaccharides, including cellulose, hemicellulose, pectin, gums and mucilages.

Disaccharide: A sugar consisting of two monosaccharides linked by a glycoside bond. The common dietary disaccharides are sucrose (cane or beet sugar), lactose, maltose and isomaltose.

Dissociation: The process whereby a molecule separates into ions on solution in water.

DNA: Deoxyribonucleic acid.

Double bond: A covalent bond in which two pairs of electrons are shared between the participating atoms.

Electrolyte: A compound that undergoes partial or complete dissociation into ions when dissolved, and so is capable of transporting an electric current. In clinical chemistry electrolyte is normally used to mean the major inorganic ions in body fluids.

Electron: The smallest unit of negative electric charge. The fundamental particles that surround the nucleus of an atom.

Electronegative: An electronegative atom exerts greater attraction for the shared electrons in a covalent bond than does its partner, so developing a partial negative charge.

Electropositive: An electropositive atom exerts less attraction for the shared electrons in a covalent bond than does its partner, so developing a partial positive charge.

Element: A substance that cannot be further divided or modified by chemical means. The basic substances from which compounds are formed.

Endergonic: A chemical reaction that will only proceed with an input of energy, usually as heat.

Endonuclease: An enzyme that hydrolyses a polynucleotide at a specific sequence within the chain, as opposed to an exonuclease.

Endopeptidase: An enzyme that hydrolyses a peptide adjacent to a specific amino acid within the sequence, as opposed to an exopeptidase.

Endothermic: A chemical reaction that will only proceed with an input of heat.

Enteral nutrition: Feeding by tube directly into the stomach or small intestine.

Enzyme: A protein that acts as a catalyst in a metabolic reaction.

Essential amino acid: The amino acids required for protein synthesis that cannot be synthesized at all in the body, but must be provided in the diet: lysine, methionine, phenylalanine, tryptophan, threonine, valine, leucine, isoleucine and histidine.

Essential fatty acids: Those polyunsaturated fatty acids that cannot be synthesized in the body and must be provided in the diet. Linoleic and linolenic acids are the only two that are dietary essentials, since the other polyunsaturated fatty acids can be synthesized from them.

Ester: The product of a condensation reaction between an alcohol and a carboxylic acid.

Exergonic: A chemical reaction that proceeds with an output of energy, usually as heat.

Exon: A region of DNA that codes for a gene (as opposed to introns).

Exonuclease: An enzyme that removes a terminal nucleotide from a polynucleotide, as opposed to an endonuclease.

Exopeptidase: An enzyme that removes a terminal amino acid from a polypeptide, as opposed to an endopeptidase.

Exothermic: A chemical reaction that proceeds with an output of heat.

Fat: Triacylglycerols, esters of glycerol with three fatty acids; fats are generally considered to be those triacylglycerols that are solid at room temperature, whereas oils are triacylglycerols that are liquid at room temperature.

Fatty acid: Aliphatic carboxylic acids (i.e. with a -COOH group). The metabolically important fatty acids have between 2 and 24 carbon atoms (always an even number) and may be completely saturated or have one (mono-unsaturated) or more (polyunsaturated) C=C double bonds in the carbon chain.

Galactose: A hexose (six-carbon) monosaccharide.

Gene: A region of DNA that carries the information for a single protein or polypeptide chain.

Genetic code: The sequence of triplets of the nucleic acid bases (purines and pyrimidines) that specifies the individual amino acids.

Glucose: A monosaccharide; a hexose (six-carbon) sugar, of empirical formula $C_6H_{12}O_6$.

Glycerol: A trihydric alcohol to which three fatty acid molecules are esterified in the formation of triacylglycerols (fats and oils). Glycerol has a sweet taste, and is hygroscopic (attracts water); it is commonly used as a humectant in food processing.

Glycogen: A branched chain polymer of glucose, linked by α1–4 links, with branch points provided by α1–6 links. The storage carbohydrate of mammalian liver and muscle.

Glycolysis: The metabolic pathway by which glucose is oxidized to pyruvate.

Hexose: A monosaccharide with six carbon atoms, and hence the empirical formula $C_6H_{12}O_6$. The nutritionally important hexoses are glucose, galactose and fructose.

Hydrocarbon: A compound of carbon and hydrogen only. Hydrocarbons may have linear, branched or cyclic structures, and may be saturated or unsaturated.

Hydrogen bond: The attraction between a partial positive charge on a hydrogen atom attached to an electropositive atom and a partial negative charge associated with an electronegative atom in another molecule or region of the same macromolecule.

Hydrolysis: The process of splitting a chemical bond between two atoms by the introduction of water, usually adding -H to one side of the bond and -OH to the other, resulting in the formation of two separate product molecules. The digestion of proteins to amino acids, polysaccharides and disaccharides to monosaccharides, and triacylglycerols to glycerol and fatty acids are all hydrolysis reactions.

Hydrophilic: A compound which is soluble in water, or a region of a macromolecule which can interact with water molecules.

Hydrophobic: A compound which is insoluble in water, but soluble in lipids, or a region of a macromolecule which cannot interact with water, although it does interact with lipids.

Induction: The initiation of new synthesis of an enzyme or other protein by activation of the transcription of the gene for the protein. Inducers are commonly metabolic intermediates or hormones. Induction results in an increase in the amount of enzyme protein in the cell.

Inhibition: Decrease in the activity of an enzyme, with no effect on the amount of enzyme protein present in the cell.

Inorganic: Any chemical compound other than those carbon compounds considered to be organic.

Insoluble fibre: Lignin and non-starch polysaccharides in plant cell walls (cellulose and hemicellulose).

International units (iu): Before vitamins and other substances were purified, their potency was expressed in arbitrary, but standardized, units of biological activity. Now obsolete, but vitamins A, D and E are still sometimes quoted in iu.

Intron: A region of DNA in between regions that code for a gene (these are exons).

Ion: An atom (or group of atoms) which has lost or gained one or more electrons and thus has an electric charge.

Isomers: Forms of the same chemical compound, but with a different spatial arrangement of atoms or groups in the molecule. D- and L-isomerism refers to the arrangement of four different substituents around a carbon atom relative to the arrangement in the triose sugar D-glyceraldehyde. *R*- and *S*-isomerism refers to the arrangement of four different substituents around a carbon atom according to a set of systematic chemical rules. *Cis*- and *trans*-isomerism refers to the arrangement of groups adjacent to a carbon–carbon double bond.

Isotope: Different forms of the same chemical element (i.e. having the same number of protons in the nucleus and the same number of electrons surrounding the nucleus as each other) differing in the number of neutrons in the nucleus, and hence in the relative atomic mass.

Joule: The SI unit of energy. One joule is the work done when the point of application of a force of 1 newton moves 1 metre in the direction of the force (1 joule = 0.239 cal, 1 cal = 4.186 joule).

Ketone: A compound with a carbonyl (C=O) group attached to two aliphatic groups.

Ketone bodies: Acetoacetate and β-hydroxybutyrate (not chemically a ketone) formed in the liver from fatty acids in the fasting state and released into the circulation as metabolic fuels for use by other tissues. Acetone is also formed non-enzymically from acetoacetate, circulates in the blood, but cannot be metabolized as a metabolic fuel.

Ketosis: An elevation of the plasma concentrations of acetoacetate, hydroxybutyrate and acetone, as occurs in the fasting state.

Kwashiorkor: A disease of protein-energy malnutrition in which there is oedema masking the severe muscle wastage, fatty infiltration of the liver, and abnormalities of hair structure and hair and skin pigmentation.

Lactose: The sugar of milk. A disaccharide composed of glucose and galactose.

Lipid: A general term including fats and oils (triacylglycerols), phospholipids and steroids.

Lipogenesis: The metabolic pathway for synthesis of fatty acids from acetyl CoA, then the synthesis of triacylglycerols by esterification of glycerol with fatty acids.

Lipolysis: The hydrolysis of triacylglycerols to yield fatty acids and glycerol.

Lower reference nutrient intake (LRNI): An intake of a nutrient, below which it is unlikely that physiological needs will be met or metabolic integrity be maintained.

Macromolecule: A term used to describe the large molecules of, for example, proteins, nucleic acids and polysaccharides.

Maltose: A disaccharide composed of two molecules of glucose linked by an α1–4-glycoside bond.

Marasmus: A disease of protein-energy malnutrition in which there is extreme emaciation as a result of catabolism of adipose tissue and protein reserves.

Metabolic fuel: Those dietary components oxidized as a source of metabolic energy: fats, carbohydrates, proteins and alcohol.

Metabolism: The processes of interconversion of chemical compounds in the body.

Mineral: Inorganic salts, so called because they can be obtained by mining.

Mitochondrion: A subcellular organelle that contains the enzymes of the citric acid cycle, fatty acid oxidation and the electron transport chain for oxidative phosphorylation of ADP to ATP.

Mol: Abbreviation for mole – the SI unit for the amount of material. The relative molecular mass of a compound, expressed in grams. One mole of any compound contains 6.0223×10^{23} molecules.

Molar: Concentration of a compound expressed in mol per L, sometimes abbreviated to M.

Molecular mass: The mass of a molecule of a compound, relative to that of carbon = 12; the sum of the relative atomic masses of the atoms that comprise the molecule.

Molecule: The smallest particle of a compound that can exist in a free state.

Monosaccharide: A simple sugar, the basic units from which disaccharides and polysaccharides are composed. The nutritionally important monosaccharides are the pentoses (five-carbon sugars) – ribose and deoxyribose; and the hexoses (six-carbon sugars) – glucose, galactose and fructose.

Neutron: One of the fundamental particles in the nucleus of an atom. Neutrons have no electric charge, and a mass approximately equal to that of a proton. Differences in the number of neutrons in atoms of the same element account for the occurrence of isotopes.

Nitrogen balance: The difference between the intake of nitrogenous compounds (mainly protein) and the output of nitrogenous products from the body. Positive nitrogen balance occurs in growth, when there is a net increase in the body content of protein; negative nitrogen balance means that there is a loss of protein from the body.

Non-essential amino acid: Those amino acids required for protein synthesis that can be synthesized in the body in adequate amounts to meet requirements, and therefore do not have to be provided in the diet. The non-essential amino acids are: glycine, alanine, serine, proline, glutamic acid, aspartic acid, glutamine, asparagine and arginine. In addition, tyrosine can be synthesized in the body, but only from the essential amino acid phenylalanine, and cysteine can be synthesized, but only from the essential amino acid methionine.

Non-starch polysaccharides: A group of polysaccharides other than starch which occur in plant foods. They are not digested by human enzymes, although they may be fermented by intestinal bacteria. They provide the major part of dietary fibre. The main non-starch polysaccharides are cellulose, hemicellulose (insoluble non-starch polysaccharides) and pectin, and the plant gums and mucilages (soluble non-starch polysaccharides).

Nucleic acid: DNA and RNA – polymers of nucleotides which carry the genetic information of the cell (DNA in the nucleus) and information from DNA for protein synthesis (RNA).

Nucleotides: Phosphate esters of purine or pyrimidine bases with ribose (ribonucleotides) or deoxyribose (deoxyribonucleotides).

Nucleus: Chemically, the central part of an atom, containing protons, neutrons and a variety of other subatomic particles. Biologically, the subcellular organelle that contains the genetic information as DNA, arranged in chromosomes.

Obesity: Excessive body weight as a result of the accumulation of adipose tissue. Obesity is generally considered to be a body mass index greater than 30; between 25 and 30 is overweight.

Oil: Triacylglycerols, esters of glycerol with three fatty acids; oils are those triacylglycerols that are liquid at room temperature, whereas fats are solid. Mineral oil and lubricating oil are chemically completely different, and consist of long-chain hydrocarbons.

Oligopeptide: A chain of 2–10 amino acids linked by peptide bonds. Longer chains of amino acids are known as polypeptides (up to about 50 amino acids) or proteins.

Oligosaccharide: A general term for polymers containing about 3–10 monosaccharides.

Orbital: An allowed energy level for an electron around the nucleus of an atom, or of two atoms in a molecule.

Organic: Chemically, all compounds of carbon, other than simple carbonate and bicarbonate salts, are called organic, since they were originally discovered in living matter. Also used to describe foods grown under specified conditions without the use of fertilizers, pesticides, etc.

Overweight: Body weight relative to height greater than is considered desirable (on the basis of life expectancy), but not so much as to be considered as obesity.

Oxidation: A chemical reaction in which the number of electrons in a compound is decreased. In organic compounds this is generally seen as a decrease in the proportion of hydrogen, an increase in the number of carbon–carbon double bonds, or an increase in the proportion of oxygen in the molecule.

Oxidative phosphorylation: The phosphorylation of ADP to ATP, linked to the oxidation of metabolic fuels in the mitochondrial membrane.

Parenteral nutrition: Feeding by tube, commonly intravenously, but also applied to any means of providing nutrients other than through the gastrointestinal tract.

Pentose: A monosaccharide sugar with five carbon atoms, and hence the empirical formula $C_5H_{10}O_5$. The most important pentose sugars are ribose and deoxyribose (in which one hydroxyl group has been replaced by hydrogen).

Peptide bond: The link between amino acids in a protein. Formed by condensation between the carboxylic acid group (-COOH) of one amino acid and the amino group ($-NH_2$) of another to give a -CO-HN- link between the amino acids.

pH: A measure of the acidity (or alkalinity) of a solution. A neutral solution has pH = 7.0; lower values are acid, higher values are alkaline. pH stands for potential hydrogen, and is the negative logarithm of the concentration of hydrogen ions (H^+) in the solution.

Phospholipid: A lipid in which glycerol is esterified to two fatty acids, but the third hydroxyl group is esterified to phosphate, and through the phosphate to one of a variety of other compounds. Phospholipids are both hydrophilic and hydrophobic, and have a central role in the structure of cell membranes.

Phosphorolysis: The cleavage of a bond between two parts of a molecule by the introduction of phosphate, yielding two product molecules. The breakdown of glycogen, to yield glucose 1-phosphate, proceeds by way of sequential phosphorolysis reactions.

Phosphorylation: The addition of a phosphate group to a compound.

Physical activity level: Energy expenditure, averaged over 24 h, expressed as a ratio of the basal metabolic rate. The sum of the physical activity ratio × time spent for each activity during the day.

Physical activity ratio: Energy expenditure in a given activity, expressed as a ratio of the basal metabolic rate.

Polypeptide: A chain of amino acids, linked by peptide bonds. Generally up to about 50 amino acids constitute a polypeptide; a larger polypeptide would be called a protein.

Polysaccharide: A polymer of monosaccharide units linked by glycoside bonds. The nutritionally important polysaccharides can be divided into starch and glycogen, and the non-starch polysaccharides.

Polyunsaturated: Fatty acids with two or more carbon–carbon double bonds in the molecule, separated by a methylene (-CH_2-) group.

PRI: Population reference intake of a nutrient, a term introduced in the 1993 EC *Tables of nutrient requirements.* An intake of the nutrient two standard deviations above the observed mean requirement, and hence greater than the requirements of 97.5 per cent of the population.

Prosthetic group: A non-protein part of an enzyme which is essential for the catalytic activity of the enzyme, and which is covalently bound to the protein.

Protein: A polymer of amino acids joined by peptide bonds.

Proton: The positively charged subatomic particle in the nucleus of atoms. The number of protons in the nucleus determines the atomic number of the element. The hydrogen ion (H^+) is a proton.

Purine: Two of the bases in nucleic acids (DNA and RNA) are purines: adenine and guanine.

Pyrimidine: Three of the bases in nucleic acids are pyrimidines: cytidine and uracil in DNA, cytidine and thymidine in RNA.

Radical: A free radical is a highly reactive molecule with an unpaired electron.

RDA: Recommended daily (or dietary) allowance (or amount) of a nutrient. An intake of the nutrient two standard deviations above the observed mean requirement, and hence greater than the requirements of 97.5 per cent of the population.

RDI: Recommended daily (or dietary) intake of a nutrient. An intake of the nutrient two standard deviations above the observed mean requirement, and hence greater than the requirements of 97.5 per cent of the population.

Reducing sugar: A sugar that has a free aldehyde (-HC=O) group, which can therefore act as a chemical reducing agent. Glucose, galactose, maltose and lactose are all reducing sugars.

Reduction: A chemical reaction in which the number of electrons in a compound is increased. In organic compounds this is generally seen as an increase in the proportion of hydrogen, a decrease in the number of carbon–carbon double bonds, or a decrease in the proportion of oxygen in the molecule. It is the opposite of oxidation.

Repression: Decreased synthesis of an enzyme or other protein, as a result of blocking the transcription of the gene for that enzyme. Metabolic intermediates, end-products of pathways and hormones may act as repressors.

Respiratory quotient (RQ): The ratio of carbon dioxide produced to oxygen consumed in the metabolism of metabolic fuels. The RQ for carbohydrates is 1.0, for fats 0.71 and for proteins 0.8.

Resting metabolic rate (RMR): The energy expenditure of the body at rest, but not measured under the strict conditions required for determination of basal metabolic rate.

Ribose: A pentose (five-carbon) sugar.

Ribosome: The subcellular organelle on which the message of messenger RNA is translated into protein. The organelle on which protein synthesis occurs.

RNI Reference nutrient intake, a term introduced in the 1992 UK Tables of dietary reference values. An intake of the nutrient two standard deviations above the observed mean requirement, and hence greater than the requirements of 97.5 per cent of the population.

Salt: The product of a reaction between an acid and an alkali. Ordinary table salt is sodium chloride.

Satiety: The state of satisfaction of hunger or appetite.

Saturated: An organic compound in which all carbon atoms are joined by single bonds, as opposed to unsaturated compounds with carbon–carbon double bonds. A saturated compound contains the maximum possible proportion of hydrogen.

Soluble fibre: Non-starch polysaccharides that are soluble in water; pectin and the plant gums and mucilages.

Starch: A polymer of glucose units. Amylose is a straight-chain polymer, with α1–4-glycoside links between the glucose units. In amylopectin there are also branch points, where chains are linked through an α1–6-glycoside bond.

Steroids: Compounds derived from cholesterol (itself also a steroid), most of which are hormones.

Substrate: The substance or substances upon which an enzyme acts.

Sugar: Chemically, a monosaccharide or small oligosaccharide. Cane or beet sugar is sucrose, a disaccharide of glucose and fructose.

Teratogen: A compound that can cause congenital defects in the developing foetus.

Transcription: The process whereby a copy of the region of DNA containing the gene for a single protein is copied to give a strand of messenger RNA.

Translation: The process of protein synthesis, whereby the message of messenger RNA is translated into the amino acid sequence.

Triacylglycerol: The main type of dietary lipid, and the storage lipid of adipose tissue. Glycerol esterified with three molecules of fatty acid. Also known as triglycerides.

Triglyceride: Alternative (and chemically incorrect) name for triacylglycerol.

Unsaturated: An organic compound containing one or more carbon–carbon double bonds, and therefore less than the possible maximum proportion of hydrogen.

Urea: The main excretory end-product of amino acid metabolism.

Valency: The number of bonds an atom must form to other atoms in order to achieve a stable electron configuration.

Van der Waals forces: Individually weak forces between molecules depending on transient charges because of transient inequalities in the sharing of electrons in covalent bonds.

Vegan: A strict vegetarian who will eat no foods of animal origin.

Vegetarian: One who does not eat meat and meat products. An ovolactovegetarian will eat milk and eggs, but not meat or fish; a lactovegetarian milk but not eggs.

Vitamin: An organic compound required in small amounts for the maintenance of normal growth, health and metabolic integrity. Deficiency of a vitamin results in the development of a specific deficiency disease, which can be cured or prevented only by that vitamin.

Bibliography

Sources of more detailed information and suggestions for further reading.

General reference books

Concise Dictionary of Biology (1990). Oxford University Press.
Concise Dictionary of Chemistry (1990). Oxford University Press.
Penguin Dictionary of Biology (1990). London: Penguin Books.
Penguin Dictionary of Chemistry (1990). London: Penguin Books.
BENDER, A.E. and BENDER, D.A. (1995) *Dictionary of Food and Nutrition.* Oxford University Press.
BENDER, D.A. and BENDER, A.E. (1997) *Nutrition: a Reference Handbook.* Oxford University Press.

General textbooks of nutrition

GARROW, J. and JAMES, W.P.T. (1993) *Human Nutrition and Dietetics,* 9th edn. Edinburgh: Churchill-Livingstone.
HERBERT, V. and SUBAK-SHARPE, G.J. (eds) (1990) *The Mount Sinai School of Medicine Complete Book of Nutrition.* New York: St Martin's Press.

General textbooks of biochemistry

ABELES, R.H., FREY, R.H. and JENCKS, W.P. (1992) *Biochemistry.* Boston: Jones & Bartlett.
CAMPBELL, P.N. and SMITH, A.D. (1994) *Biochemistry Illustrated,* 3rd edn. Edinburgh: Churchill-Livingstone.
CHAMPE, P.C. and HARVEY, R.A. (1994) *Lippincott's Illustrated Reviews, Biochemistry,* 2nd edn. Philadelphia: J B Lippincott Co.
FRAYN, K.N. (1996) *Metabolic Regulation: a Human Perspective.* London: Portland Press.
GILLHAM, B., PAPACHRISTODOULOU, D.K. and THOMAS, J.H. (1997) *Will's Biochemical Basis of Medicine,* 3rd edn. Oxford: Butterworth-Heinemann.
SMITH, C.A. and WOOD, E.J. (1991) *Biological Molecules.* London: Chapman & Hall.
STRYER, L. (1995) *Biochemistry,* 4th edn. New York: Freeman.

VOET, D. and VOET, J.G. (1995) *Biochemistry*, 2nd edn. New York: Wiley.

WOOD, E.J. and MYERS, A. (1991) *Essential Chemistry for Biochemistry*, 2nd edn. London: Biochemical Society.

Food composition tables

BENDER, A.E. and BENDER, D.A. (1986) *Food Tables.* Oxford University Press.

BENDER, A.E. and BENDER, D.A. (1991) *Food Labelling: a Companion to Food Tables.* Oxford University Press.

DAVIES, J. and DICKERSON, J.W.T. (1991) *Nutrient Content of Food Portions.* London: Royal Society of Chemistry.

HOLLAND, B., WELCH, A.A., UNWIN, I.D., BUSS, D.H., PAUL, A.A. and SOUTHGATE, D.A.T. (1991) *McCance and Widdowson's Composition of Foods*, 5th edn. London: Royal Society of Chemistry and Ministry of Agriculture, Fisheries and Food.

Diet and health, reference nutrient intakes

ANDERSON, D. (ed.) (1986) *A Diet of Reason: Sense and Nonsense in the Healthy Eating Debate.* London: Social Affairs Unit.

BRITISH MEDICAL ASSOCIATION (1986) *Diet, Nutrition and Health: Report by the Board of Science and Education.* London: BMA.

Department of Health and Social Security Report on Health and Social Subjects no 28: *Diet and Cardiovascular Disease* (1984). London: HMSO.

Department of Health Report on Health and Social Subjects no 37: *Dietary Sugars and Human Disease* (1989). London: HMSO.

Department of Health Report on Health and Social Subjects no 41: *Dietary Reference Values for Food Energy and Nutrients for the United Kingdom* (1991). London: HMSO.

GIBNEY, M.J. (1986) *Nutrition, Diet and Health.* Cambridge University Press.

NATIONAL RESEARCH COUNCIL (1989) *Recommended Dietary Allowances*, 10th edn. Washington DC: National Academy Press.

OLIVER, M.E. (1981) Diet and coronary heart disease. *British Medical Bulletin*, **37**: 49–58.

SCIENTIFIC COMMITTEE FOR FOOD (1993) *Nutrient and Energy Intakes for the European Community.* Luxembourg: Commission of the European Communities.

WORLD HEALTH ORGANIZATION (1985) WHO Technical reports Series no. 724: *Energy and Protein Requirements.* Geneva: WHO.

WORLD HEALTH ORGANIZATION (1990) WHO Technical Reports Series no. 797: *Diet, Nutrition and the Prevention of Chronic Diseases.* Geneva: WHO.

Energy balance, obesity and anorexia nervosa

BENDER, A.E. and BROOKES, L.J. (eds) (1987) *Bodyweight Control: the Physiology, Clinical Treatment and Prevention of Obesity.* Edinburgh: Churchill-Livingstone.

BRAY, G.A. (1985) Complications of obesity. *Annals of Internal Medicine*, **103**, 1052–1062.

CRISP, A.H. (1980) *Anorexia Nervosa: Let Me Be.* London: Academic Press.

GARROW, J.S. (1988) *Obesity and Related Disorders,* 2nd edn. Edinburgh: Churchill-Livingstone.

JAMES, W.P.T. and SCHOFIELD, E.C. (1990) *Human Energy Requirements.* Oxford: FAO/Oxford University Press.

ROYAL COLLEGE OF PHYSICIANS OF LONDON 1983. Obesity. *Journal of the Royal College of Physicians of London,* **17**, 1–58.

Vitamins

BARKER, B.M. and BENDER, D.A. (eds) (1980 – Vol. 1; 1982 – Vol. 2). *Vitamins in Medicine.* London: William Heinemann Medical Books.

BENDER, D.A. (1992) *Nutritional Biochemistry of the Vitamins.* Cambridge University Press.

DIPLOCK, A.T. (ed.) (1985) *Fat Soluble Vitamins.* London: William Heinemann Medical Books.

FRIEDRICH, W.F. (1988) *Vitamins.* Berlin: Walter de Gruyter.

GABY, S.K., BENDICH, A., SINGH, V.N. and MACHLIN, L.J. (1991) *Vitamin Intake and Health.* New York: Marcel Dekker.

MARKS, J. (1968) *The Vitamins in Health and Disease: a Modern Reappraisal.* London: J & A Churchill.

Clinical nutrition

DICKERSON, J.W.T. and BOOTH, E.M. (1985) *Clinical Nutrition for Nurses, Dietitians and Other Health Care Professionals.* London: Faber & Faber.

FRANCIS, D.E.M. (1974) *Diets for Sick Children.* Oxford: Blackwell Scientific Publications.

GIBSON, R.S. (1990) *Principles of Nutritional Assessment.* New York: Oxford University Press.

LEEDS, A.R., JUDD, P. and LEWIS, B. (1990) *Nutrition Matters for Practice Nurses: a Handbook on Dietary Advice for Use in the Community.* London: John Libbey.

Food intolerance and allergy

BROSTOFF, J. and CHALLACOMBE, S.J. (1987) *Food Allergy and Intolerance.* London: Baillière Tindall.

METCALFE, D.P., SAMPSON, H.A. and SIMON, R.A. (1991) *Food Allergy: Adverse Reactions to Foods and Food Additives.* Boston: Blackwell Scientific Publications.

Sources of research reviews on nutritional topics

Annual Reviews of Nutrition, Annual Reviews Inc., Palo Alto, California.
Nutrition Research Reviews, CAB International, Oxford.
Advances in Nutrition Research, Plenum Press, New York.
Nutrition Reviews, The Nutrition Foundation Inc., New York.
World Review of Nutrition and Dietetics, Karger, Basel.
Nutrition Abstracts and Reviews, CAB International, Oxford.
Proceedings of the Nutrition Society, CAB International, Oxford.

Index